Pharynx - Diagnosis and Treatment

Edited by Xiaoying Zhou and Zhe Zhang

Published in London, United Kingdom

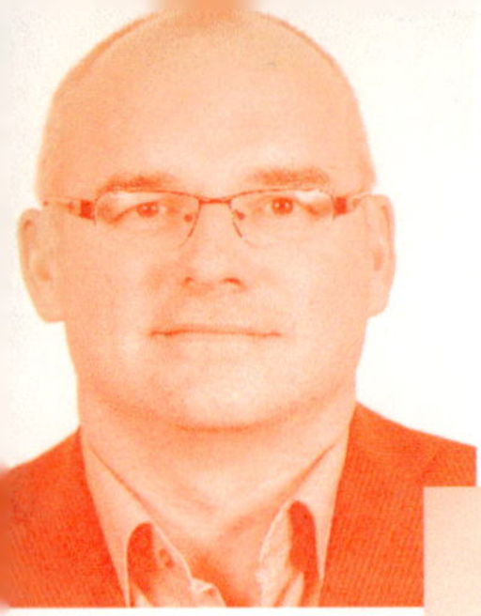
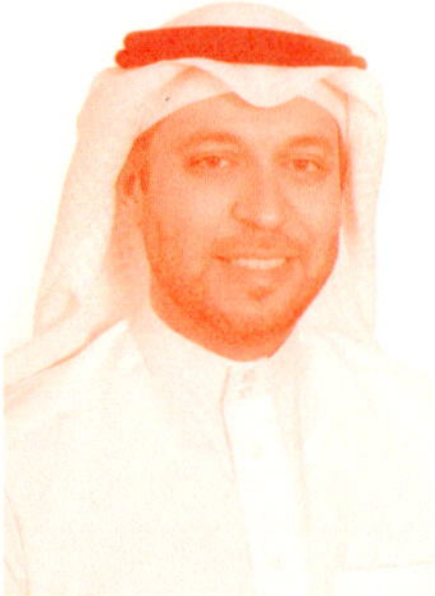
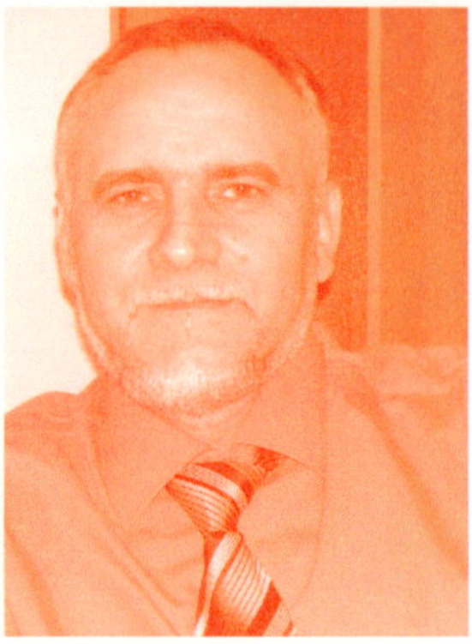
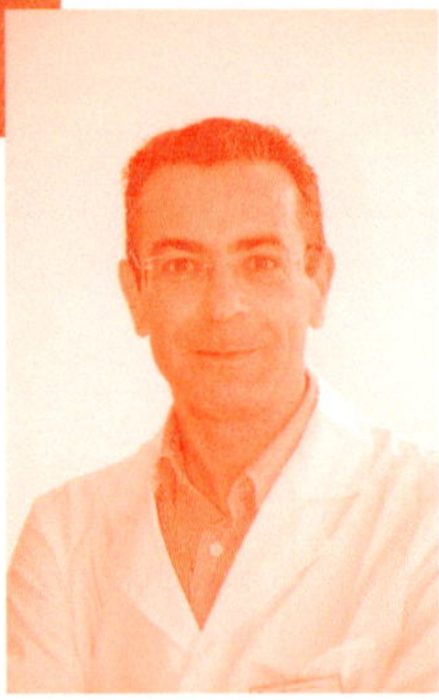
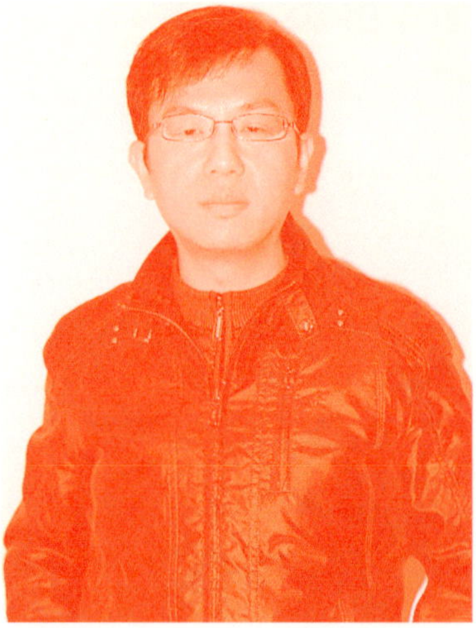
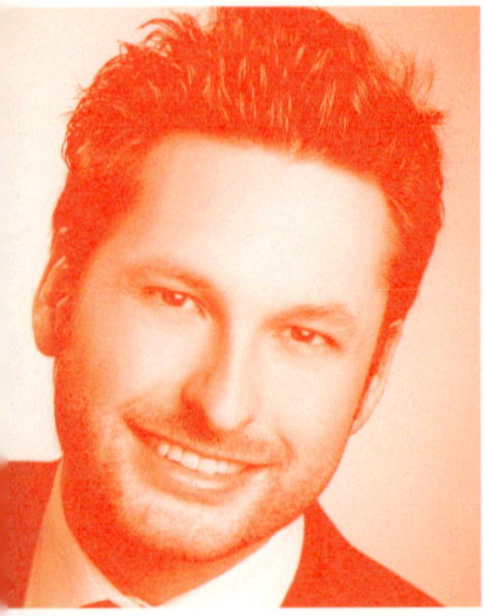
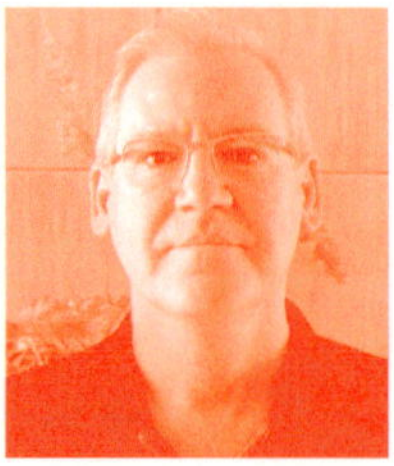

IntechOpen

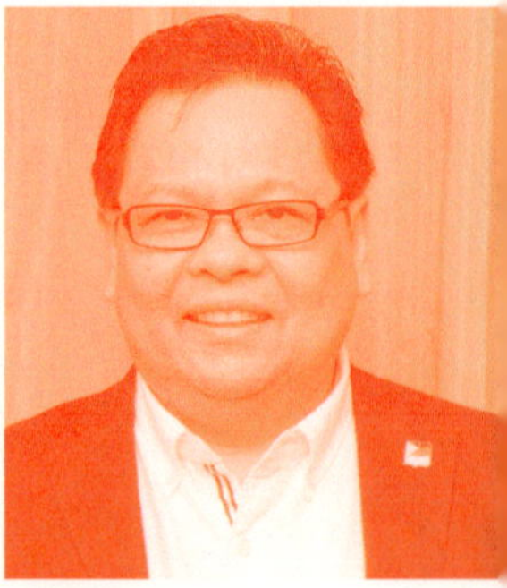
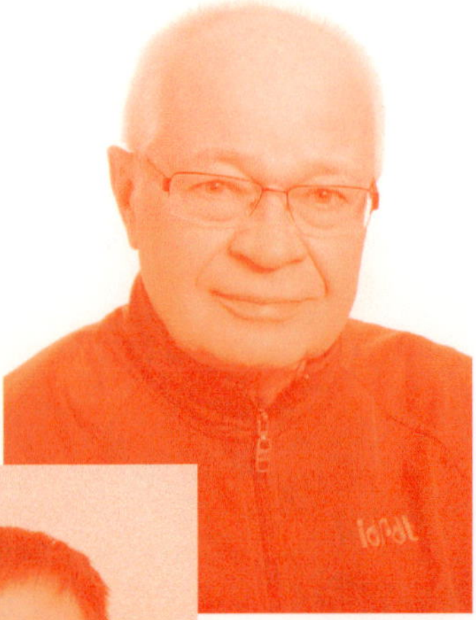
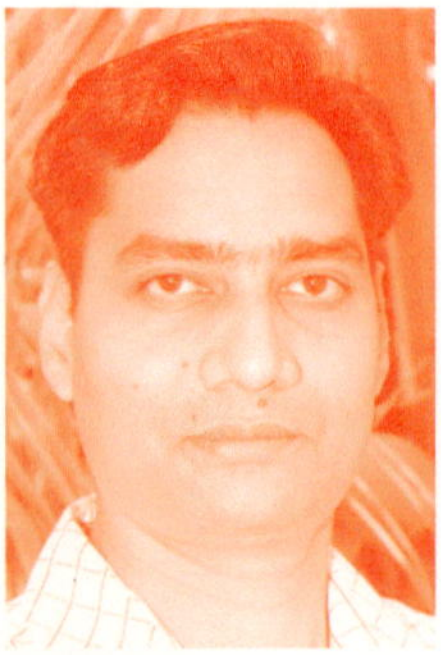
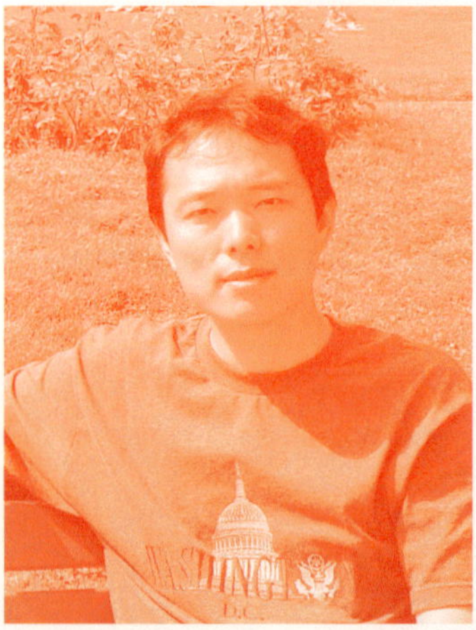
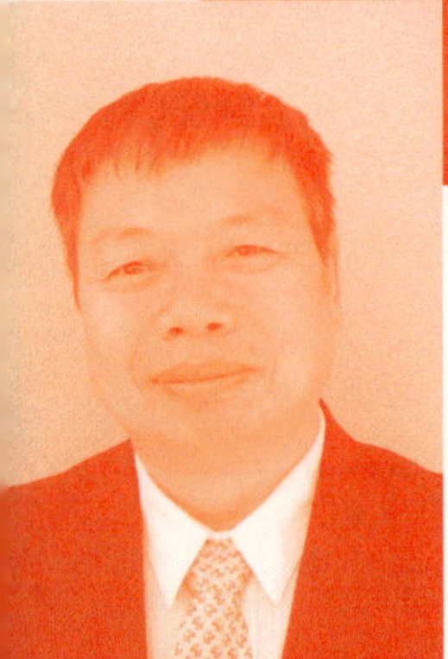
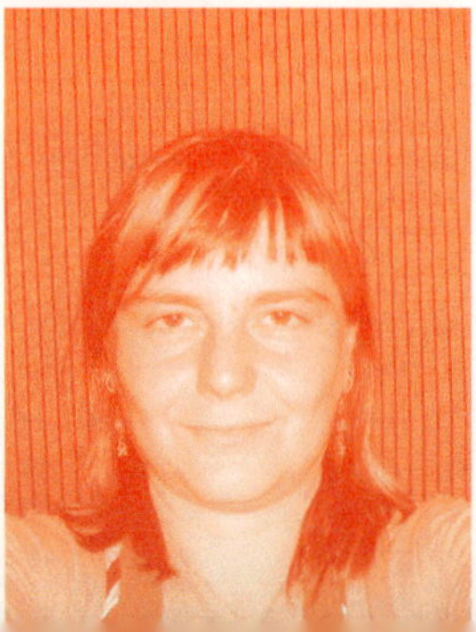

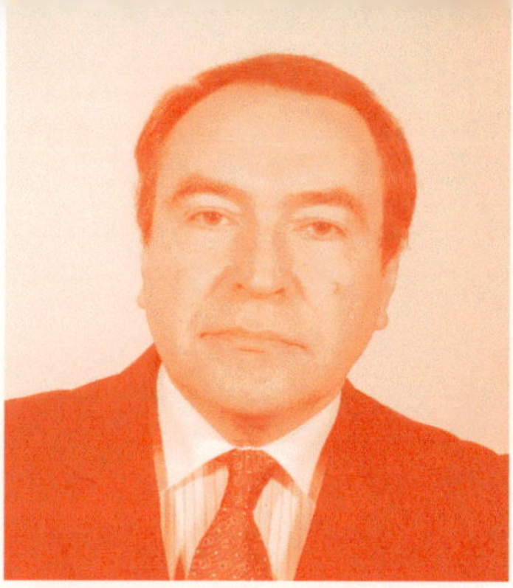
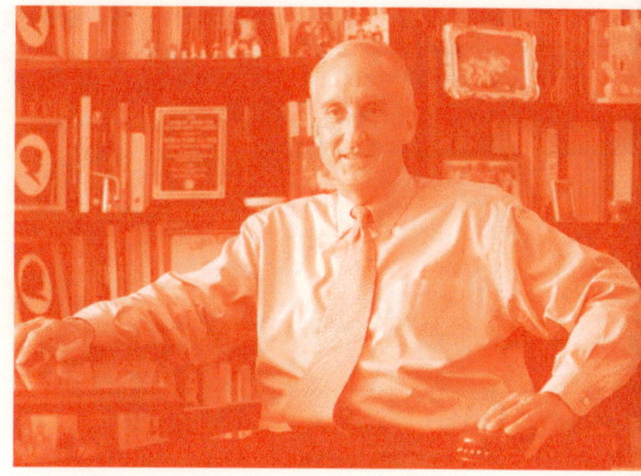
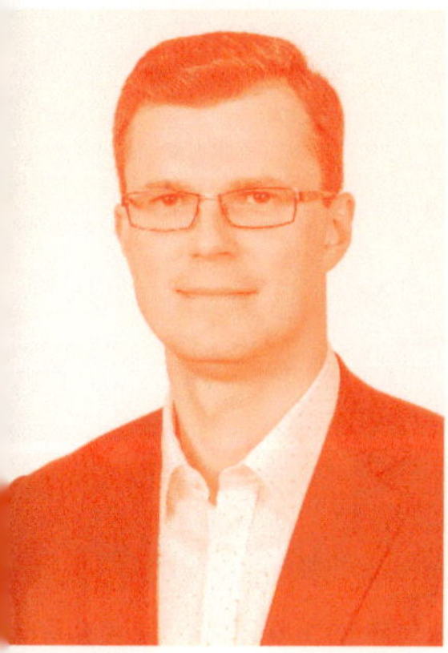
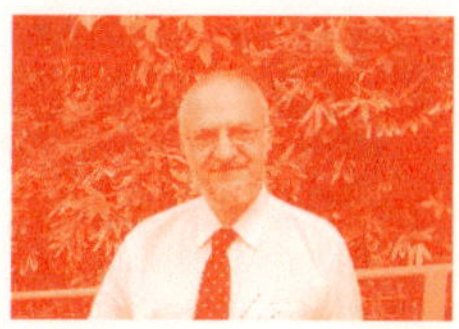
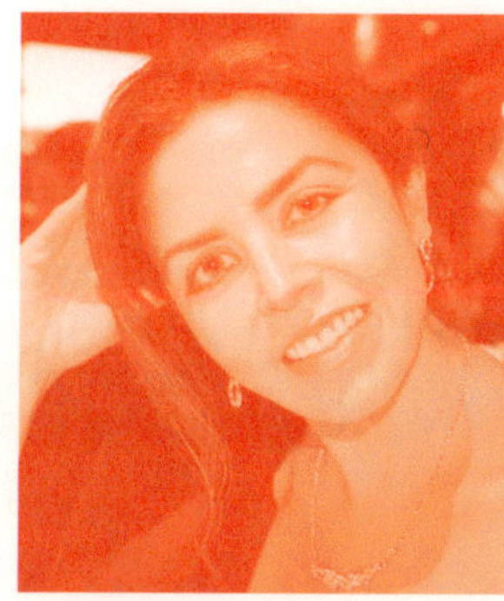

Supporting open minds since 2005

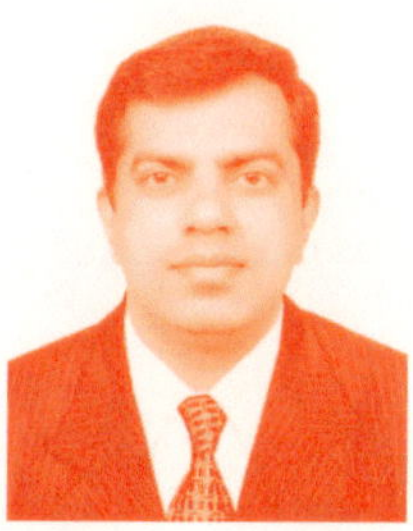
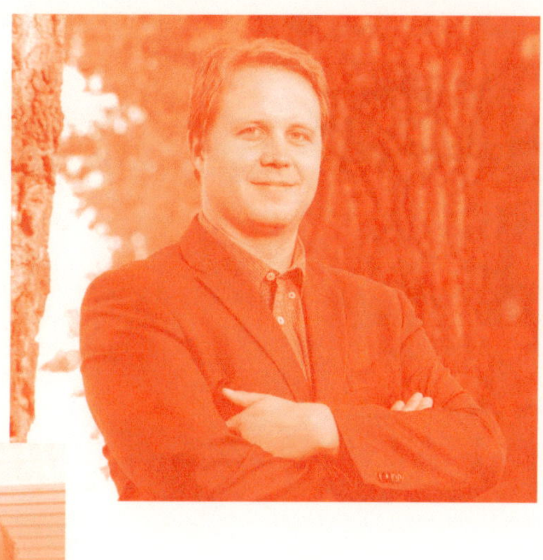
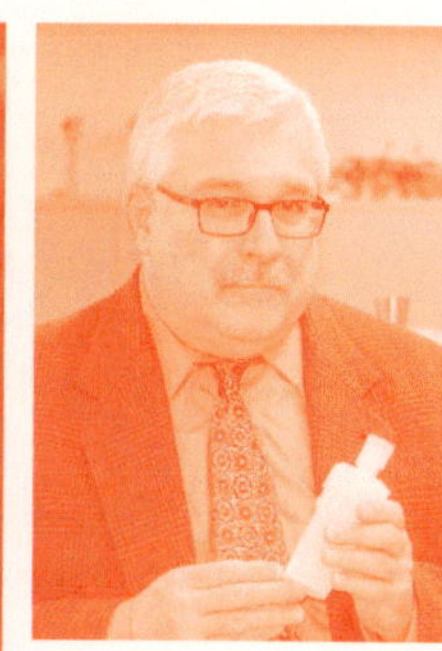
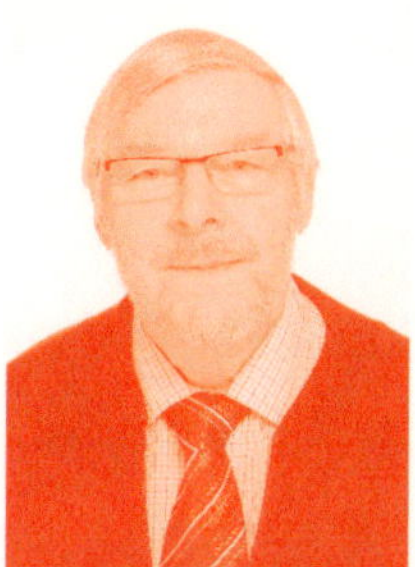
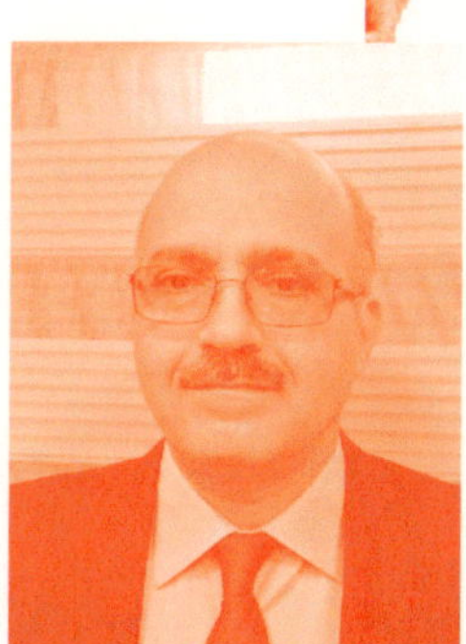
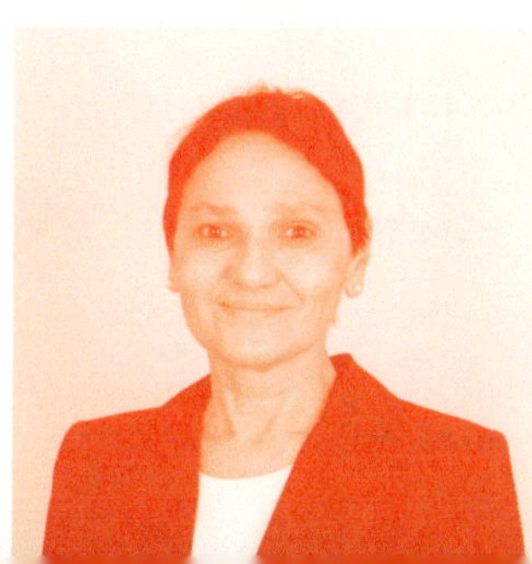
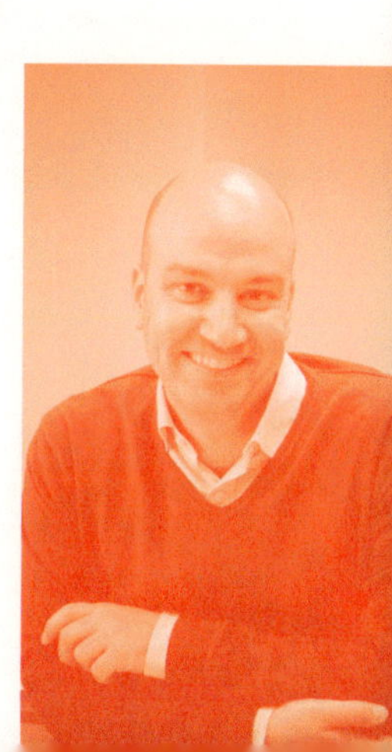

Pharynx - Diagnosis and Treatment
http://dx.doi.org/10.5772/intechopen.91522
Edited by Xiaoying Zhou and Zhe Zhang

Contributors
Nitika Mehta, Saima Tabassum, Anukaran Mahajan, Karunesh Gupta, Anna Staniszewska, Barbara Jamróz, Magdalena Milewska, Joanna Chmielewska-Walczak, Kazimierz Niemczyk, Anna Brytek-Matera, Magdalena Arcimowicz, Magdalena Lachowska, Marta Dąbrowska-Bender, Jaime Bustos-Martínez, Samuel González-García, Aida Hamdan-Partida, Anaíd Bustos-Hamdan, Koji Araki, Akihiro Shiotani, Kainickal Cessal Thommachan, Mullangath Prakasan Aparna, Kunnambath Ramadas, Ravi Rejnish Kumar, Malu Rafi, Geethu Babu, Pradeep Naveen Kumar, Abdullah Alhelali, Xiaoying Zhou, Tingting Huang, Zhe Zhang, Gamal Abdul Hamid, Yonglin Cai, Yanping Yang, Xue Xiao, zhou wang, Weilin Zhao, Yi Huang, Yushan Liang, Lekha Madhavan Nair, Rejnish Ravi Kumar, Farida Nazeer

First published in London, United Kingdom, 2021 by IntechOpen
IntechOpen is the global imprint of INTECHOPEN LIMITED, registered in England and Wales, registration number: 11086078, 5 Princes Gate Court, London, SW7 2QJ, United Kingdom
Printed in Croatia

British Library Cataloguing-in-Publication Data
A catalogue record for this book is available from the British Library

Additional hard and PDF copies can be obtained from orders@intechopen.com

Pharynx - Diagnosis and Treatment
Edited by Xiaoying Zhou and Zhe Zhang
p. cm.
Print ISBN 978-1-78985-264-6
Online ISBN 978-1-78985-609-5
eBook (PDF) ISBN 978-1-78985-610-1

For EU product safety concerns:
IN TECH d.o.o., Prolaz Marije Krucifikse Kozulić 3, 51000 Rijeka, Croatia, info@intechopen.com or visit our website at intechopen.com.

Meet the editors

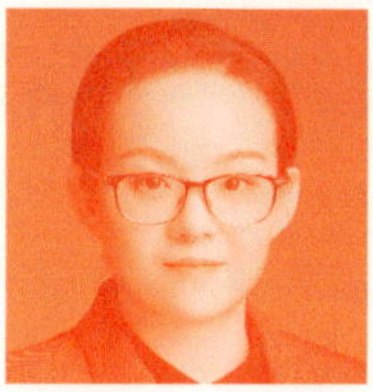

Xiaoying Zhou is an associate researcher at Guangxi Medical University, China. In 2009, she obtained a master's degree in Otolaryngology Head and Neck Surgery from Guangxi Medical University. She obtained a Ph.D. from the Karolinska Institutet, Sweden, in 2016. Her research focuses on the pathogenesis of nasopharyngeal carcinoma. She has published twenty-seven papers and participated in the compilation of four books.

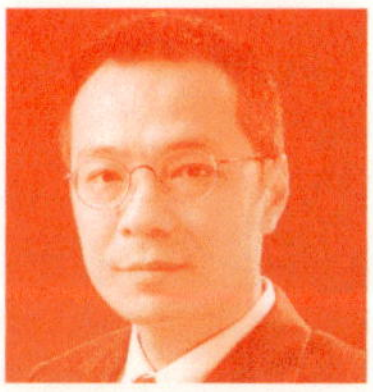

Zhe Zhang studied in Sweden as a postdoc and in Japan as a visiting researcher. He completed training at the Affiliated Cancer Hospital and served as a professor in the Department of Otolaryngology Head and Neck Surgery, First Affiliated Hospital, Guangxi Medical University, China. He is skillful at thyroid cancer surgery and reconstruction of head and neck surgical defects. His research focuses on the pathogenesis and etiology of nasopharyngeal carcinoma and he has published more than fifty papers.

Contents

Preface XI

Section 1
Pharyngeal Carcinoma 1

Chapter 1 3
Oral Cancer
by Xue Xiao and Zhou Wang

Chapter 2 13
Human Papillomavirus Associated Oropharyngeal Carcinoma-Diagnosis and Management
by Mullangath Prakasan Aparna, Ravi Rejnish Kumar, Malu Rafi, Geethu Babu, Pradeep Naveen Kumar, Kunnambath Ramadas and Kainickal Cessal Thomachan

Chapter 3 29
Screening of Nasopharyngeal Carcinoma
by Yanping Yang and Yonglin Cai

Chapter 4 43
Epidemiology and Outcomes of Nasopharyngeal Carcinoma
by Gamal Abdul Hamid

Chapter 5 59
Diagnosis and Therapy of Nasopharyngeal Carcinoma
by Tingting Huang, Zhe Zhang and Xiaoying Zhou

Chapter 6 75
Chemotherapy in Nasopharyngeal Carcinoma
by Lekha Madhavan Nair, Rejnish Ravi Kumar, Malu Rafi, Farida Nazeer, Kainickal Cessal Thommachan and Kunnambath Ramadas

Chapter 7 89
Hypopharyngeal Cancer: Staging, Diagnosis, and Therapy
by Yi Huang, Yushan Liang and Weilin Zhao

Chapter 8 113
Role of Organ Preservation in Locally Advanced Hypopharyngeal Carcinoma
by Farida Nazeer, Rejnish Ravi Kumar, Malu Rafi, Lekha M. Nair, Kainickal Cessal Thommachan and Kunnambath Ramadas

Chapter 9 125
Premalignant Conditions of Larynx
by Nitika Mehta and Saima Tabassum

Chapter 10 141
Transoral Videolaryngoscopic Surgery (TOVS)
by Koji Araki and Akihiro Shiotani

Section 2
Other Pharyngeal Diseases 161

Chapter 11 163
Factors of Nasopharynx that Favor the Colonization and Persistence of *Staphylococcus aureus*
by Samuel González-García, Aída Hamdan-Partida, Anaíd Bustos-Hamdan and Jaime Bustos-Martínez

Chapter 12 185
The Evaluation and Treatment of Obstructive Sleep Apnea Syndrome
by Abdullah Alhelali

Chapter 13 195
Assessment of Dysphagia as a Risk Factor of Chronic Cough
by Barbara Jamróz, Magdalena Milewska, Joanna Chmielewska-Walczak, Magdalena Lachowska, Marta Dąbrowska-Bender, Magdalena Arcimowicz, Anna Staniszewska, Anna Brytek-Matera and Kazimierz Niemczyk

Chapter 14 209
Juvenile Nasopharyngeal Angiofibroma
by Anukaran Mahajan and Karunesh Gupta

Preface

Diagnosis is an ordinary and commonplace topic for all diseases, and correct diagnosis is the premise of correct treatment, suggesting a key role of diagnosis and treatment in clinics. In recent years, the achievements of advanced technologies and their application in clinics has prompted the rapid progress of otolaryngology. As an important branch of otorhinolaryngology head and neck surgery, there are few books devoted to pharyngeal diseases. *Pharynx - Diagnosis and Treatment* introduces the most advanced diagnosis and treatment techniques, clinical application principles, indication selection, and operation norms in pharynx diseases. The chapters provide updated scientific views from international experts on the latest advances in pharyngeal diseases, including pharyngeal carcinomas (e.g., oral cancer, nasopharyngeal carcinoma, hypopharyngeal carcinoma, and laryngeal carcinoma) and non-cancerous diseases (e.g., nasopharyngeal angiofibroma and obstructive sleep apnea syndrome). The book also includes reviews concerning nasopharyngeal microflora and research work evaluating dysphagia as a risk factor for chronic cough.

I am confident this book will enhance readers' understanding and knowledge of the differential diagnosis and therapeutic options of pharyngeal diseases. I sincerely appreciate my co-editor Professor Zhe Zhang and the publishing managers at IntechOpen as well as all the contributing authors for their help, support, and patience throughout the process of creating and publishing this book.

Xiaoying Zhou
Life Science Institute,
Guangxi Medical University,
Nanning, China

Zhe Zhang
First Affiliated Hospital of Guangxi Medical University,
China

Section 1

Pharyngeal Carcinoma

Chapter 1

Oral Cancer

Xue Xiao and Zhou Wang

Abstract

Oral cancer is a frequent head and neck cancer in developing countries and some developed world. According to the World Health Organization classification 2017, oral cancer influences the anatomical subsites including buccal mucosa, the anterior two-third of the tongue, lip, palate, vestibule, alveolus, floor of the mouth, and gingivae. A variety of premalignant lesions are related with the development of oral cancer, such as leukoplakia, erythroplakia, et al. The predominant histological type of oral cancer is squamous cell carcinoma (SCC). Tobacco and alcohol consumption are regarded as critical etiological factors. Due to the unspecific symptoms in early stage, the majority are diagnosed in advanced stages. Despite the development of medicine over decades, the mortality rate of oral cancer remains high, indicating the importance of optimized treatment and screening strategies.

Keywords: oral cancer, etiology, diagnosis, treatment, prognosis

1. Introduction

Oral cancer is a malignant head and neck disease, and it accounts for 2–5% of cancer types and around 30% of head and neck cancers [1, 2]. According to the World Health Organization classification 2017, oral cancer is defined to tumors in the buccal mucosa, the anterior two-third of the tongue, the lip, palate, vestibule, alveolus, floor of the mouth, and gingivae [3]. Cancers of salivary glands or oropharynx will not be discussed in this chapter.

Oral cancer is distributed high in countries such as India, Pakistan, Taiwan China, and Germany [4]. It is more frequent in men than women [5]. It has a complicated etiology and it is related to many risk factors like tobacco, alcohol, betel nut, human papillomavirus (HPV) infection, et al. Around 90% of oral cancers are squamous cell carcinoma. In early stage of oral cancer, signs are unspecific and not easy to be recognized. As a result, most of the patients are diagnosed at a late stage, dropping down the survival rate from 80–90% to 20–50% [6]. Thus, the prognosis of oral cancer is poor and it is urgent to raise the awareness of public health education. The major management of oral cancer is surgery, supplemented with/without adjuvant radiochemotherapy. However, for better survival, personalized and multidisciplinary treatment strategies are needed.

2. Incidence of oral cancer

Despite the development of modern treatment methods, no significant achievement was reported in the prognosis, survival and mortality of oral cancer. According to the GLOBOCAN 2018 project, there is 354,864 new cases and 177,382 deaths due to oral cancer worldwide [7]. Geographically speaking, oral cancer is highly prevalent in South and Southeast Asia (India, Pakistan, etc.), West, Middle and Eastern of Europe (France, Germany, Hungary, etc.), and Oceania [4, 8, 9]. It is important to notice that the incidence of oral cancer is high in transitioning countries, particularly in India [10]. The incidence rate for the male is higher than female, approximately 10:1 to 2:1 [5, 7]. It is noted that oral cancer patients are usually aged from 50 to 70 years. However, increasing numbers of oral cancer patients have been observed at younger age, possibly due to a distinct etiology and pathogenesis [11].

3. Pathology of oral cancer

More than 90% of oral cancers are squamous cell carcinoma (SCC) arising from the mucosal epithelium, namely oral squamous cell carcinoma (OSCC). A majority of them are moderate to well-differentiated. According to the WHO 2017 classification, eight kinds of subtypes are identified, including basaloid squamous cell carcinoma, spindle cell squamous cell carcinoma, adenosquamous carcinoma, carcinoma cuniculatum, verrucous squamous cell carcinoma, lymphoepithelial carcinoma, papillary squamous cell carcinoma, and acantholytic squamous cell carcinoma [12]. Each different subtype indicates different outcome.

Furthermore, a variety of oral potentially malignant disorders (OPMDs) have been reported to increase the potential of developing into oral cancer. Generally speaking, the common OPMDs, including erythroplakia, leukoplakia, oral submucous fibrosis, oral lichen planus, et al., increase the risk of malignant transformation, and they also serve as premalignant indicators in clinical works [12, 13].

4. Etiology of oral cancer

Numerous studies have demonstrated a multifactoral etiology in the development and carcinogenesis of oral cancer, involving tobacco, alcohol, betel quid, high-risk human papillomavirus (HPV) 16/18, poor nutrition, poor oral hygiene, immune system suppression, bacterial infection, and so on.

4.1 Tobacco

Tobacco is a well-established risk factor for lots of cancers as well as oral cancer. There are more than 80% of oral cancer patients with a habit of tobacco use. All types of tobacco products, for example cigarettes, pipe tobacco, chewing tobacco, contain many carcinogenic molecules, especially nitrosamines, benzopyrenes and polycyclic hydrocarbons, raising the risk of generating cancers. For tobacco smoking, it has a combined odds ratio of 4.65 (95% CI, 3.19–6.77) related with oral cancer [14]. For smokeless tobacco such as paan chewing and gutkha swallowing, it would lead to oral submucous fibrosis (OSMF) and ultimately increase the potential to transform into oral cancer. According to a nested case–control study in India, tobacco chewing was found the most potent high-risk factor linked to oral cancer, with adjusted odds ratios (ORs) of 3.1 for males and 11.0 for females [15].

4.2 Alcohol

Alcohol is also a well-defined significant risk factor for oral cancer [16–18]. An updated analysis based on cohort and case–control studies from 1988 to 2009 shows that, a consumption of 60 g per day or more than 4 drinks per day would raise the risk of oral cancer by 3–9 times when adjusted for smoking and other potential confounding variables [19]. The risk between alcohol and oral cancer is not only dose–response, but also related with the type of alcoholic beverage, meaning those consuming hard liquor or beer have a higher risk than those consuming wine. Besides, a greater significance is observed in both heavy smoker and heavy drinker [18].

4.3 HPV infection

Human papillomavirus (HPV) is a kind of small DNA virus that causes cervix cancer in females and anal cancer in males [20]. As a sexually transmitted pathogen, HPV also infects the human oral cavity in forms of oral sex behaviors and open-mouthed kissing. HPV, especially high-risk subtypes 16 and 18, is reported to have its role in the carcinogenesis of around one-third of oral cancer [21, 22]. Further, oncoprotein p16 is found over-expressed in oral cancer patients with high-risk HPV infection. Meanwhile, the relationship between HPV and oral cancer is not so strong when compared with oropharynx cancer, as studies showed that HPV-16 is found in 10–25% and HPV-18 in 14% of oral cancers [23]. Interestingly, HPV-positive oral cancers generate a more favorable outcome, possibly due to an enhanced anti-virus immune reaction. However, the role of HPV in oral cancer is far from clear [24].

4.4 Others

Besides, carcinogenesis of oral cancer is influenced by other factors namely betel quid chewing [25], poor diet and nutrition such as lack of fresh fruits and vegetables [26], poor oral hygiene [27], oral microbiome alteration [28], and genetic susceptibility [29].

5. Clinical presentations, diagnosis and staging of oral cancer

5.1 Clinical presentations

The most common symptoms of oral cancer patients may include ulceration (57.7%), induration (44.3%), and rupture (14.1%) [30]. However, due to the asymptomatic and unspecific signs, more than half of the patients went to a doctor in advanced stages when the discomforts worsen or appearance of new symptoms. In this situation, patients may present with an enlarged lesion, no improvement after the first treatment, onset of pain, inflexible movement of the tongue, discomfort in the mouth, difficulty in speaking and swallowing, bleeding, neck mass, et al.

5.2 Diagnosis

The physical examination of oral cancer is usually performed by inspection and palpation. The examination lasts around several minutes and does not require special equipment or technique. Dentists are the ideal position to perform examination and alarm suspected changes. Clinical investigation include assessment of primary tumor and the surrounded structures, such as deep muscle invasion, fixation to bone, and cranial neuropathies. Once a suspicious lesion is discovered, it is important for clinicians to perform biopsy, which is the gold standard for diagnosis.

An appropriate imaging detection is a complement of physical examination. It provides proper evaluation for patients. Initial examinations of the primary site are usually done with computed tomography (CT) scan and/or magnetic resonance imaging (MRI). CT scan is good at evaluating the larynx, neck nodes and invasion of bone or cartilage. In comparison, MRI is preferred in patients concerning tumor involvement of soft tissue, perivascular, perineural, skull base, and intracranial. In addition, dental films or panoramic X-rays can be used in the assessment of cortical bone involvement and ultrasound (US) can be used to evaluate the metastasis of lymph nodes. As distant metastasis evaluation, FDG-PET/CT works more excellent [31]. However, in case of a concerned specific anatomic site, further contrast-enhanced CT and/or MRI should be performed. All the imaging measures mentioned above could help to describe the margins and invasion of the primary tumor, lymph node involvement, local and distant metastasis, thereby providing evidence for clinical TNM (cTNM) staging identification.

5.3 Staging

Nowadays, more and more studies realize that the malignant behavior of oral cancer is not only determined by tumor size but also invasive depth. Based on this, pathologic examination is further performed to identify pT (an actual measurement of unfixed fresh surgical tumor specimens) and/or pN. As an improvement of the previous oral cancer TNM staging algorithm, the eighth edition of American Joint Committee on Cancer (AJCC) Staging Manual highlights depth of invasion (DOI) for T stages and extranodal extension (ENE) for N stages. These alterations improve the discrimination ability of disease-free survival (DFS) between overall stages as well as T categories [32]. A comparison between the seventh and eighth edition is shown below in **Table 1**.

6. Treatment of oral cancer

Treatment of oral cancer patients, especially with invasive condition, is best determined by a multidisciplinary team of medical experts, which may include head and neck surgeons, pathologists, radiation oncologists, chemotherapy oncologists, neuroradiologists, reconstructive surgeons, dentists, nurse specialists and nutritionists. Managements include surgical resection, radiotherapy and chemotherapy, depending on anatomic site and size of the primary tumor, lymph node metastasis and distant metastasis, the patient's risk as well as benefit from the treatment, namely a personalized treatment.

6.1 Surgery

Surgery is the main option for oral cancer patients. There are series of choices: conventional/laser/thermal/robotic surgery, et al. Small tumors located in the anterior part of the oral cavity could be accessed via transoral approach. While for those advanced and/or located in the posterior part of oral cavity, routes of lip-splitting and/or mandibulotomy are suggested. As the first-line treatment strategy, the primary principle of surgery is adequate clearance of tumor and functional preservation (speech, swallowing, deglutition). A positive surgical margin increases the risk of recurrence and generates poor survival outcomes [34]. Thus, complete ablation is demanded, usually a 1-cm macroscopic resection margins around the tumor tissue are suggested for conventional surgery [35–37]. As an adjuvant technique, iodine vital staining supports evidence distinguishing dysplastic or tumorigenic tissues from benign mucosa [38].

However, difficulties of reconstruction come with enough resection margins. The most acceptable reconstruction scheme should take many factors into consideration, including the anatomic site and invasive condition of the primary

	AJCC (7th edition)	AJCC (8th edition) [33]
Primary tumor		
Tx: T0: Tis:	Primary tumor cannot be assessed. No evidence of primary tumor. Carcinoma in situ.	The same as the 7th edition. The same as the 7th edition. The same as the 7th edition.
T1:	Primary tumor <2 cm in biggest dimension.	Primary tumor≤2 cm, DOI ≤ 5 mm.
T2:	Primary tumor is 2–4 cm in biggest dimension.	Primary tumor ≤2 cm, 5 mm<DOI ≤ 10 mm; or 2 cm<tumor≤4 cm, and DOI ≤ 10 mm.
T3:	Primary tumor >4 cm in biggest dimension.	Primary tumor>4 cm or any tumor DOI>10 mm
T4: T4a: T4b:	Moderately or very advanced local disease Moderately advanced local disease. (lip) Tumor invades through cortical bone, inferior alveolar nerve, floor of mouth, or skin of face; (oral cavity) Tumor invade adjacent structures only. Very advanced local disease, tumor invades masticator space, pterygoid plates, or skull base and/or encases internal carotid artery.	The same as the 7th edition.
Regional lymph node status		
 Nx: N0:	**N** Regional lymph node cannot be assessed. No regional lymph node metastasis.	**pN** The same as the 7th edition. The same as the 7th edition.
N1:	Metastasis to a single ipsilateral lymph node (≤3 cm).	New introduction of negative extranodal extension, based on the 7th edition.
N2a:	Metastasis to a single ipsilateral lymph node (3–6 cm).	Metastasis to one single ipsilateral lymph node (3–6 cm) and extranodal extension (−); metastasis to a single ipsilateral or contralateral lymph node ≤3 cm and extranodal extension (+).
N2b:	Metastasis to multiple ipsilateral lymph nodes (<6 cm)	New introduction of negative extranodal extension, based on the 7th edition.
N2c:	Metastasis to bilateral or contralateral lymph nodes (<6 cm)	New introduction of negative extranodal extension, based on the 7th edition.
N3:	Metastasis to any lymph node (>6 cm)	N3a: Metastasis to one lymph node >6 cm and extranodal extension (−); N3b: Metastasis in one single ipsilateral node >3 cm and extranodal extension (+); or metastasis in multiple ipsilateral, contralateral, or bilateral lymph node, with any extranodal extension (+)
Distant metastasis		
Mx:	Cannot be assessed.	The same as the 7th edition.
M0:	No distant metastasis.	The same as the 7th edition.
M1:	Distant metastasis.	The same as the 7th edition.

Table 1.
A comparison of the 7th and 8th edition of AJCC/TNM staging of oral cancer.

tumor, the general healthy and social economic condition of the patient, and the surgeon team's skills. There are many soft tissue reconstructive techniques such as local flaps, regional pedicled flaps and microvascular free flap, depending on the defection. For hard tissue defection, autologous bone grafts from the iliac crest, fibula, radius or scapula are common choices.

Elective neck dissection (END) is suggested for all oral cancer patients [37]. It is reported that around 15–30% of cN0 patients have inapparent lymph node invasion (pN) [1], suggesting the importance of prophylactic dissection for N0 patients. Though recent evidence shows that sentinel node biopsy can be a reliable indicator for N0 oral cancer patients, more data is needed to support its function [39]. Additionally, patients with a DOI of more than 4 mm or T2/3/4 stage should undergo neck dissection to improve overall and disease-free survival rate [40].

6.2 Radiotherapy and chemotherapy

For patients with pathologically positive lymph nodes, occult neck metastasis or existence of extra-capsular spread (ECS), radiotherapy should be initiated. Disadvantages of radiotherapy are many which influence the quality of patients, introducing alteration in skin color, oral cavity mucositis, xerostomia, osteoradionecrosis of the mandible, as well as late toxic symptoms such as dysphagia and dehydration [41]. With the development of intensity-modulated radiotherapy (IMRT), side effects are reduced significantly [42].

Chemotherapy has been applied as an adjuvant approach in oral cancer, especially for patients with locally advanced stage. It can be performed before surgery (known as induction chemotherapy), and also as a combination with radiotherapy (known as chemoradiotherapy) before or after surgery which helps effectively controlling the progression of patients with extracapsular extension in lymph nodes and positive resection margin. As a radiosensitizer, cisplatin is the first-line agent to combine with radiotherapy. What's more, the application of anti-programmed cell death-ligand 1 (PD-L1) antibody is found to improve the prognosis of oral cancer patients with metastasis after chemotherapy using platinum [43].

7. Survival and prognosis of oral cancer

With the development of diagnosis and adjuvant therapy, a retrospective database study involving 16,020 cases of oral cancer patients between 1973 and 2014 showed that the 3-year survival rate for early stage patients increased from 78% to 92.9%, and for those with late stage disease increased from 51.9% to 70.3% [44]. Another study including 2082 patients in a tertiary cancer care center from 1985 to 2015 found that the 5-year over survival (OS) rate of oral cancer was 64.4% and disease special survival (DSS) rate was 79.3% [45].

Age, surgical margin clearance, vascular and perineural invasion situation, pT and pN are factors affecting prognosis. Among these, lymph node involvement strongly indicates poor prognosis, especially for those with extracapsular spread [46]. Increased tumor size and advanced tumor stage also have their roles on prognosis [47]. However, tumor differentiation, number of metastasis nodes, ethnicity are found to have no relationship with prognosis. Due to variation in the geography and studied population, more evidence is needed.

8. Screening of oral cancer

More than 50% of oral cancer patients are diagnosed at the state of regional or distant metastasis. Thus, a proper screening is urgently needed for earlier detection and prevention. A primary screening for oral cancer is visual inspection combined with palpation. Any abnormality that with a history longer than fourteen days should be reevaluated, and a tissue biopsy is required. There are other adjunctive techniques providing subjective interpretations, including toluidine blue staining, brush cytopathology, salivary diagnosis, tissue autofluorescence and chemiluminescence [48]. Alteration of the oral microbial community has its role in predicting oral cancer too, such as the carcinogenic Porphyromonas gingivalis and F nucleatum [49]. Although there is increasing clues showing HPV infection in oral cancer, no screening project has been approved by the U.S. Food and Drug Administration (FDA). Furthermore, a recommendation from the U.S. Preventive Services Task Force (USPSTF) suggested that more evidence is needed to access the value of screening for oral cancer between benefits and drawbacks [50].

9. Conclusion

In spite of advancement of reconstruction surgery and adjuvant therapy in recent decades, oral cancer remains a public social healthy problem because of its high incidence and mortality rate. To better control this malignant disease, the key principle lies in early diagnosis and prevention such as social education about lifestyle. Finally but not lastly, a personalized treatment should be made by a multidisciplinary team for every patient.

Acknowledgements

This work was supported by grants from the National Natural Science Foundation of China (81560439 and 82060511).

Conflict of interest

The authors declare no conflict of interest.

Author details

Xue Xiao[1]* and Zhou Wang[2]

1 Department of Otolaryngology-Head and Neck Surgery, First Affiliated Hospital of Guangxi Medical University, Nanning, China

2 Department of Geriatric Cardiology, the People's Hospital of Guangxi Zhuang Autonomous Region, Nanning, China

*Address all correspondence to: pearxiaoxue@gmail.com

References

[1] Kademani D. Oral cancer. Mayo Clin Proc. 2007;82(7):878-87.

[2] The world health report 2004: Changing history. World Health Organization. 2004.

[3] Tahir A, Nagi AH, Ullah E, Janjua OS. The role of mast cells and angiogenesis in well-differentiated oral squamous cell carcinoma. J Cancer Res Ther. 2013;9(3):387-91.

[4] Ghantous Y, Abu Elnaaj I. [Global Incidence and Risk Factors of Oral Cancer]. Harefuah. 2017;156(10):645-9.

[5] Vissink A, Burlage FR, Spijkervet FK, Jansma J, Coppes RP. Prevention and treatment of the consequences of head and neck radiotherapy. Crit Rev Oral Biol Med. 2003;14(3):213-25.

[6] van der Waal I. Are we able to reduce the mortality and morbidity of oral cancer; some considerations. Med Oral Patol Oral Cir Bucal. 2013;18(1):e33-7.

[7] Bray F, Ferlay J, Soerjomataram I, Siegel RL, Torre LA, Jemal A. Global cancer statistics 2018: GLOBOCAN estimates of incidence and mortality worldwide for 36 cancers in 185 countries. CA Cancer J Clin. 2018;68(6):394-424.

[8] Khan Z, Tonnies J, Muller S. Smokeless tobacco and oral cancer in South Asia: a systematic review with meta-analysis. J Cancer Epidemiol. 2014;2014:394696.

[9] de Camargo Cancela M, Voti L, Guerra-Yi M, Chapuis F, Mazuir M, Curado MP. Oral cavity cancer in developed and in developing countries: population-based incidence. Head Neck. 2010;32(3):357-67.

[10] Shrestha AD, Vedsted P, Kallestrup P, Neupane D. Prevalence and incidence of oral cancer in low- and middle-income countries: A scoping review. Eur J Cancer Care (Engl). 2020;29(2):e13207.

[11] Hussein AA, Helder MN, de Visscher JG, Leemans CR, Braakhuis BJ, de Vet HCW, et al. Global incidence of oral and oropharynx cancer in patients younger than 45 years versus older patients: A systematic review. Eur J Cancer. 2017;82:115-27.

[12] EI-Naggar A.K. CJ, K, C., Grandis J. R., Takata T., Slootweg P.J. WHO Classification of Head and Neck Tumours (4th edition) International Agency for Research on Cancer. Lyon 2017.

[13] Walsh T, Liu JL, Brocklehurst P, Glenny AM, Lingen M, Kerr AR, et al. Clinical assessment to screen for the detection of oral cavity cancer and potentially malignant disorders in apparently healthy adults. Cochrane Database Syst Rev. 2013(11):CD010173.

[14] Sadri G, Mahjub H. Tobacco smoking and oral cancer: a meta-analysis. J Res Health Sci. 2007;7(1):18-23.

[15] Muwonge R, Ramadas K, Sankila R, Thara S, Thomas G, Vinoda J, et al. Role of tobacco smoking, chewing and alcohol drinking in the risk of oral cancer in Trivandrum, India: a nested case-control design using incident cancer cases. Oral Oncol. 2008;44(5):446-54.

[16] Neville BW, Day TA. Oral cancer and precancerous lesions. CA Cancer J Clin. 2002;52(4):195-215.

[17] D'Souza S, Addepalli V. Preventive measures in oral cancer: An overview. Biomed Pharmacother. 2018;107:72-80.

[18] Blot WJ, McLaughlin JK, Winn DM, Austin DF, Greenberg RS,

Preston-Martin S, et al. Smoking and drinking in relation to oral and pharyngeal cancer. Cancer Res. 1988;48(11):3282-7.

[19] Goldstein BY, Chang SC, Hashibe M, La Vecchia C, Zhang ZF. Alcohol consumption and cancers of the oral cavity and pharynx from 1988 to 2009: an update. Eur J Cancer Prev. 2010;19(6):431-65.

[20] Palefsky JM. Human papillomavirus-related disease in men: not just a women's issue. J Adolesc Health. 2010;46(4 Suppl):S12-9.

[21] zur Hausen H. Papillomaviruses and cancer: from basic studies to clinical application. Nat Rev Cancer. 2002;2(5):342-50.

[22] Doorbar J, Quint W, Banks L, Bravo IG, Stoler M, Broker TR, et al. The biology and life-cycle of human papillomaviruses. Vaccine. 2012;30 Suppl 5:F55-70.

[23] Sugerman PB, Shillitoe EJ. The high risk human papillomaviruses and oral cancer: evidence for and against a causal relationship. Oral Dis. 1997;3(3):130-47.

[24] Hubbers CU, Akgul B. HPV and cancer of the oral cavity. Virulence. 2015;6(3):244-8.

[25] Islam S, Muthumala M, Matsuoka H, Uehara O, Kuramitsu Y, Chiba I, et al. How Each Component of Betel Quid Is Involved in Oral Carcinogenesis: Mutual Interactions and Synergistic Effects with Other Carcinogens-a Review Article. Curr Oncol Rep. 2019;21(6):53.

[26] Soler M, Bosetti C, Franceschi S, Negri E, Zambon P, Talamini R, et al. Fiber intake and the risk of oral, pharyngeal and esophageal cancer. Int J Cancer. 2001;91(3):283-7.

[27] Oji C, Chukwuneke F. Poor oral Hygiene may be the Sole Cause of Oral Cancer. J Maxillofac Oral Surg. 2012;11(4):379-83.

[28] Healy CM, Moran GP. The microbiome and oral cancer: More questions than answers. Oral Oncol. 2019;89:30-3.

[29] Ali J, Sabiha B, Jan HU, Haider SA, Khan AA, Ali SS. Genetic etiology of oral cancer. Oral Oncol. 2017;70:23-8.

[30] Rutkowska M, Hnitecka S, Nahajowski M, Dominiak M, Gerber H. Oral cancer: The first symptoms and reasons for delaying correct diagnosis and appropriate treatment. Adv Clin Exp Med. 2020;29(6):735-43.

[31] Rohde M, Nielsen AL, Johansen J, Sorensen JA, Nguyen N, Diaz A, et al. Head-to-Head Comparison of Chest X-Ray/Head and Neck MRI, Chest CT/Head and Neck MRI, and (18)F-FDG PET/CT for Detection of Distant Metastases and Synchronous Cancer in Oral, Pharyngeal, and Laryngeal Cancer. J Nucl Med. 2017;58(12):1919-24.

[32] Pollaers K, Hinton-Bayre A, Friedland PL, Farah CS. AJCC 8th Edition oral cavity squamous cell carcinoma staging - Is it an improvement on the AJCC 7th Edition? Oral Oncol. 2018;82:23-8.

[33] Lydiatt WM, Patel SG, O'Sullivan B, Brandwein MS, Ridge JA, Migliacci JC, et al. Head and Neck cancers-major changes in the American Joint Committee on cancer eighth edition cancer staging manual. CA Cancer J Clin. 2017;67(2):122-37.

[34] Sutton DN, Brown JS, Rogers SN, Vaughan ED, Woolgar JA. The prognostic implications of the surgical margin in oral squamous cell carcinoma. Int J Oral Maxillofac Surg. 2003;32(1):30-4.

[35] Mistry RC, Qureshi SS, Kumaran C. Post-resection mucosal margin shrinkage in oral cancer: quantification and significance. J Surg Oncol. 2005;91(2):131-3.

[36] McMahon J, O'Brien CJ, Pathak I, Hamill R, McNeil E, Hammersley N, et al. Influence of condition of surgical margins on local recurrence and disease-specific survival in oral and oropharyngeal cancer. Br J Oral Maxillofac Surg. 2003;41(4):224-31.

[37] Kerawala C, Roques T, Jeannon JP, Bisase B. Oral cavity and lip cancer: United Kingdom National Multidisciplinary Guidelines. J Laryngol Otol. 2016;130(S2):S83-S9.

[38] Xiao T, Kurita H, Shimane T, Nakanishi Y, Koike T. Vital staining with iodine solution in oral cancer: iodine infiltration, cell proliferation, and glucose transporter 1. Int J Clin Oncol. 2013;18(5):792-800.

[39] Govers TM, Hannink G, Merkx MA, Takes RP, Rovers MM. Sentinel node biopsy for squamous cell carcinoma of the oral cavity and oropharynx: a diagnostic meta-analysis. Oral Oncol. 2013;49(8):726-32.

[40] Asakage T, Yokose T, Mukai K, Tsugane S, Tsubono Y, Asai M, et al. Tumor thickness predicts cervical metastasis in patients with stage I/II carcinoma of the tongue. Cancer. 1998;82(8):1443-8.

[41] Mallick S, Benson R, Rath GK. Radiation induced oral mucositis: a review of current literature on prevention and management. Eur Arch Otorhinolaryngol. 2016;273(9):2285-93.

[42] Brennan PA, Bradley KL, Brands M. Intensity-modulated radiotherapy in head and neck cancer - an update for oral and maxillofacial surgeons. Br J Oral Maxillofac Surg. 2017;55(8):770-4.

[43] Marta GN, William WN, Jr., Feher O, Carvalho AL, Kowalski LP. Induction chemotherapy for oral cavity cancer patients: Current status and future perspectives. Oral Oncol. 2015;51(12):1069-75.

[44] Cheraghlou S, Schettino A, Zogg CK, Judson BL. Changing prognosis of oral cancer: An analysis of survival and treatment between 1973 and 2014. Laryngoscope. 2018;128(12):2762-9.

[45] Zanoni DK, Montero PH, Migliacci JC, Shah JP, Wong RJ, Ganly I, et al. Survival outcomes after treatment of cancer of the oral cavity (1985-2015). Oral Oncol. 2019;90:115-21.

[46] Johnson JT, Barnes EL, Myers EN, Schramm VL, Jr., Borochovitz D, Sigler BA. The extracapsular spread of tumors in cervical node metastasis. Arch Otolaryngol. 1981;107(12):725-9.

[47] Ghani WMN, Ramanathan A, Prime SS, Yang YH, Razak IA, Abdul Rahman ZA, et al. Survival of Oral Cancer Patients in Different Ethnicities. Cancer Invest. 2019;37(7):275-87.

[48] Jitender S, Sarika G, Varada HR, Omprakash Y, Mohsin K. Screening for oral cancer. J Exp Ther Oncol. 2016;11(4):303-7.

[49] Chattopadhyay I, Verma M, Panda M. Role of Oral Microbiome Signatures in Diagnosis and Prognosis of Oral Cancer. Technol Cancer Res Treat. 2019;18:1533033819867354.

[50] Moyer VA, Force USPST. Screening for oral cancer: U.S. Preventive Services Task Force recommendation statement. Ann Intern Med. 2014;160(1):55-60.

Chapter 2

Human Papillomavirus Associated Oropharyngeal Carcinoma-Diagnosis and Management

Mullangath Prakasan Aparna, Ravi Rejnish Kumar, Malu Rafi, Geethu Babu, Pradeep Naveen Kumar, Kunnambath Ramadas and Kainickal Cessal Thomachan

Abstract

Head and neck squamous cell carcinomas arise from the mucosa of the upper aerodigestive tract and is often driven by risk factors like tobacco and alcohol consumption. Most of the time patients present with locally advanced stages and the outcome is poor, despite recent advances in multi-modality treatment. The epidemiology of the disease has changed over the last decade with the introduction of a separate clinical entity; Human Papillomavirus (HPV) associated head and neck cancer. The tumorigenesis is different from that of tobacco and alcohol-driven malignancies. These tumors have a better response to treatment owing to their inherent genetic makeup and carry an excellent prognosis. The current school of thought is to reduce the long-term morbidities associated with various treatment modalities, as these patients tend to survive longer. The best management of HPV-associated oropharyngeal cancer is under active investigation.

Keywords: human papilloma virus, oropharyngeal cancer, squamous cell carcinoma, treatment, prognosis

1. Introduction

HPV is currently a well-recognized and emerging risk factor for head and neck squamous cell carcinoma. HPV associated oropharyngeal carcinoma have distinct clinical behavior and outcome. This led to a paradigm shift in the research and trend towards De-escalating treatment strategies. The rationale of these trials is to prove that the de-intensified treatment modality has same efficacy with less morbidity compared to standard of treatment. This chapter tries to elaborate on the epidemiology, oncogenesis, testing for HPV, treatment approaches and different clinical trials addressing the issue.

2. Epidemiology

Oropharyngeal carcinoma represents 0.9% of all cancers and its incidence is increasing with an estimate of 173,495 new cases in 2018 [1]. Epidemiological studies have demonstrated that there has been a reduction in the incidence of laryngeal, hypopharyngeal, and oral cavity cancers since 1980, following a reduction in tobacco use in developed countries [2]. Oropharyngeal cancer incidence initially remained constant, then started rising [2, 3]. Later it was correlated to HPV-associated cancers in the tonsillar region and base of the tongue. There is a geographical variation in the incidence of oropharyngeal carcinoma with the increasing incidence of HPV associated cancers in the developed countries [4]. Among men the rising incidence of HPV associated oropharyngeal cancer was noticed in the United States, Australia, Canada, Japan and Slovakia and among women it was noticed in Denmark, Estonia, France, Netherlands, Poland, Slovakia and United Kingdom [4]. These patients tend to be younger and follow a biphasic distribution, which peaks around 30 and 55 years [5]. Male gender preponderance has been noted in many studies. In the ICON-S database median age of the HPV positive cases was 57 years and 84% of patients were male [5].

3. Clinical characteristics of HPV associated oropharyngeal cancer

HPV-associated Oropharyngeal Squamous cell Carcinoma (OPSCC) has different demographic and biological features when compared to HPV negative cancers [6]. These patients tend to be younger, with little or no tobacco exposure, and associated with certain sexual behaviors like oral sex. They have different molecular alterations. **Table 1** shows a comparison between clinical and biological profiles of HPV positive and HPV negative oropharyngeal carcinoma. The synergetic mechanism of HPV with tobacco and alcohol is unknown. The subset of OPSCC patients with significant smoking history may harbor TP53 and EGFR mutations and their outcomes are similar to HPV negative head and neck cancers.

Characteristics	HPV positive	HPV negative
Age	younger	older
Gender	3:1 men	3:1 men
Socioeconomic status	high	low
Risk factors	sexual behavior	tobacco, alcohol
Co factors	immunosuppression, marijuana use	diet, hygiene
Incidence	increasing	decreasing
Survival	better	worse
Predilection site	tonsil, base of tongue	none
Histology	basaloid/poorly differentiated	keratinized
T-Stage	lower T-stage	higher T stage
Nodal status	higher, often cystic nodes	lower
Field cancerization	unknown	present
Genetics	P53 inactivated by E6	P53 is mutated
	Rb inactivated by E7	Rb inactivated by cyclin D1Amplification
	P 16 over expressed	Inactivation of p 16

Table 1.
Major differences between HPV positive and negative oropharyngeal cancers.

4. Human papillomavirus and carcinogenesis

A systematic review by Kriemer et al. has described the presence of HPV DNA in head and neck cancers [7]. Approximately 150 HPV subtypes have been reported. HPV 16 is associated with >90% of HPV associated oropharyngeal cancers [7]. HPV is a circular, double stranded DNA virus of 55 nm. Multiple sexual partners and/or higher frequency of oral sex may increase the risk of HPV infection and later malignant transformation. Tonsillar crypts provide large epithelial surface and deep invaginations of the mucosal surface are thought to favor the capture and processing of viral antigens. The epithelial basal cells are the target cells of the virus, where the viral DNA undergoes uncoating and is transported to the nucleus. In high risk HPV infection E6 and E7 proteins are produced from the supra basal layers. In HPV induced carcinogenesis, E6 and E7 oncoproteins deregulates cell cycle and apoptosis by acting on p53 [8]. P53 is a tumor suppressor gene which controls G1 transition to S phase in the cell cycle at G1 check point by inducing the expression of cyclin inhibitors p16, p21 and p27 which in turn will block cyclin dependent kinases and progression of the cell cycle at G1/S transition. Inactivation, of p53 gene causes increased cell proliferation. Rb family of proteins governs the check point between G1 and S Phase. In normal cell cycle hypo phosphorylated Rb forms a complex with E2F and makes it unavailable for the DNA synthesis. E7 oncoprotein inactivate Rb family of proteins that causes over expression of E2F thereby produces increased cell proliferation [9].

5. Principles of HPV testing for oropharyngeal carcinoma

All patients diagnosed with OPSCC should undergo testing for HPV status. Biopsy from the primary lesion or FNAC from an involved node is sufficient for HPV testing. The gold standard is the demonstration of HPV E6/E7 mRNA expression in clinical specimens, which is often impractical. Demonstration of HPV DNA, by polymerase chain reaction (PCR), has high sensitivity, but specificity is low as cross-contamination can occur. In situ hybridization (ISH) technique allows the identification of a single viral copy and is more specific. In the HPV carcinogenesis, E7 mediated Rb inhibition leads to induction of demethylases resulting in overexpression of $p16^{INK4A}$, which is a cyclin-dependent kinase inhibitor. Hence the immunohistochemistry (IHC) test for P 16 is used as a surrogate marker for HPV status. Various methods for testing the HPV status is summarized in **Table 2**. Infection with non-HPV subtypes or low viral copy numbers cannot be detected by IHC and there can be a 7% disparity between HPV ISH and IHC reports. In the case of an equivocal P16, further testing by ISH can clarify the HPV status. Work up for patients includes thorough history taking, with documentation on pack-years smoked, and clinical examination (inspection, palpation, and endoscopy evaluation to see the extent of the lesion). Imaging using CT or MRI

Tumor tissue	Serum
• Testing for viral load(Viral DNA) In situ-hybridization	• Antibody testing (Cumulative viral load) L1
Polymerase Chain Reaction	Capsid protein
• Gene expression E6,E7 mRNA	• Expressed oncoprotein E6, E7
• Surrogate Immunohistochemistry-P_{16}	

Table 2.
Various methods used for testing HPV status.

neck aids in staging detects regional lymphadenopathy including retropharyngeal nodes. MRI neck in treatment position is particularly useful in delineation of the primary lesion for radiotherapy planning. The primary lesions of HPV positive OPSCC often had well-defined borders on imaging with a cystic nodal disease with or without necrosis. A chest X-ray is advisable to assess the baseline pulmonary function. Additionally, they need a dental evaluation for radiotherapy planning. All patients should undergo nutrition, speech, and swallowing evaluation, and smoking cessation counseling should be given if needed. Pre-anesthesia workup is needed if planning for surgery.

6. New staging system

As the number of HPV-associated OPSCC increased the 7th AJCC staging system lost its ability to differentiate between stages. There was an overlap of survival among different stages of HPV positive oropharyngeal carcinoma. Based on

Clinical and Pathological T categories
• T1 Tumour 2 cm or less in greatest dimension
• T2 Tumour more than 2 cm but not more than 4 cm
• T3 Tumour more than 4 cm in or extension to lingual surface of epiglottis
• T4 Tumour invades any of the following: larynx, deep/extrinsic muscle of tongue(genioglossus, hyoglossus, palatoglossus, and styloglossus), medial pterygoid, hard palate, mandible, lateral pterygoid muscle, pterygoid plates, lateral nasopharynx, skull base; or encases carotid artery
Clinical N categories
N0 No regional lymph node metastasis
N1 Unilateral metastasis, in lymph node(s), all 6 cm or less
N2 Contralateral or bilateral metastasis in lymph node(s), all 6 cm or less in greatest dimension
N3 Metastasis in lymph node(s) greater than 6 cm in dimension
Clinical
Stage I T1,T2 N0,1 M0
Stage II T1,T2 N2 M0
T3 N0,N1,N2M0
Stage III T1-T4 N3 M0
T4 Any N M0
Stage IV Any T Any N M1
Pathological N categories
Nx-regional nodes cannot be assessed
pN0-No regional lymph node metastasis
pN1-Metastasis in 4 or few lymphnodes
pN2-Metastasis in more than 4 lymphnodes
There is no T4b in the current classification and carcinoma in-situ is removed as there is absence of a distinct basement membrane in the epithelium of Waldeyers ring.
Extra capsular extension is not included in the pathological classification and there is no pN3 status.

Table 3.
New classification for HPV positive carcinoma oropharynx based on AJCC Cancer Staging Manual, 8th [11].

accumulating evidence of prognostic value for HPV-positive OPSCC new staging system was refined [5, 10]. The new AJCC 8th staging system for HPV positive oropharyngeal carcinoma is summarized in **Table 3** [11].

7. HPV status and treatment response

There are many factors attributed to the survival advantage for p16 positive oropharyngeal carcinoma. Many of the patients are younger, they have fewer comorbidities and less chance of field cancerization given reduced smoking history. HPV-positive tumours may harbour fewer or different genetic alterations. HPV-positive tumours have higher radio sensitivity, due to compromised DNA repair capacity [12]. Other studies have reported intrinsic radiation sensitivity and increased apoptosis following radiation exposure [13]. The immunologic response may play a role in the improved response to radiotherapy and chemotherapy in HPV-positive tumors.

The survival advantage noted for HPV positive OPSCC in the radiotherapy setting has been summarized in **Table 4**. Retrospective analysis of the HPV positive subgroup in the RTOG 0129 trial reported a strong association between HPV status and good survival [19]. They risk stratified the patients as having a low, intermediate, or high risk of death based on the combination of tumor HPV status, pack-years of tobacco smoking, and cancer stage. In the low-risk group, which included

Study	N	Subsite	% HPV	Treatment	Survival HPV + ve	Survival HPV − ve	P value
ECOG 2399 [14]	96	oropharynx + larynx	40	induction chemotherapy + chemo radiation	95%	62%	0.005
DAHANCA 5 [15]	156	all head and neck sites	22	radiotherapy + concurrent Nimorazole	62%	26%	0.003
TROG 02.02 [16]	172	oropharynx	57	chemo radiation with or without Tirapazamine	91%	74%	0.004
TAX 324 [17]	111	oropharynx	50	induction chemotherapy + chemo radiation	79%	31%	0.0001
RTOG 9003 [18]	190	oropharynx	39	standard fractionation versus altered fractionation radiotherapy	49%	19.6%,	<0.0001
RTOG 0129 [19]	323	oropharynx	64	accelerated RT vs. Standard RT + concurrent chemotherapy	82.4%,	57.1%	<0.001
DAHANCA6, 7 [20]	769	all head and neck sites	23	five or six fractions of radiotherapy per week +Nimorazole	62%	47%	0.0001

Table 4.
Major randomized trials that have reported survival benefit for HPV positive subset.

HPV positive and non-smokers, 3-year disease-free survival (DFS) was 93% when compared to<50% in the high-risk group which included the HPV negative and smokers. The intermediate-risk group included HPV positive patients with smoking history and HPV negative non -smokers. This led to the thought for de-intensification of the multimodality approach for low-risk category patients. In the post-op setting, the German radiation oncology group study showed a better correlation of HPV positive status with oropharyngeal carcinoma subsite and better outcomes in the patients undergoing adjuvant chemoradiation for locally advanced head and neck cancers [21]. Retrospective analysis of IMCL-9815 study, where patients were treated with radiotherapy with or without Cetuximab, the overall survival was better for p16 positive patients [22]. In the abovementioned trials, a better prognosis for HPV positive oropharyngeal carcinoma was independent of treatment modality. The association of HPV positive status with improved outcome was restricted to the oropharyngeal primary site [23].

8. De-escalating treatment intensity

The treatment options for early-stage OPSCC includes radical radiotherapy versus surgery (resection of the primary+/_ ipsilateral or bilateral neck dissection). For locally advanced oropharyngeal carcinoma primary treatment is radical chemoradiation or induction chemotherapy followed by radical chemoradiation with or without salvage surgery. The primary lesion and involved node with a margin are treated to a dose of 66-70Gy in 33–35 fractions and prophylactic nodal stations will receive 54 Gy in 30 fractions. With the introduction of intensity-modulated radiotherapy (IMRT) dose to dysphagia aspiration, related structures can be minimized. Cisplatin 80–100 mg/m2 once in 3 weeks is the standard concurrent chemotherapy schedule. For primary lesions of the oropharynx, surgical clearance is an issue, considering the complex anatomy and proximity to critical structures. Reconstruction is difficult and retropharyngeal nodes cannot be surgically removed. Bilateral neck dissection should be considered for lesions over the base of the tongue, soft palate, posterior pharyngeal wall, or tonsillar lesion invading the base of the tongue. Functional outcome is better with radiotherapy. In advanced-stage disease, surgery is often followed by adjuvant therapy which will lead to increased morbidity and decreased quality of life. Major factors deciding the treatment modality include performance status of the patient, location of the primary lesion, expertise available, morbidities associated with each treatment option, and patient preference. Since HPV-positive oropharyngeal carcinoma patients tend to be younger and have prolonged survival, there is a potential to improve the quality of life through reducing the treatment-related toxicities. Application of this knowledge has led to multiple de-escalating strategies.

8.1 Minimally invasive surgery

The development of minimally invasive surgical techniques like transoral laser microsurgery (TLM) and transoral robotic surgery (TORS) has changed the surgical management for early oropharyngeal carcinoma. No prospective randomized studies are supporting the use of TORS over conventional surgery for oropharyngeal carcinoma. Small series report better swallowing outcomes in selected oropharyngeal carcinoma patients treated with less invasive surgery with or without neck dissection, followed by adjuvant therapy [24]. Complications include postoperative haemorrhage and the need for temporary tracheostomy.

ORATOR trial is the first phase 2 randomized trial comparing radiotherapy with transoral robotic surgery and neck dissection for early stage oropharyngeal squamous cell carcinoma [25]. Patients with T1–T2, N0–2 (≤4 cm) OPSCC tumor types were randomized to radiotherapy arm (70 Gy, with chemotherapy, if N1–2) or TORS plus neck dissection (with or without adjuvant chemoradiotherapy, based on pathology). In the surgery arm, 24% of patients received postoperative chemoradiotherapy. The initial report showed swallowing related quality of life score was better in the radiotherapy group after one year follow up. The ongoing ORATOR II trial is testing the overall survival between radiotherapy arm versus surgery [26].

Few other trials are assessing whether the swallowing function can be improved following minimally invasive surgery like Trans Oral Robotic Surgery (TORS) and to prove non-inferiority of reducing the intensity of adjuvant treatment in terms of overall survival. **Table 5** shows de-intensification trials after surgical intervention. The aim of the ECOG 3311 study was to find out whether the dose of adjuvant radiotherapy can be reduced in the intermediate risk patients [27]. 2-year Progression free survival was not affected by observation alone in the low risk group and reduced dose radiotherapy in the intermediate risk group. Pathos trial examines whether swallowing function is better in patients undergoing transoral resection of HPV-positive OPSCC with reduced adjuvant treatment and results are awaited [28]. The rationale behind ADEPT trial is to find out is it safe to avoid concurrent chemotherapy in patients with extracapsular extension following minimally invasive surgery [29].

In the ECOG 3311 trial, the negative margin was defined as 3 mm or greater and adjuvant radiotherapy was offered to those with, <3 mm margin [27]. For transoral resection, the chance of positive margin is likely for the base of tongue tumors than Tonsillar tumors. In transoral laser microsurgery, the tumor may be removed in multiple pieces and it may be difficult to commend on the margin status. In many recent studies, the margin is generally considered clear unless involved [24].

Trial	Phase	N	Inclusion criteria (HPV + ve OPSCC)	Intervention (following TORS+ neck dissection)	Outcome
ECOG 3311 [27]	II	511	resectable stage III–IVB	A.Low risk-observation B.Intermediate risk-50Gy/25 fractions or 60Gy/30 fractions C.High risk–Chemo radiation 66Gy/33 fractions	2-year PFS A-93.9% B- 95.0% C- 95.9%
PATHOS trial [28]	III	1100	resectable T1–T3, N0–2b. excludes active smokers with N2b disease	Intermediate risk-50Gy/25 fractions or 60Gy/30 fractions High risk–60Gy/30 fractions or 60Gy/30 fractions + weekly Cisplatin	Awaited
ADEPT [29] (NCT01687413)	III	500	resectableT1–4a with negative margin pN positive with ECE	RT 60Gy/30 fractions or RT 60Gy/30 fractions + weekly Cisplatin	Awaited

TORS:Trans oral robotic surgery; ECE: extracapsular extension.

Table 5.
Trials addressing the role of minimal invasive surgery and reduced dose radiotherapy.

Currently, it is proven that the number of involved nodes is more prognostic than extranodal extension in resected oropharyngeal carcinoma and has been incorporated in the pathological staging of AJCC 8th edition [30]. Some authors have tried omitting chemotherapy in high-risk patients with extranodal extension, to reduce the toxicity associated with triple modality treatment [31]. In the absence of evidence, this practice is not recommended. Routman has reported resected oropharyngeal cancer patients without high-risk features have an 11% risk of failure, whereas those with ECE had a 53% risk of recurrence [32]. This implicates the role of adjuvant radiotherapy in this setting. The role of adjuvant radiotherapy in resected HPV positive oropharyngeal cancer with intermediate-risk patients (PNI, LVI, T3 to T4, or N2 diseases) needs further clarification. The basic principle of oncology is to limit the number of modalities used for treatment to reduce long term morbidities. Long-term data are needed for further refinement of the best management strategy.

8.2 Non-surgical de-intensification strategies

De-intensification strategies employing reducing the dose or volume of radiation therapy have the potential to reduce gastric tube dependence, osteoradionecrosis, dysphagia, xerostomia, dental decay, hypothyroidism, carotid stenosis, etc. which include the following

a. Replace Cisplatin with Cetuximab (along with radiotherapy).

b. Neoadjuvant chemotherapy followed by decreased radiotherapy dose/volume

c. Chemo-radiation with decreased radiotherapy and chemotherapy doses.

d. Omitting chemotherapy.

e. Protons instead of photons.

8.2.1 Replace cisplatin with cetuximab

In the subset analysis of Bonners trial, the benefit of Cetuximab plus RT was restricted to the oropharyngeal subsite [33]. It was later hypothesized to replace Cisplatin with Cetuximab in this favorable group. The three major trials which looked into this aspect were RTOG1016, De-Escalate HPV, and the TROG study (Summarized in **Table 6**).

Results from both RTOG 1016 trial and De-Escalate HPV trial show that HPV positive disease has a good prognosis, there was no difference of toxicity between the two arms, better overall survival and less recurrence with Cisplatin plus RT arm and Cisplatin plus RT remains the standard of care in low-risk HPV positive disease. The result of the TROG 12.01 study is awaiting [36].

8.2.2 Neoadjuvant chemotherapy followed by decreased radiotherapy dose/volume

E1308 was a phase II trial, in which patients were selected to reduced RT dose based on complete clinical response to neoadjuvant chemotherapy with Cisplatin + Paclitaxel + Cetuximab [37]. Those who achieved complete clinical response was treated to an RT dose of 54Gy in 27 fractions, 5 days a week with concurrent cetuximab for 6 weeks, and those patients who achieved a partial response or stable disease was treated to a

Trial	Phase	N	Inclusion criteria (HPV-positive OPSCC)	Intervention	Results
RTOG 1016 [34]	III	706	T1–2, N2a–3 or T3–4, any N	Accelerated RT(70Gy) + cetuximab vs. RT+ 3 weekly Cisplatin	5 year survival 77·9% vs. 84·6% p = 0.5056(non-inferiority)
De-ESCALaTE HPV [35]	III	334	T3N0–T4N0, T1N1 –T4N3 excludes > N2b, >10 PY	Conventional RT+ Cetuximab vs. RT + weekly Cisplatin	2-year survival 89·4% vs. 97·5% (p = 0.001)
TROG 12.01 [36]	III	200	Stage III (excluding T1–2, N1) or IV (excluding T4, N3, or M1) if ≤10 PY. If >10 PY, only N0 – 2A	RT+cetuximab vs. RT+ weekly Cisplatin	Awaited

PY: pack years.

Table 6.
Trials replacing Cisplatin with Cetuximab.

dose of 69.3 Gy in 33 fractions, 5 days a week with concurrent Cetuximab for 7 weeks. After a median follows up of 35.4 months, the 2-year progression-free survival was 80% in the reduced RT group with improved swallowing and nutritional status.

The Quarterback trial is another trial that is looking into this aspect. It is a phase III randomized trial comparing reduced dose (IMRT,56Gy in 28 fractions with concurrent Carboplatin weekly) and standard-dose radiotherapy (IMRT,70Gy in 35 fractions with concurrent Carboplatin weekly) for locally advanced HPV oropharyngeal carcinoma after neoadjuvant chemotherapy with TPF (Cisplatin, Docetaxel, and 5-Fluorouracil) regimen [38]. The primary endpoint is progression-free survival and results are awaited.

Another study has tried reducing the radiation therapy volume, keeping the radiation dose unchanged [39]. Following induction chemotherapy (Cisplatin, Paclitaxel, Cetuximab ± Everolimus), patients with >50% reduction received radiotherapy to gross disease only. Whereas patients with <50% reduction received radiotherapy to gross disease and next elective nodal station. Two -year PFS was 93.1% in the responders versus 74% in the non-responders.

In the OPTIMA trial, both dose reduction and volume de-escalation were tried where radiation was limited to the first echelon of uninvolved nodes [40]. After 3 cycles of neoadjuvant chemotherapy (Carboplatin+ nab-Paclitaxel), low-risk patients with ≥50% response received 50 Gy RT, low-risk patients with 30%–50% response, and high-risk patients with ≥50% response received 45 Gy RT + concurrent chemotherapy and patients with the lesser response received 75Gy + concurrent chemotherapy. Two-year progression survival was not compromised compared to historical control.

8.2.3 Chemoradiation with decreased radiotherapy and chemotherapy doses

In a phase II trial, favourable risk HPV associated oropharyngeal carcinoma patients were randomized to receive 60Gy intensity-modulated radiation therapy with concurrent weekly Cisplatin (30 mg/m^2) followed by biopsy from the primary site and planned neck dissection of the initially involved site [41]. The primary endpoint of the study, pathological complete response was 86% and was associated with less toxicity. Few drawbacks of this study are that they included early-stage cases, short follow-up (14 months), and planned neck dissection which was unnecessary in some patients. In the follow up study, with the same IMRT dose 60 Gy in 30 fractions, multiple chemotherapy options were there (weekly regimens with Cisplatin 30 to 40 mg/m2 (first choice), Cetuximab 250 mg/m^2 (second choice), Carboplatin AUC 1.5 and paclitaxel 45 mg/m^2) and chemotherapy was omitted for patients with T0-2 N0-1 disease, ≤ 10 pack-years smoking history [42]. The neck dissection was advised based on positive PET/CT done after 10–16 weeks. The results are awaited.

8.2.4 Omitting chemotherapy

In the HN 002 trial, patients with stage T1- T2, N1-N2b or T3, N0-N2b, p16 positive oropharyngeal carcinoma patients were randomized to receive either IMRT 60 Gy/30 fractions over 6 weeks, or IMRT with concurrent weekly Cisplatin 40 mg/m^2 [43]. Estimated 2-year survival and late toxicity were similar and acute toxicity were more in the chemotherapy arm.

8.2.5 Protons instead of photons

The goal of the trial was to compare the side effects of 2 radiation treatments; intensity-modulated photon beam therapy 70Gy(RBE) in 33 fractions, with intensity-modulated proton beam therapy, 70Gy(RBE) in 33 fractions. The estimated study completion date is 2024 [44].

9. Unknown primary with cervical node metastasis

If p16 positive in lymph node specimen, it is staged as per p16 positive oropharynx carcinomas and treated accordingly.

10. Immunotherapy

Immunotherapy as sole therapy has reported a delay in progression in metastatic HPV positive oropharyngeal carcinoma [45]. Combining Checkpoint inhibitors like anti-programmed cell death 1 (PD-1) with tumor vaccine has some shown benefit in a recurrent setting in phase II trials [46].

11. Post-treatment surveillance

Following the completion of treatment, the patient should be evaluated clinically once in 3 months for the initial 2 years, once in 6 months for 5 years, and yearly thereafter. Persisting symptoms, radiating pain to the ear, etc. warrants local recurrence. Negative PET/CT scan obtained between 3 and 6 months after completion of treatment and at 12 months post-treatment is associated with a good prognosis. Considering the low recurrence rate in HPV positive OPSCC and the cost involved, it's not a routine investigation that is followed.

DOI: http://dx.doi.org/10.5772/intechopen.96234

12. Treatment of recurrent and metastatic disease

Salvage surgery or irradiation if feasible should be considered for recurrent disease. Palliative chemotherapy with platinum doublets can be considered if local treatment not feasible. Clinical trials are ongoing with targeted agents, immunotherapy as sole treatment versus combination therapy.

13. Conclusion

HPV associated oropharyngeal carcinoma is on the rise. A lot of research is happening in this field to refine the best treatment for this separate clinical entity with the vision to reduce long term morbidities. Mature data with long term follow up is needed to change the current practice. At present, HPV-positive oropharyngeal carcinoma patients should not be treated with de-intensification protocols outside the clinical trial setting.

Conflict of interest

"The authors declare no conflict of interest."

Author details

Mullangath Prakasan Aparna, Ravi Rejnish Kumar, Malu Rafi, Geethu Babu, Pradeep Naveen Kumar, Kunnambath Ramadas and Kainickal Cessal Thomachan*
Department of Radiation Oncology, Regional Cancer Centre, Thiruvananthapuram, Kerala, India

*Address all correspondence to: drcessalthomas@gmail.com

References

[1] F. Bray, J. Ferlay, I. Soerjomataram, R. L. Siegel, L. A. Torre, and A. Jemal. Global cancer statistics 2018: GLOBOCAN estimates of incidence and mortality worldwide for 36 cancers in 185 countries, CA: A Cancer Journal for Clinicians 2018; 68: 394-424.

[2] Sturgis EM, Ang KK. The epidemic of HPV-associated oropharyngeal cancer is here: is it time to change our treatment paradigms? J Natl Compr Canc Netw 2011; 9:665.

[3] Chaturvedi AK, Engels EA, Pfeiffer RM, et al. Human papillomavirus, and rising oropharyngeal cancer incidence in the United States. J Clin Oncol 2011; 29:4294

[4] Chaturvedi AK, Anderson WF, Lortet-Tieulent J, et al. Worldwide trends in incidence rates for oral cavity and oropharyngeal cancers. J Clin Oncol 2013; 31:4550.

[5] O'Sullivan B, Huang SH, Su J, et al. Development and validation of a staging system for HPV-related oropharyngeal cancer by the International Collaboration on Oropharyngeal cancer Network for Staging (ICON-S): a multicenter cohort study. Lancet Oncol. 2016; 17:440.

[6] Maura L. Gillison, Gypsyamber D'Souza, William Westra et al. Distinct Risk Factor Profiles for Human Papillomavirus Type 16–Positive and Human Papillomavirus Type 16–Negative Head and Neck Cancers. Journal of the National Cancer Institute. *2008;* 100: 6, 407-420.

[7] Kreimer, A.R.; Clifford, G.M.; Boyle, P.; Franceschi, S. Human papillomavirus types in head and neck squamous cell carcinomas worldwide: A systematic review. Cancer Epidemiol 2005; 14, 467-475.

[8] Boscolo-Rizzo P, Del Mistro A, Bussu F, et al. New insights into human papillomavirus-associated head and neck squamous cell carcinoma. Acta OtorhinolaryngolItal.2013; 33: 77-87

[9] Kumaraswamy KL1, Vidhya M. Human papillomavirus, and oral infections: an update. J Cancer Res Ther. 2011 Apr-Jun; 7(2):120-127

[10] Shao Hui Huang, Wei Xu, John Waldron et al. Refining American Joint Committee on Cancer/Union for International Cancer Control TNM Stage and Prognostic Groups for Human Papillomavirus-Related Oropharyngeal Carcinomas. J.ClinOncol. 2015; 33(8):836-845.

[11] O'Sullivan B, Lydiatt WM, Haughey BH, et al. HPV-Mediated (p16+) Oropharyngeal Cancer. In: AJCC Cancer Staging Manual, 8th, Amin MB (Ed), Springer, New York 2017. p.113.

[12] Thorsten Rieckmann, SilkeTribius, Tobias J Grob, et al.HNSCC Cell Lines Positive for HPV and p16 Possess Higher Cellular Radiosensitivity Due to an Impaired DSB Repair Capacity. RadiotherOncol. 2013; 107(2):242-246.

[13] Randall J Kimple, Molly A Smith, Grace C Blitzer et al. Enhanced Radiation Sensitivity in HPV-positive Head and Neck Cancer.Cancer Res.2013; 73(15):4791-4800.

[14] Carole Fakhry, William H. Westra, Sigui Li etal.Improved Survival of Patients With Human Papillomavirus–Positive Head and Neck Squamous Cell Carcinoma in a Prospective Clinical Trial. *Journal of the National Cancer Institute.2008; 100(4): 261*-269, https://doi.org/10.1093/jnci/djn011

[15] Pernille Lassen , Jesper G Eriksen, Stephen Hamilton-Dutoit, et al. Effect of HPV-associated p16INK4A

Expression on Response to Radiotherapy and Survival in Squamous Cell Carcinoma of the Head and Neck. J ClinOncol. 2009; 27(12):1992-1998.

[16] Danny Rischin, Richard J Young, Richard Fisher et al. Prognostic Significance of p16INK4A and Human Papillomavirus in Patients with Oropharyngeal Cancer Treated on TROG 02.02 Phase III Trial. J ClinOncol. 2010 Sep 20; 28(27):4142-8.

[17] MR Posner, JH Lorch, O Goloubevaet al. Survival and Human Papillomavirus in Oropharynx Cancer in TAX 324: A Subset Analysis From an International Phase III Trial. AnnOncol .2011; 22(5):1071-7.

[18] M. L. Gillison, Q. Zhang, K. Ang, K. K. Fu et al. Analysis of the effect of p16 and tobacco pack-years (p-y) on overall (OS) and progression-free survival (PFS) for patients with oropharynx cancer (OPC) in Radiation Therapy Oncology Group (RTOG) protocol 9003.Journal of Clinical Oncology. 2010; 28:5510-5510.

[19] K. Kian Ang, M.D., Ph.D., Jonathan Harris, M.S., Richard Wheeler, M.D. et al. Human Papillomavirus and Survival of Patients with Oropharyngeal Cancer. N Engl J Med. 2010 Jul 1; 363(1): 24-35. DOI: 10.1056/NEJMoa0912217

[20] Lassen P, Eriksen JG, Krogdahl et al. Danish Head, and Neck Cancer Group (DAHANCA). The influence of HPV-associated p16-expression on accelerated fractionated radiotherapy in head and neck cancer: evaluation of the randomized DAHANCA 6&7 trial. Radiotherapy and Oncology 2011; 100:49-55.

[21] Fabian Lohaus, Annett Linge, IngeTinhofer et al.HPV16DNA Status Is a Strong Prognosticator of Loco-Regional Control After Postoperative Radio chemotherapy of Locally Advanced Oropharyngeal Carcinoma: Results From a Multicenter Explorative Study of the German Cancer Consortium Radiation Oncology Group (DKTK-ROG).RadiotherOncol. 2014; 113(3):317-323.

[22] David I Rosenthal, Paul M Harari, JordiGiralt, Bell et al. Association of Human Papillomavirus and p16 Status With Outcomes in the IMCL-9815 Phase III Registration Trial for Patients With Locoregionally Advanced Oropharyngeal Squamous Cell Carcinoma of the Head and Neck Treated With Radiotherapy With or Without Cetuximab. J ClinOncol. 2016; 34(12):1300-1308.

[23] Pernille Lassen, Hanne Primdahl, Jorgen Johansen et al. Impact of HPV-associated p16-expression on Radiotherapy Outcome in Advanced Oropharynx and Non-Oropharynx Cancer.RadiotherOncol. 2014; 113(3):310-316.

[24] Hinni ML, Zarka MA, Hoxworth JM. Margin mapping in transoral surgery for head and neck cancer. Laryngoscope. 2013; 123:1190-1198.

[25] Anthony C Nichols, Julie Theurer, EitanPrismanetal. Radiotherapy versus transoral robotic surgery and neck dissection for oropharyngeal squamous cell carcinoma (ORATOR): an open-label, phase 2, randomized trial. Lancet Oncol 2019; 20: 1349-1359

[26] David Palma et al Primary Radiotherapy Versus Primary Surgery for HPV-Associated Oropharyngeal Cancer (ORATOR2). ClinicalTrials.gov Identifier: NCT03210103

[27] Transoral Surgery Followed by Low-Dose or Standard-Dose Radiation Therapy with or Without Chemotherapy in Treating Patients with HPV Positive Stage III-IVA Oropharyngeal Cancer. A trial of the ECOG-ACRIN Cancer Research Group (E3311). J.ClinOncol. 2020; 38:15

[28] Mererid Evans, Terrence Jones et al.PATHOS: a phase II/III trial of

risk-stratified, reduced intensity adjuvant treatment in patients undergoing transoral surgery for Human papillomavirus (HPV) positive oropharyngealcancer.ClinicalTrials.gov Identifier: NCT02215265

[29] Post-Operative Adjuvant Therapy De-Intensification Trial for Human Papillomavirus-related, p16+ Oropharynx Cancer (ADEPT). ClinicalTrials.gov Identifier: NCT01687413.

[30] Sinha P, Kallogjeri D, Gay H, et al. High metastatic node number, not extracapsular spread or N-classification is a node-related prognosticator in transorally-resected, neck-dissected p16-positive oropharynx cancer. Oral Oncol. 2015; 51:514-520.

[31] Su W, Liu J, Miles BA, et al. Adjuvant radiation therapy alone for HPV related oropharyngeal cancers with high-risk features. PLoS One. 2016; https://doi.org/10.1371/journal.pone.0168061

[32] Routman DM, Funk RK, Tangsriwong K, et al. Relapse rates with surgery alone in human papillomavirus-related intermediate- and high-risk group oropharynx squamous cell cancer: a multi-institutional review. Int J RadiatOncolBiol Phys. 2017; 99:938-946.

[33] James A Bonner, Paul M Harari, JordiGiralt et al. Radiotherapy Plus Cetuximab for Loco regionally Advanced Head and Neck Cancer: 5-year Survival Data From a Phase 3 Randomised Trial, and Relation Between Cetuximab-Induced Rash and Survival.LancetOncol. 2010; 11(1):21-28.

[34] Gillison ML, Trotti AM, Harris J et al. Radiotherapy plus cetuximab or cisplatin in human papillomavirus-positive oropharyngeal cancer (NRG Oncology RTOG 1016): a randomized, multicentre, non-inferiority trial. Lancet.2019; 39: 40-50.

[35] Mehanna H, Robinson M, Hartley A et al. Radiotherapy plus cisplatin or cetuximab in low-risk human papillomavirus-positive oropharyngeal cancer (De-ESCALaTE HPV): an open-label randomized controlled Phase III trial. Lancet .2019; 393: 51-60.

[36] Weekly Cetuximab/RT versus Weekly Cisplatin/RT in HPV-Associated Oropharyngeal Squamous Cell Carcinoma (HPVOropharynx)ClinicalTrials.gov Identifier: NCT01855451.

[37] ShanthiMarur, Shuli Li, Anthony J Cmelak et al. E1308: Phase II Trial of Induction Chemotherapy Followed by Reduced-Dose Radiation and Weekly Cetuximab in Patients With HPV-Associated Resectable Squamous Cell Carcinoma of the Oropharynx- ECOG-ACRIN Cancer Research Group. J ClinOncol.2017; 35(5):490-497.

[38] Marshall Posner et al.The Quarterback Trial: A Randomized Phase III Clinical Trial Comparing Reduced and Standard Radiation Therapy Doses for Locally Advanced HPV Positive Oropharynx Cancer.https://clinicaltrials.gov/ct2/show/NCT01706939.

[39] V M Villaflor, J M Melotek, T G Karrison et al.Response-adapted volume de-escalation (RAVD) in locally advanced head and neck cancer. Ann Oncol. 2016 May; 27(5):908-13. DOI: 10.1093/annonc/mdw051.

[40] T Y Seiwert, C C Foster, E A Blair et al. OPTIMA: A Phase II Dose and Volume De-Escalation Trial for Human Papillomavirus-Positive Oropharyngeal Cancer. Ann Oncol. 2019; 30(2):297-302.

[41] Bhishamjit S Chera, Robert J Amdur, Joel Tepper et al. Phase 2 Trial of De-intensified Chemoradiation Therapy for Favorable-Risk Human Papillomavirus-Associated Oropharyngeal Squamous Cell Carcinoma. Int J RadiatOncolBiol Phys. 2015; 93(5):976-985.

[42] De-intensification of Radiation and Chemotherapy for Low-Risk HPV-related Oropharyngeal SCC: Follow-up Study.ClinicalTrials.gov Identifier: NCT02281955.

[43] S.S. Yom, P. Torres-Saavedra, J.J. Caudell et al. NRG-HN002: A Randomized Phase II Trial for Patients With p16-Positive, Non-Smoking-Associated, Loco regionally Advanced Oropharyngeal Cancer.Int J RadiatOncolBiol Phys. 2019; 105:3.

[44] Steven J. Frank, MD et al.Randomized Trial of Intensity-Modulated Proton Beam Therapy (IMPT) Versus Intensity-Modulated Photon Therapy (IMRT) for the Treatment of Oropharyngeal Cancer of the Head and Neck.ClinicalTrials.gov Identifier: NCT01893307.

[45] Nieto K., Gissmann L., Schadlich L et al.Human papillomavirus-specific immune therapy: failure and hope. Antivir. Ther. 2010; 15(7):951-957.

[46] Massarelli E. Combining immune checkpoint blockade and tumor-specific vaccine for patients with incurable human papillomavirus 16-related cancer: a phase 2 clinical trial. JAMA Oncol. 2019; 5(1):67-73.

Chapter 3

Screening of Nasopharyngeal Carcinoma

Yanping Yang and Yonglin Cai

Abstract

Nasopharyngeal carcinoma (NPC) is one of head and neck cancer. It has a complicated etiology involving Epstein–Barr virus (EBV) infection, environment changes, and genetic susceptibility. Early symptoms of NPC are unspecific, so most NPC patients are diagnosed at a late stage. An effective population screening strategy could increase the early detection and early diagnosis rate. As far, serological detection of EBV antibodies such as VCA-IgA, EA-IgA, and EBNA1-IgA, are widely used in NPC mass screening; EBV DNA load detection in plasma or nasopharyngeal swab was applied to screen in endemic populations for assessing the feasibility. However, the current screening schemes still have disadvantages such as lowly positive predictive value, unclear effectiveness of screening and cost-effectiveness. In the present chapter, we try to review the different screening strategies for NPC to understand the future direction of development.

Keywords: Nasopharyngeal carcinoma, Screening, Early diagnosis, Biomarker, Epstein–Barr virus, Antibody, DNA load

1. Introduction

Screening is primary measure of secondary prevention of cancer. It mainly regularly monitor the asymptomatic high-risk population to achieve the purpose of early detection and early treatment of malignant tumors. Cancer carring out the secondary prevention should have the following conditions: 1) great harm to the health and life of the population; 2) long enough pre-clinical period; 3) better effect of both the early treatment and intervention of precancerous lesions; 4) screening methods with effective sensitivity and specificity.

Nasopharyngeal carcinoma (NPC) is a one of head and neck cancer. At present, the etiology of NPC has not remained completely elucidated, generally considered involving Epstein–Barr virus (EBV) infection, environment changes, and genetic susceptibility. There are no feasible preventive measures for NPC. However, it has secondary prevention. First, NPC exhibiting marked racial and geographical differences, is epidemic in the population of Southern China, Southeast Asia, and North Africa, which is extremely harmful to human life and health [1]. In 2014, the incidence and mortality of NPC were 2.48 per 100,000 and 1.23 per 100,000 in China respectively [2]. At the same time, the morbidity and mortality of males were higher than females. The morbidity was mainly in the young while the mortality was mainly in middle and old age. Besides, the occurrence and development of NPC is a multi-stage process, which includes initiation, promotion, malignant transformation, and advanced stage of disease [3]. It takes a certain amount of time to develop into a malignant tumor. In addition, the clinical stage of NPC is an important factor affecting therapeutic outcome. The 10-year survival rate for NPC with stages I and II can reach up to over 90%, whereas for patients with stage III and IV is less than 50% [4]. At last, there are effective methods to detect pre-clinical patients, and the level of antibody against EBV antigens is significantly related to the risk of NPC [5, 6].

NPC first occurs in the epithelium of the nasopharynx, which can invade the base of the skull and metastasize to the cervical lymph nodes. It has the characteristics of complex manifestations, hidden onset, non-specificity of the initial symptoms, and difficulty in early diagnosis. According to statistics, patients with NPC at an early stage who came to the hospital accounted for only about 20% of the total [7]. Strengthening secondary prevention - early detection, early diagnosis, and early treatment - is an important part of the prevention and treatment of NPC. At the same time it is the key to improve the cure rate and obtain a better prognosis of NPC patients.

2. EBV specific antibodies-based serologic testing

EBV belonging to γ-herpesvirus is a human herpesvirus with B lymphocytes. Nearly 95% of adults worldwide are infected with this virus. EBV in infected cells can be divided into two states: EBV latent infection and EBV lytic infection. Only a few virus genes are expressed in EBV latent infection, which can ensure the basic replication function of the virus but lossing infection ability. In EBV lytic infection, EBV needs to be activated about 80 ~ 100 viral genes to complete host-to-host propagation, and finally produce and form infectious virions (or viral particles). After the initial infection, EBV can establish a lifelong latent infection in the host, and persistent EBV lysis replication state infection can lead to a series of human malignant tumors [8].

EBV infection is closely related to the occurrence and development of NPC. EBV latent infection of nasopharyngeal epithelial cells is considered to be a key step in the carcinogenesis of epithelial cells. After EBV infection, the expressed virus genes can produce different antigens, such as EBV nuclear antigen (EBNA), membrane antigen (MA), early antigen (EA), viral capsid antigen (VCA), BZLF1 transcription activator protein (Zta), BRLF1 transcription activator protein (Rta), etc. [9].

The detection of antibodies against EBV antigens in the sera of NPC patients was reported as early as 1966. Helen W et al. first proposed the view that immunoglobulin A (IgA) antibodies against EBV can be used for the diagnosis of NPC [10]. Studies also confirmed that the expression of IgA antibodies against VCA (VCA-IgA) in NPC patients was higher than in healthy people and the antibody titer was related to the stage of NPC. The idea of using this antibody for NPC screening also was proposed [11]. In 1977, Y Zeng et al. established a prospective prevention and treatment site for NPC in Cangwu, Guangxi province China, in order to carry out research on early diagnosis and etiology analysis. The first NPC mass screening was carried out in Cangwu County by the application of the immunoenzymatic (IE) method to detect VCA-IgA and EA-IgA [12]. Therefore, the NPC screening model suitable for the population in the high-risk areas was established by Zeng's team. Then this mass screening model was promoted to three high-risk areas in China, including Guangxi, Guangdong, and Hainan province; and more than four hundred thousand people were screened for NPC [13–16]. In the 1980s, similar methods were used to screen and follow up large populations in Guangdong and Taiwan provinces [17, 18]. SM Cao et al. performed a prospective screening study of 18,986 subjects with a 20-year follow-up in Guangdong province using the same method [6].

This study showed that both VCA-IgA and EA-IgA antibodies were effective serum markers for NPC screening in high-risk areas. Thus, this method was considered as the standard tool for NPC mass screening in China. However, the IE method for detecting EBV antibodies also has disadvantages, such as tedious operation, long time consuming, no quality control standard, and subjective influence on manual interpretation results. These characteristics made it difficult to consistently perform in a large population.

Enzyme-linked immunoassay (ELISA) with many advantages compared with the IE method, such as simple operation, automatic detection, and interpretation of results by a microplate reader, which have subsequently been applied in NPC screening. Many studies about using ELISA for NPC screening were reported. The detection of ZEBRA-IgG by ELISA was applied to screen NPC, but it's specificity and sensitivity were lower compared with the detection of VCA-IgA based on IE [19]. ELISA-based detection of EBV-related antibodies, such as VCA-IgA, EBNA1-IgA have also found to be a marker for NPC screening [20–22]. The detection rate of one single marker was found to be not ideal, and issues such as the combination of indicators for joint detection, the setting of thresholds, and the strategy of screening intervals were discussed.

In Indonesia, the two-step approach employed the EBV IgA ELISA based on a combination of VCA p18- and EBNA1-derived synthetic peptides as an initial screening test and the EA-IgA ELISA as a confirmation test. The sensitivity and specificity for diagnosing NPC using it significantly increased, as well as positive predictive value and negative predictive value [23].

JY Guo et al. evaluated the diagnostic effect of VCA-IgA, EA-IgA and Rta-IgG antibody detection alone or Combiningly in NPC. The triple-positive of VCA-IgA, EA-IgA and Rta-IgG antibodies suggested the highest risk of NPC, and the triple-negative of them showed the lowest risk [24].

In Taiwan, the ability of anti-EBV-IgA antibody to detect NPC in a high-risk population was evaluated. These markers targeted at the following EBV peptides including EBNA1, VCAp18, EAp138, Ead_p47 and VCAp18 + EBNA1 peptide mixture. The result showed that EBNA1-IgA was a sensitive biomarker for differential diagnosis of NPC. At the same time they identified 80% of the high-risk individuals who developed to NPC during follow-up (80% sensitivity) during measuring at baseline [25].

SM Cao's team developed a prediction formula to calculate Logit P-value with VCA-IgA and EBNA1-IgA as variables ($\text{Logit } P = -3.934 + 2.203 \times VCA/IgA + 4.797 \times EBNA1/IgA$). The specificity of the new screening scheme is equivalent to traditional screening scheme with the IE method (estimated at 98.5%), but the sensitivity of former (75.0%) is significantly higher than the latter (25.0%) [26]. A total of 28,688 Guangdong residents aged 30–59 years were screened by the combination of two EBV antibodies tests in addition to indirect mirror examination in the nasopharynx and/or lymphatic palpation (IMLP) in Sihui and Zhongshan, Guangdong province China. After one year of follow-up, the total detection rate of NPC was 0.14% (41/28,688), and the early diagnosis rate was as high as 68.3% (28/41) [27]. After six-year follow-up, the sensitivity of the new scheme was 95.7%, with AUC = 0.926 (95% CI: 0.885–0.966). The new screening scheme for NPC is verified to be the preferred serum diagnostic strategy for long-term screening in high-incidence areas of NPC [28]. For the best interval, studies have shown that the incidence of NPC was low in the first few years after the negative screening and then it would increase to the general population level. Therefore, the screening interval of 4–5 years may be more appropriate than 9–10 years after VCA-IgA negative detection in NPC screening [29]. The above research results were adopted by the Chinese Technical Program of Cancer Early

Diagnosis and Early Treatment --Technical Scheme of NPC Screening to guide the annual routine population screening in NPC high-risk areas (**Figure 1**).

However, there are still limitations in NPC screening using EBV antibodies as tumor markers. The false-positive rate of EBV serological screening is relatively high. The positive rate of EBV antibody in the high-risk areas of NPC is 3% ~ 10%. High-risk groups require further examinations, such as nasopharyngeal fibroscopy

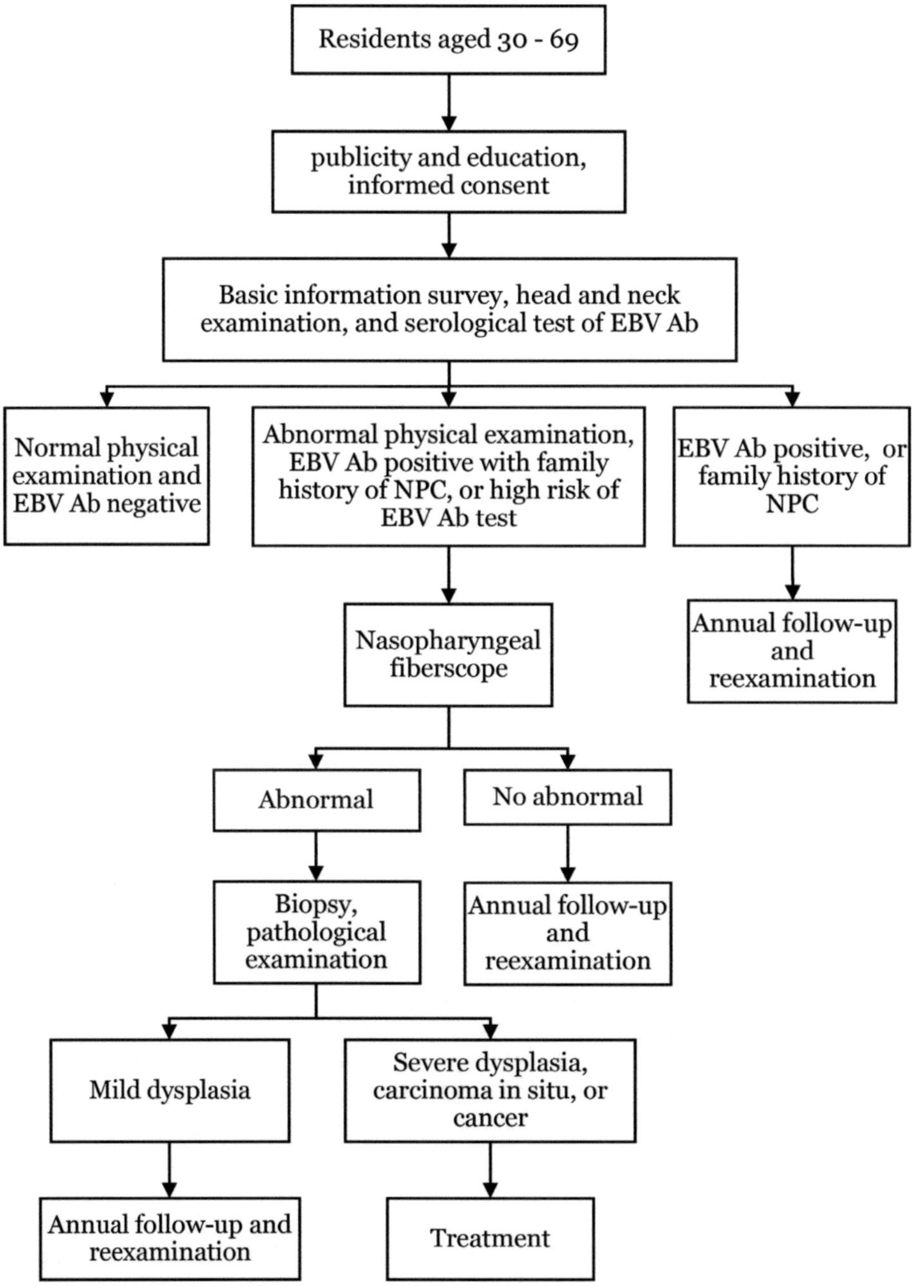

Figure 1.
Flowchart of NPC screening procedure for nasopharyngeal carcinoma (NPC). EBV, Epstein–Barr virus; ab, antibody. Cited by expert group of NPC screening project, expert committee on early diagnosis and treatment of cancer project, China. The technical scheme of NPC screening, early diagnosis and early treatment (2015 edition).

and nasopharyngeal tissue biopsy. Pathologically diagnosed NPC only accounts for 1.5% ~ 3.3% of the high-risk population at the initial screening, which further leads to a higher false positive rate [27, 30, 31].

3. EBV DNA load detection in plasma or nasopharyngeal swab/brushing

Plasma EBV DNA load detected with polymerase chain reaction (PCR) has been also explored to detect early-stage NPC in asymptomatic patients. Research has demonstrated that EBV DNA could be quantitatively measured in the blood of NPC patients by PCR [32]. A study of 175 patients in New York City found that EBV DNA test had much higher specificity and positive predictive value than IgA test alone [33]. A systematic review reported that the EBV DNA load test had the largest area of 0.932 under the summary receiver operator curve with high sensitivity (73%) and specificity (89%), which suggested that EBV DNA detection in plasma could be an efficient marker in NPC screening [34].

In Hong Kong, a prospective study of 20,174 participants revealed that EBV DNA load in plasma samples was particularly useful in screening for early asymptomatic NPC [35]. The participants were ethnically Chinese men at 40 to 60 years of age. The subjects with initial positive results were detected again after about four weeks, while the subjects with persistent positive EBV DNA in plasma were performed to check by nasal endoscopy and magnetic resonance imaging (MRI). The median duration of follow-up was 22 months (range, 12 to 44 months). This study showed that the sensitivity and specificity of this method in NPC screening were 97.1% and 98.6% respectively.

However, a study reported that EBV DNA load had a little poor sensitivity and specificity for NPC screening among high-risk family members compared with EBV-IgA serology [36].

The patients with early NPC may only release a limited amount of viral DNA to the blood, making it impossible to detect blood circulation. The potential value of plasma EBV DNA detection in screening for early NPC remains controversial. NPC mainly originates from epithelial cells in the nasopharynx fossa or posterior wall of the nasopharynx. EBV genome can be detected in almost all tumor cells of NPC cases [37]. Clonal EBV genome can be continuously detected in invasive cancer and precancerous high-grade dysplasia [38]. It is suggested that direct detection of EBV genome from nasopharyngeal brushing or swab specimens had highly predictive value for screening asymptomatic NPC.

In the 1990s, a prospective study was designed to assess the feasibility of a new method for NPC screening by using of PCR coupled with nasopharyngeal swab [39]. In this study, 55 patients were enrolled. The result showed that this method had a similar sensitivity to serological methods, indicating this new method was a good supplement to NPC screening. Nasopharyngeal swab is a quite simple procedure with little discomfort. SP Hao et al. detected the expression of EBV-derived latent membrane protein 1 (LMP-1) by nasopharyngeal swab, and he found that this strategy could serve as part of a screening program for high-risk populations with a sensitivity of 87.3% and a specificity of 98.4% [40]. Raymond's study has also confirmed the effectiveness of this new method of screening for NPC. This study performed on 578 patients yielded a sensitivity of 98.9% and a specificity of 99.3% with a positive predictive value of 96.9% and a negative predictive value of 99.7% [41]. In a prospective and population-based study, the detection of EBV load in the nasopharynx by nasopharyngeal swab was demonstrated to be a useful tool as a supplement to serological tests [42]. Studies of both Zheng and Zhang also verified the same conclusion [43, 44]. Notably, Nasopharyngeal swab detection of EBV load alone should not be used as a mean of NPC screening because of its high false-positive rate [42]. However, nasopharyngeal swab serving as an applicable sampling method for NPC screening is great feasible, but more research will be needed in the future.

4. Novel biomarkers/technology for NPC screening

As mentioned above, EBV-related test has been widely used for early NPC screening, especially the combination of EBV-antibody VCA-IgA and EBNA1-IgA. With the development of research technologies, other biomarkers also develope for NPC screening. Liu et al. reported that a combination of PCR and MWCNT-Fe3O4 nanocomposites had the higher detection rate and higher sensitivity compared with the traditional ELISA method [45]. MWCNT-Fe3O4 nanocomposites are a combination of multi-walled carbon nanotubes and iron oxide nanoparticles, which can provide a large surface areas for antigen–antibody binding. A nested case–control study including 20 patients with NPC and 88 normal control showed that EBV microRNA BART2-5p had been proved to be a valuable biomarker for NPC screening with a sensitivity of 90.9% [46]. Thirteen genes including DNAAF1, PARPBP, TTC18, GSTA3, RCN1, MUC5AC, POU2AF1, FAM83B, SLC22A16, SPEF2, ERICH3, CCDC81, and IL33 have been associated with NPC detection based on comprehensive bioinformatics analyses [47]. A recent study showed that higher methylation rates of EGFR and ZNF6671 in circulating cell-free DNA (ccfDNA) could predict NPC, which was a potential novel molecular marker for NPC screening [48]. However, all these researches need more evidence and more data to demonstrate their effectiveness in NPC screening.

Many studies have shown that intestinal flora disruption was associated with malignant tumors. C. ramosum bacteria that promotes the secretion of 5-HT was found to be a strong risk factor for NPC. The establishment of a disease prediction model based on C. ramosum might be used for the prediction of disease risk in a high-risk population and early non-invasive screening of NPC [49].

Raman spectroscopy combined with multivariate analysis technology has been reported to analyze the sera of NPC patients and healthy individuals. In NPC samples, the lipid content, phenylalanine, and β-carotene decreased while amide III, tyrosine and tryptophan increased. The changes in these biomolecular concentrations may be applied for NPC diagnosis [50]. A unmodified nanotechnology based on surface-enhanced Raman spectroscopy was used to detect the blood circulating DNA; and the diagnostic sensitivity and specificity for differentiating the NPC patients from the normal control were 83.3% and 82.5% respeactively. Nanotechnology which was sensitive, rapid, and easy-to-use may have the potential to become a better method for NPC detection and screening based on liquid biopsy [51].

5. Cost-effectiveness of NPC screening

A Markov stimulation model was constructed to evaluate the cost-effectiveness of different screening strategies for serological tests in China. In this study, NPC detection rate, cost, quality-adjust life, and incremental cost-effectiveness ratio were considered. Results showed that strategy (annual screening for EBV-seropositive subject, triennial screening for seronegative subjects) was the economical and practical option [52]. In 2019, a Markov cohort model was also reported to use to estimate the screening for NPC with plasma EBV DNA for

50-year-old Asian American men in the United States. The study suggested that because of its high false-positive results in high-risk regions and its uncertain clinical value in non-endemic areas this method wasn't the most cost-effective, despite its specificity and sensitivity were high [53]. Therefore more research will be required in the future.

Studies about NPC screening based on EBV-related test have been widely reported, but there are few studies on the association between EBV-antibody screening and NPC mortality. Recently a study about prospective, cluster-randomized, controlled trial in southern China for NPC screening was revealed that the combination of EBV antibody EBNA1-IgA and VCA-IgA could effectively identify the high-risk population and improve diagnosis of NPC in the interim analysis. Although the mortality of the screening group was not significantly reduced, the specific mortality of NPC in the screening participants was significantly reduced [54]. That was the first report which presented a mortality reduction by NPC screening. It is expected to further improve the participation rate in the future, and finally confirm the effectiveness of NPC screening based on EBV detection.

6. Conclusions and future directions

Due to the hidden location of NPC, it is difficult to diagnose early. Strengthening the publicity of NPC prevention and control, popularizing basic knowledge of it, and making residents cooperate with screening projects will be way helpful to improve the accuracy of early diagnosis rate of NPC. At present, the above screening methods have positive significance, but they also have limitations regrettably. How to make better use of their advantages and disadvantages to carry out local screening schemes in different regions is worthy to further exploration. And developing faster, simpler, higher true-positive rate and lower false-positive rate screening methods and more effective treatment were important ways to improve the survival rate and life quality of NPC patients.

Currently, there are few reports from randomized controlled trials (RCT) and controlled clinical trials (CCT) to determine the efficacy of screening for NPC or the cost-effectiveness of a screening strategy. Future studies with long-term follow-up need to systematically assess the impact of the screening methods in mortality, assess their ability to detect NPC, evaluate the impact on quality of life and cost-effectiveness.

Acknowledgements

This work was supported by grants from the National Natural Science Foundation of China (grant number: 81860601, recipient: YLC).

Conflict of interest

The authors declare no conflict of interest.

Author details

Yanping Yang[1] and Yonglin Cai[2*]

1 Department of Otolaryngology-Head and Neck Surgery, Guangxi Medical University, Nanning, China

2 Guangxi Health Commission Key Laboratory of Molecular Epidemiology of Nasopharyngeal Carcinoma, Wuzhou Red Cross Hospital, Wuzhou, China

*Address all correspondence to: cylzen@163.com

References

[1] Tang L L, Chen W Q, Xue W Q, He Y Q, Zheng R S, Zeng Y X, Jia W H. Global trends in incidence and mortality of nasopharyngeal carcinoma. Cancer Lett. 2016:1:22-30. DOI:10.1016/j.canlet.2016.01.040

[2] Fu Z T, Guo X L, Zhang S W, Zeng H M, Sun K X, Chen W Q, He J. Incidence and mortality of nasopharyngeal carcinoma in China, 2014. Zhonghua Zhong Liu Za Zhi. 2018:8:566-571. DOI:10.3760/cma.j.issn.0253-3766.2018.08.002

[3] Chen Y P, Chan A, Le QT, Blanchard P, Sun Y, Ma J. Nasopharyngeal carcinoma. Lancet. 2019:10192:64-80. DOI:10.1016/S0140-6736(19)30956-0

[4] Mao Y, Li W, Chen L, Sun Y, Liu L, Tang L, Cao S, LinAi-Hua, Hong M, Lu T, Liu M, Li L, Ma J. A clinical verification of the Chinese 2008 staging system for nasopharyngeal carcinoma. Ai Zheng. 2009:10:1022-1028.

[5] Deng H, Zeng Y, Liang J, Zheng Y, Zhang Z, Zhong J, Ou B, Zhang F, Lin J, Cheng J, Tang M, Huang B. The basic screening project in 488 683 persons for nasopharyneal carcinoma. Zhong Liu. 2005:2:152-154.

[6] Cao S M, Liu Z, Jia W H, Huang Q H, Liu Q, Guo X, Huang T B, Ye W, Hong M H. Fluctuations of epstein-barr virus serological antibodies and risk for nasopharyngeal carcinoma: a prospective screening study with a 20-year follow-up. PLoS One. 2011:4:e19100. DOI:10.1371/journal.pone.0019100

[7] Yang S, Wu S, Zhou J, Chen X Y. Screening for nasopharyngeal cancer. Cochrane Database Syst Rev. 2015:11:CD008423. DOI:10.1002/14651858.CD008423.pub2

[8] Shannon-Lowe C, Rickinson A. The Global Landscape of EBV-Associated Tumors. Front Oncol. 2019:713. DOI:10.3389/fonc.2019.00713

[9] Young L S, Dawson C W. Epstein-Barr virus and nasopharyngeal carcinoma. Chinese Journal of Cancer. 2014:12:581-590. DOI:10.5732/cjc.014.10197

[10] Henle W, Henle G, Ho H C, Burtin P, Cachin Y, Clifford P, de Schryver A, De-Thé G, Diehl V, Klein G. Antibodies to Epstein-Barr virus in nasopharyngeal carcinoma, other head and neck neoplasms, and control groups. J Natl Cancer Inst. 1970:1:225-31.

[11] Henle W, Ho J H, Henle G, Chau J C, Kwan H C. Nasopharyngeal carcinoma: significance of changes in Epstein-Barr virus-related antibody patterns following therapy. Int. J. Cancer. 1977:5:663-72. DOI:10.1002/ijc.2910200504

[12] Yi Z, Yuxi L, Chunren L, Sanwen C, Jihneng W, Jisong Z, Huijong Z. Application of an immunoenzymatic method and an immunoauto radiographic method for a mass survey of nasopharyngeal carcinoma. Intervirology. 1980:3:162-8. DOI:10.1159/000149121

[13] Deng H, Zhao Z, Zhang Z. Serologic screening on nasopharyngeal cancer in 338,868 persons in 21 cities and counties of Guangxi Region, China. Zhong hua Yu Fang Yi Xue Za Zhi. 1995:6:342-3.

[14] Zeng Y, Zhang L G, Li H Y, Jan M G, Zhang Q, Wu Y C, Wang Y S, Su G R. Serological mass survey for early detection of nasopharyngeal carcinoma in Wuzhou City, China. Int. J. Cancer. 1982:2:139-41. DOI:10.1002/ijc.2910290204

[15] Zeng Y, Zhang L G, Wu Y C, Huang Y S, Huang N Q, Li J Y, Wang Y B, Jiang

M K, Fang Z, Meng N N. Prospective studies on nasopharyngeal carcinoma in Epstein-Barr virus IgA/VCA antibody-positive persons in Wuzhou City, China. Int. J. Cancer. 1985:5:545-7. DOI:10.1002/ijc.2910360505

[16] Zeng Y, Zhong J M, Li L Y, Wang P Z, Tang H, Ma Y R, Zhu J S, Pan W J, Liu Y X, Wei Z N, Et A. Follow-up studies on Epstein-Barr virus IgA/VCA antibody-positive persons in Zangwu County, China. Intervirology. 1983:4:190-4. DOI:10.1159/000149391

[17] Chien Y C, Chen J Y, Liu M Y, Yang H I, Hsu M M, Chen C J, Yang C S. Serologic markers of Epstein-Barr virus infection and nasopharyngeal carcinoma in Taiwanese men. N Engl J Med. 2001:26:1877-82. DOI:10.1056/NEJMoa011610

[18] Ji M F, Wang D K, Yu Y L, Guo Y Q, Liang J S, Cheng W M, Zong Y S, Chan K H, Ng S P, Wei W I, Chua D T, Sham J S, Ng M H. Sustained elevation of Epstein-Barr virus antibody levels preceding clinical onset of nasopharyngeal carcinoma. Br J Cancer. 2007:4:623-30. DOI:10.1038/sj.bjc.6603609

[19] Zhang X, Zhong J, Tang M, Zhang X, Liao J, Zheng Y, Deng H, Zeng Y. Comparison of IgA/VCA, IgA/EA, IgG/EA in immunoenzyme methods and ZEBRA ELISA in early diagnosis of nasopharyngeal carcinoma. Zhong Hua Shi Yan He Lin Chuang Bing Du Xue Za Zhi. 2006:3:263-265.

[20] Hsu M M, Hsu W C, Sheen T S, Kao C L. Specific IgA antibodies to recombinant early and nuclear antigens of Epstein-Barr virus in nasopharyngeal carcinoma. Clin Otolaryngol Allied Sci. 2001:4:334-8. DOI:10.1046/j.1365-2273.2001.00489.x

[21] Ng M H, Chen H L, Luo R X, Chan K H, Woo P C, Sham J S, Huang J, Seto W H, Smith P, Griffin B E. Serological diagnosis of nasopharyngeal carcinoma by enzyme linked immunosorbent assay: optimization, standardization and diagnostic criteria. Chin Med J (Engl). 1998:6:531-6.

[22] Foong Y T, Cheng H M, Sam C K, Dillner J, Hinderer W, Prasad U. Serum and salivary IgA antibodies against a defined epitope of the Epstein-Barr virus nuclear antigen (EBNA) are elevated in nasopharyngeal carcinoma. Int. J. Cancer. 1990:6:1061-4. DOI:10.1002/ijc.2910450614

[23] Paramita D K, Fachiroh J, Haryana S M, Middeldorp J M. Two-step Epstein-Barr virus immunoglobulin A enzyme-linked immunosorbent assay system for serological screening and confirmation of nasopharyngeal carcinoma. Clin. Vaccine Immunol. 2009:5:706-11. DOI:10.1128/CVI.00425-08

[24] Guo J, Cui Z, Zheng Y, Li X, Chen Y. Comparison of Epstein-Barr Virus Serological Tools for the Screening and Risk Assessment of Nasopharyngeal Carcinoma: a Large Population-based Study. Pathol. Oncol. Res. 2020:4:2185-2190. DOI:10.1007/s12253-020-00808-0

[25] Coghill A E, Hsu W L, Pfeiffer R M, Juwana H, Yu K J, Lou P J, Wang C P, Chen J Y, Chen C J, Middeldorp J M, Hildesheim A. Epstein-Barr virus serology as a potential screening marker for nasopharyngeal carcinoma among high-risk individuals from multiplex families in Taiwan. Cancer Epidemiol Biomarkers Prev. 2014:7:1213-9. DOI:10.1158/1055-9965.EPI-13-1262

[26] Liu Y, Huang Q, Liu W, Liu Q, Jia W, Chang E, Chen F, Liu Z, Guo X, Mo H, Chen J, Rao D, Ye W, Cao S, Hong M. Establishment of VCA and EBNA1 IgA-based combination by enzyme-linked immunosorbent assay as preferred screening method for nasopharyngeal carcinoma: a two-stage design with a preliminary performance study and a mass screening in southern

China. Int. J. Cancer. 2012:2:406-16. DOI:10.1002/ijc.26380

[27] Liu Z, Ji M F, Huang Q H, Fang F, Liu Q, Jia W H, Guo X, Xie S H, Chen F, Liu Y, Mo H Y, Liu W L, Yu Y L, Cheng W M, Yang Y Y, Wu B H, Wei K R, Ling W, Lin X, Lin E H, Ye W, Hong M H, Zeng Y X, Cao S M. Two Epstein-Barr virus-related serologic antibody tests in nasopharyngeal carcinoma screening: results from the initial phase of a cluster randomized controlled trial in Southern China. Am. J. Epidemiol. 2013:3:242-50. DOI:10.1093/aje/kws404

[28] Yu X, Ji M, Cheng W, Wu B, Du Y, Cao S. Assessment of the Long-term Diagnostic Performance of a New Serological Screening Scheme in Large-scale Nasopharyngeal Carcinoma Screening. J. Cancer. 2018:12:2093-2097. DOI:10.7150/jca.23755

[29] Chen F, Huang Q H, Fang F, Liu Z W, Liu K, Xie S H, Liu Q, Hong M H, Liao Z E, Ye W M, Zeng Y X, Cao S M. Interval cancers in nasopharyngeal carcinoma screening: comparing two screening intervals after a negative initial screening result. J. Med. Screen. 2012:4:195-200. DOI:10.1258/jms.2012.012068

[30] Lian S, Ji M, Wu B, Yu X. The following-up study of high-risk and moderate-risk groups defined by EB virus serology test at the nasopharyngeal carcinoma screening programme. Zhong hua Yu Fang Yi Xue Za Zhi. 2015:1:26-30.

[31] Deng H, Zeng Y, Zheng Y, Jianping L, Liao J, Zhou W, Huang B, Cheng J, Zhong W. Studies on mass survery of 413 164 persons for nasopharyneal carcinoma. Zhong Guo Ai Zheng Za Zhi. 2003:2:109-111.

[32] Lo Y M, Chan L Y, Chan A T, Leung S F, Lo K W, Zhang J, Lee J C, Hjelm N M, Johnson P J, Huang D P. Quantitative and temporal correlation between circulating cell-free Epstein-Barr virus DNA and tumor recurrence in nasopharyngeal carcinoma. Cancer Res. 1999:21:5452-5.

[33] O T M, Yu G, Hu K, Li J C. Plasma Epstein-Barr virus immunoglobulin A and DNA for nasopharyngeal carcinoma screening in the United States. Otolaryngol Head Neck Surg. 2007:6:992-7. DOI:10.1016/j.otohns.2006.11.053

[34] Han B L, Xu X Y, Zhang C Z, Wu J J, Han C F, Wang H, Wang X, Wang G S, Yang S J, Xie Y. Systematic review on Epstein-Barr virus (EBV) DNA in diagnosis of nasopharyngeal carcinoma in Asian populations. Asian Pac J Cancer Prev. 2012:6:2577-81. DOI:10.7314/apjcp.2012.13.6.2577

[35] Chan K, Woo J, King A, Zee B, Lam W, Chan S L, Chu S, Mak C, Tse I, Leung S, Chan G, Hui E P, Ma B, Chiu R, Leung S F, van Hasselt A C, Chan A, Lo Y. Analysis of Plasma Epstein-Barr Virus DNA to Screen for Nasopharyngeal Cancer. N Engl J Med. 2017:6:513-522. DOI:10.1056/NEJMoa1701717

[36] Tay J K, Chan S H, Lim C M, Siow C H, Goh H L, Loh K S. The Role of Epstein-Barr Virus DNA Load and Serology as Screening Tools for Nasopharyngeal Carcinoma. Otolaryngol Head Neck Surg. 2016:2:274-80. DOI:10.1177/0194599816641038

[37] Wu H C, Lin Y J, Lee J J, Liu Y J, Liang S T, Peng Y, Chiu Y W, Wu C W, Lin C T. Functional analysis of EBV in nasopharyngeal carcinoma cells. Lab. Invest. 2003:6:797-812. DOI:10.1097/01.lab.0000074896.03561.fb

[38] Pathmanathan R, Prasad U, Sadler R, Flynn K, Raab-Traub N. Clonal proliferations of cells infected with Epstein-Barr virus in preinvasive lesions related to nasopharyngeal carcinoma. N

Engl J Med. 1995:11:693-8. DOI:10.1056/NEJM199509143331103

[39] Sheen T S, Ko J Y, Chang Y L, Chang Y S, Huang Y T, Chang Y, Tsai C H, Hsu M M. Nasopharyngeal swab and PCR for the screening of nasopharyngeal carcinoma in the endemic area: a good supplement to the serologic screening. Head Neck. 1998:8:732-8. DOI:10.1002/(sici)1097-0347(199812)20:8<732::aid-hed12>3.0.co;2-a

[40] Hao S P, Tsang N M, Chang K P. Screening nasopharyngeal carcinoma by detection of the latent membrane protein 1 (LMP-1) gene with nasopharyngeal swabs. Cancer-Am. Cancer Soc. 2003:8:1909-13. DOI:10.1002/cncr.11312

[41] Ng R H, Ngan R, Wei W I, Gullane P J, Phillips J. Trans-oral brush biopsies and quantitative PCR for EBV DNA detection and screening of nasopharyngeal carcinoma. Otolaryngol Head Neck Surg. 2014:4:602-9. DOI:10.1177/0194599813520136

[42] Chen Y, Zhao W, Lin L, Xiao X, Zhou X, Ming H, Huang T, Liao J, Li Y, Zeng X, Huang G, Ye W, Zhang Z. Nasopharyngeal Epstein-Barr Virus Load: An Efficient Supplementary Method for Population-Based Nasopharyngeal Carcinoma Screening. PLoS One. 2015:7:e0132669. DOI:10.1371/journal.pone.0132669

[43] Zheng X H, Lu L X, Li X Z, Jia W H. Quantification of Epstein-Barr virus DNA load in nasopharyngeal brushing samples in the diagnosis of nasopharyngeal carcinoma in southern China. Cancer Sci. 2015:9:1196-201. DOI:10.1111/cas.12718

[44] Zhang P F, Zheng X H, Li X Z, Tian T, Zhang S D, Hu Y Z, Jia W H. Nasopharyngeal brushing: a convenient and feasible sampling method for nucleic acid-based nasopharyngeal carcinoma research. Cancer Commun (Lond). 2018:1:8. DOI:10.1186/s40880-018-0278-z

[45] Chia-Ching L, Subramaniam S, Sivasubramanian S, Feng-Huei L. MWCNT-Fe3O4-based immuno-PCR for the early screening of nasopharyngeal carcinoma. Mater Sci Eng C Mater Biol Appl. 2016:422-8. DOI:10.1016/j.msec.2015.12.055

[46] Jiang C, Chen J, Xie S, Zhang L, Xiang Y, Lung M, Kam N W, Kwong D L, Cao S, Guan X Y. Evaluation of circulating EBV microRNA BART2-5p in facilitating early detection and screening of nasopharyngeal carcinoma. Int. J. Cancer. 2018:12:3209-3217. DOI:10.1002/ijc.31642

[47] Zhang J Z, Wu Z H, Cheng Q. Screening and identification of key biomarkers in nasopharyngeal carcinoma: Evidence from bioinformatic analysis. Medicine (Baltimore). 2019:48:e17997. DOI:10.1097/MD.0000000000017997

[48] Xu Y, Zhao W, Mo Y, Ma N, Midorikawa K, Kobayashi H, Hiraku Y, Oikawa S, Zhang Z, Huang G, Takeuchi K, Murata M. Combination of RERG and ZNF671 methylation rates in circulating cell-free DNA: A novel biomarker for screening of nasopharyngeal carcinoma. Cancer Sci. 2020:7:2536-2545. DOI:10.1111/cas.14431

[49] Jiang H, Li J, Zhang B, Huang R, Zhang J, Chen Z, Shang X, Li X, Nie X. Intestinal Flora Disruption and Novel Biomarkers Associated with Nasopharyngeal Carcinoma. Front Oncol. 2019:1346. DOI:10.3389/fonc.2019.01346

[50] Khan S, Ullah R, Javaid S, Shahzad S, Ali H, Bilal M, Saleem M, Ahmed M. Raman Spectroscopy Combined with Principal Component Analysis for Screening Nasopharyngeal Cancer in Human Blood Sera. Appl.

Spectrosc. 2017:11:2497-2503. DOI:10.1177/0003702817723928

[51] Lin D, Wu Q, Qiu S, Chen G, Feng S, Chen R, Zeng H. Label-free liquid biopsy based on blood circulating DNA detection using SERS-based nanotechnology for nasopharyngeal cancer screening. Nanomedicine-UK. 2019:102100. DOI:10.1016/j.nano.2019.102100

[52] Rao D, Qing L, Cao S. Cost-effectiveness evaluation of seven strategies for nasopharyngeal carcinoma. Zhong Hua Zhong Liu Za Zhi. 2012:7:549-553.

[53] Harris J P, Saraswathula A, Kaplun B, Qian Y, Chan K, Chan A, Le QT, Owens D K, Goldhaber-Fiebert J D, Pollom E. Cost-effectiveness of Screening for Nasopharyngeal Carcinoma among Asian American Men in the United States. Otolaryngol Head Neck Surg. 2019:1:82-90. DOI:10.1177/0194599819832593

[54] Ji M F, Sheng W, Cheng W M, Ng M H, Wu B H, Yu X, Wei K R, Li F G, Lian S F, Wang P P, Quan W, Deng L, Li X H, Liu X D, Xie Y L, Huang S J, Ge S X, Huang S L, Liang X J, He S M, Huang H W, Xia S L, Ng P S, Chen H L, Xie S H, Liu Q, Hong M H, Ma J, Yuan Y, Xia N S, Zhang J, Cao S M. Incidence and mortality of nasopharyngeal carcinoma: interim analysis of a cluster randomized controlled screening trial (PRO-NPC-001) in southern China. Ann. Oncol. 2019:10:1630-1637. DOI:10.1093/annonc/mdz231

Chapter 4

Epidemiology and Outcomes of Nasopharyngeal Carcinoma

Gamal Abdul Hamid

Abstract

Nasopharyngeal carcinoma (NPC) is a rare head and neck neoplasm worldwide. It is common among the southern Chinese with significant geographical variation with the highest incidence being in Southeast Asia up to 6.4/100,000 males and 2.4/100,000 females in these regions and the Epstein Barr virus (EBV) is associated closely with NPC. This disease has peculiarities in its etiopathogenesis, presentation, risk of nodal and distant metastasis, response to therapy and overall survival (OS) outcomes that stand out as compared to other head and neck cancer subsites. NPC is mainly treated by RT and is profoundly radiosensitive and radiotherapy treatment is the spine of treatment for all stages of NPC without far off metastases. Many advances in RT techniques and schedules are attempted to improve outcomes of the disease starting from intracavitary brachytherapy, intensity modulated RT to simultaneous modulated accelerated RT, all showing some promise with most significant benefit seen with addition of chemotherapy, especially in intermediate (Stage II) and advanced (Stage III, IVA, IVB) cases. At a time when modern radiation treatment like *intensity-modulated radiotherapy* (IMRT) are accomplishing great good local control, distant metastases are getting to be the transcendent design of treatment failure, particularly in patients with locally progressed illness. There are numerous results from clinical trials looking at combined radiation treatment (RT) and chemotherapy for NPC. Survival rates significantly differ between NPC patients according to stages of disease.

Keywords: nasopharyngeal carcinoma, epidemiology, risk factors, Epstein-Barr virus, clinical outcomes

1. Introduction

Nasopharyngeal carcinoma (NPC) is a rare disease and one of the most common types of malignancies that appear in the nasopharynx, which is the narrow tube passage behind the nasal cavity and one of the malignancies associated with the Epstein-Barr virus (EBV) and is considered one of the malignant and rare tumors in most parts of the world and is distinguished by distribution geographical and ethnic [1]. In southern China, it is one of the leading causes of death and morbidity. Notwithstanding the common burden of NPC in some endemic areas, the etiology and prevention of NPC is relatively unknown.

In 1978 the histopathological classification of nasopharyngeal carcinoma proposed by the World Health Organization was adopted, which divided tumors into three types. Type 1 was typical of squamous cell carcinoma, similar to the rest of the upper gastrointestinal tract. The second type included non-keratinized squamous cell carcinoma and the third type was undifferentiated carcinoma. In epidemiological research this classification is more applicable and has been shown to have a predictive effect. Undifferentiated carcinomas have a higher rate of localized tumor control during treatment and a higher rate of distant metastases.

Among cancers of the head and neck, nasopharyngeal carcinoma is one of the most common type of cancers [2]. It is also a virulent disease that has been accounted for to occur in many parts of the world with a uniform incidence rate for age and sex, one of every 100,000 every year [3]. This malignant growth has an unequal geographical distribution with the incidence rate on one continent higher than on other continents, which was very high in Asia (80%) and 10% in Africa. The rest 10% have been accounted for somewhere in the world, and Southeast Asian nations represent 67% of cancer burden worldwide. In addition to geographical differences, some ethnic gatherings might be in danger of creating nasopharyngeal malignancy. For example: Bidayuh on Borneo Island, Inuit in the Arctic and Nagas in Northern India, with an old norm of more than 16 for every 100,000 every year for men [4].

In non endemic regions, during last 50 years, incidence of poorly or undifferentiated NPC raised [5, 6]. However, this was supposed to be mostly related to the increase of migration flows towards these areas from endemic regions rather than an augmented exposure of residents to risk factors for NPC development. Indeed, in low incidence countries, the risk of development of NPC in immigrants is estimated to be around 30-fold greater than in residents. The association between Epstein-Barr virus (EBV) and nasopharyngeal carcinoma (NPC), has marked geographic and ethnic differences in its incidence [7]. The Over population in Asia, responsible for the increased rate of death by NPC, from 45,000 (in 1990) to 65,000 (in 2010) [8]. In Africa and some regions of East Asia, the nasopharyngeal carcinoma is more common and the incidence rate is generally lower from 1 for every 100,000 persons [9]. However, there are around 25 per 100,000 people in southern China, which is 18% of all cancers [10]. In Asia, NPC occurs in all ages but more common in the middle-aged population, although there is a high incidence of cases in children in Africa. A study on NPC and EBV showed a particular association between natural factors such as viral antibody factors, genetic factors and diet [11].

NPC is one of the highly invasive neoplasia and malignancies that spread early to regional lymph nodes [12]. Radiation therapy (RT) is also seen as an essential supportive treatment for management because of the sensitivity of the radiation to the type of disease. In advanced stages of disease, chemotherapy (CT) has been used for more than 20 years and some studies confirmed the benefit of chemoradiotherapy (CRT) in stages II to IV [13].

2. Global trends

In 2012, 86,691 nasopharynx cancer cases occurred in the world and 50,831 nasopharynx death cases, and in 2018 there were around 130,000 accidents and more than 73,000 deaths from nasopharyngeal carcinoma (NPC) worldwide [14]. The global NPC incidence and mortality distribution reported very high rates (more than 20-30/100,000 men and 10/100,000 women) in Southeast Asia [15], some regions of southern China, [16], Singapore, [17] Hong Kong, [18] Taiwan, [19] Selected Chinese immigrants (mainly to North America), [20, 21] and the Middle East [22]. In most of the western countries, Latin America and Japan that are non-endemic areas, the incidence rate of NPC showed less than 1/100,000 [23]. Recent studies have shown the incidence of NPC is high in cities like Zhongshan, Zhuhai, Hong Kong, and Jiangmen (standard age: 12.8-25 per 100,000 per year for men) in southern China [24–26] (**Figure 1**).

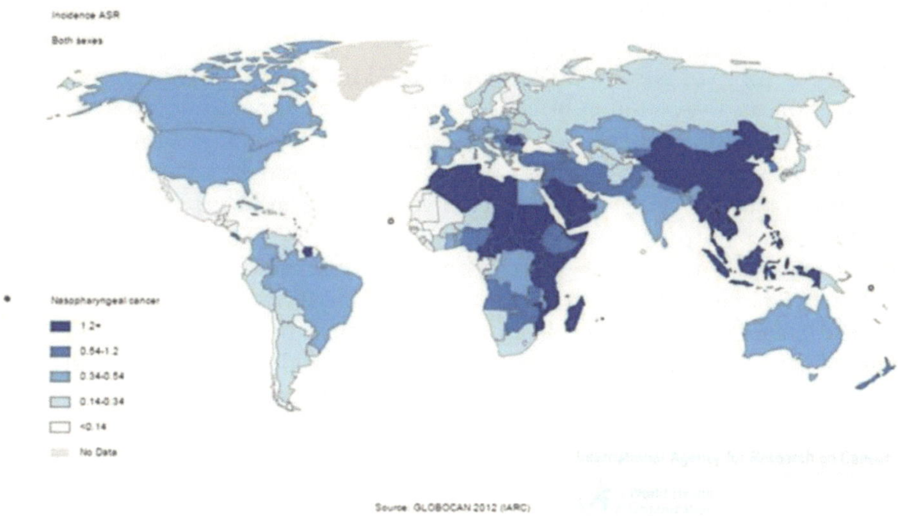

Figure 1.
Incidence of Nasopharyngeal carcinoma (2012) (GLOBOCAN 2012) [26].

3. Age and gender

The incidence of nasopharyngeal carcinoma increases two to three times more frequently in men than in women [27]. Male predominance in the population is a common trait among NPC patients. Male dominance in the incidence of NPC can be partly explained by biological or gender differences or different lifestyles in the prevalence of some environmental risk factors, such as smoking and hazardous occupational exposure [28].

The nasopharyngeal carcinoma incidence in most low-risk groups is consistent with increasing age [29]. On the other hand, in the 50 to 59 age group, the incidence of NPC increases because these groups are more susceptible, and then decreases [30], which is related to the exposure of these groups to carcinogens in the early life stages [31].

It can take several decades for nasopharyngeal carcinoma to develop malignant cells. After that, the signs appear. Therefore, the outcome of carcinogens exposure in early life will have a sizeable effect on the development of this cancer [28].

4. Risk factors

Since the first case of this malignancy was recorded in 1901 [32], the etiology of the NPC has not been identified as a mystery. Risk factors for NPC, most commonly in men [33], include a family history of NPC, EBV infection, low intake of fresh vegetables and fruits, high consumption of salt-canned fish, smoking and Cantonese races [34]. On the other side, a reduced risk may be associated with a history of infectious mononucleosis (IM) and HLA genotypes [35]. Other potential risk factors are the genetic polymorphism in glutathione S-transferase M1 (*GSTM1*), *GSTT1*, cytochrome P450 2E1 (CYP2E1) and CYP2A6 [36], possibly high consumption of other preserved foods [37, 38] and the history of chronic respiratory diseases. The exposures to dust and formaldehyde, nickel exposure and consumption of herbal medicine are less established risk factors [39].

4.1 Epstein-Barr virus (EBV)

The relationship of NPC to EBV-associated is known and proven, and EBV infection is one of the common infectious agents in the population. This relationship concluded the hypothesis that an EBV subtype of NPC plays a role in increasing the incidence of NPC in the epidemic regions. The association between EBV infection and nasopharyngeal carcinoma is very strong and has been demonstrated in several studies [40].

In the nucleus of malignant cells there are approximately 30 copies of the EBV gene. Most versions refer to the presence of "small circular chromosomes" called episomes. In some cases, these episomes are adjacent to the viral DNA releases. The use of serological and virological tests is recommended to diagnose and study the populations at risk. In areas with an increased incidence of nasopharyngeal carcinoma, high levels of IgA antibodies with EBV capsid antigen and Epstein-Barr nuclear antigen are considered to be a valuable screening test or the new prediction model combining VCA/IgA and EBNA1/IgA which will improve diagnosis of NPC and could identify high-risk population [41].

4.2 Familial history and genetic susceptibility

It is known that families with a history of cancer, particularly nasopharyngeal carcinoma, are 4 to 10 times more likely to develop nasopharyngeal carcinoma. Some studies have reported that familial clustering is stable in areas with a high incidence of NPC [42] and in areas with low to moderate incidence [43]. In southern China, where NPC is endemic, more than 5% reported NPC with a positive family history of NPC in cases with first-degree family history [44]. Evidence and studies of previous case control studies have shown indifferent populations that the odds ratios for people between 2 and 20 with history of NPC and history of first-degree family were compared to people without such a medical history [45]. This size of association is among the highest in any malignant disease. In nasopharyngeal carcinoma the genetic research focuses on genes of human leukocyte antigen. Where it occurred in subjects with presence of EBV and weak HLA allele, the antigens likely increased the risk of developing nasopharyngeal carcinoma. The development of NPC less likely in people with the presence of EBV associated with strong HLA allele. In etiology of NPC, it is possible that genetics and environmental exposure play a common role. Four correlation studies with susceptibility sites of 4p15.1_q12, 6p2153, 3p21.31e21.2 and 5p13 in NPC families of a single major susceptibility gene were observed and reported, supported by the results of NPC complex family segregation analysis, indicating that this the pathogens of NPC includes the interaction of many environmental and genetic factors [46, 47].

The genetic factor is one of the notable features of the race distribution in the cantonese population. The shared roles of environmental factors, lifestyle and genetics should not be ignored. Whether familial NPC cases differ significantly from sporadic cases in terms of clinical features (such as histopathology, stage of disease, and prognosis), gender, race, age, EBV sera, genetic risk factors, and environmental risk factors [48].

4.3 Exposure to carcinogens

4.3.1 Salt-preserved foods and fish

Several studies have reported that eating fish with salt is considered a risk factor for cancer. For the Chinese, the relative risk of developing pharyngeal cancer is lower among weekly consumers than those who use very little or no salt-canned fish. Overall it was about 1.4 to 3.2 [36, 37]. The relative risks are between 1.8 and 7.5 for those who consume daily [49, 50]. The risk of developing nasopharyngeal carcinoma is higher with other canning foods such as fruits, vegetables, eggs and meat in Southeast Asia, Southern China, the Middle East, North Africa and the Arctic [51]. This preservative food is also implicated in people found in low-incidence areas of northern China and the United States [52].

4.3.2 Exposure to smoking and occupational products

The direct relationship between nasopharyngeal carcinoma and smoking was confirmed by reports that people who had smoked cigarettes for ten years or more were more likely to develop NPC [53]. Several studies have confirmed that cigarette smoking is linked to nasopharyngeal carcinoma. The relationship pattern between the risk of developing nasopharyngeal carcinoma and smoking depends on the dose, especially in well-differentiated nasopharyngeal carcinoma [54]. Lin et al. [55] compared the surroundings of NPC patient with those of neighboring controls in Taiwan and found that cigarettes were smoking and working in poorly ventilated rooms was closely related to the NPC.

Another study found that long-term cigarette smoking was linked to the NPC, but only to a minor extent exposure to cigarette smoke through passive exposure to smoking and alcohol consumption is not associated with a disease risk [56].

4.3.3 Oral hygiene

There is a connection between poor oral hygiene in the elderly and cancers of the head, neck, esophagus and stomach [57]. In NPC, periodontal disease can increase recurrent inflammation and thus increase possibility of developing NPC as the inflammatory response may be on the way to promoting carcinogenesis, Zhiwei Liu et al 2016 suggested poor oral health may increase risk of NPC [58]. In addition, When more teeth are lost, the bacterial load also increases. Some types of bacteria are involved in the increased production of nitrosamine, which is thought to be carcinogenic and has been linked to the development of NPC. Poor oral hygiene can also increase the risk of NPC by EBV stimulation and proliferation, as evidenced by higher viral loads in people with periodontitis more than others [59].

4.3.4 Other risk factors

The relationship between alcohol consumption and nasopharyngeal carcinoma has been documented in complicated ways. Several studies have documented that there is no clear confirmation of a relationship between the risk of nasopharyngeal carcinoma and alcohol consumption [60]. Other studies confirmed the relation between nasopharyngeal carcinoma and the exposure to wood dust. Several studies have shown an increased risk of developing nasopharyngeal carcinoma after exposure to formaldehyde [61]. Exposure to other chemicals or stimuli such as smoke, steam, cotton dust, chemicals, flammable products, or solvents such as chlorophenol and phenoxy acid increases the risk of developing nasopharyngeal carcinoma [62]. An association between nasal cavity and sinus cancer and the textile work has also been reported [63]. In addition, several other non-dietary risk factors for nasopharyngeal carcinoma have been included [64]. It has been reported that occupational exposure to combustion products and cotton dust is independently related to NPC risk. The risk of developing NPC also increases through occupational exposure to formaldehyde and not through exposure to wood dust [65]. However, this association appears to be specific to squamous cell carcinoma. In addition, eating canned foods has been linked to NPC at a young age and risk in all population groups [33]. Studies and data on inhalation of different types of smoke/fumes/dust show that inhalants can play an important role, although they can secondary as a catalyst is the high incidence of NPC in various geographic regions of the world.

5. Treatment

5.1 Radiation therapy

Radiation therapy is the first type of cancer treatment method for non-invasive nasopharyngeal carcinoma (NPC) due to anatomical limitations and high sensitivity to radiation. One of the treatment method is with two-dimensional radiation therapy (2DRT), which has been converted to 3D compliant radiation therapy, and particularly highly modified radiation therapy (IMRT), is an important step forward in the treatment of NPC.

IMRT use was first reported in 2000 by the University of California at San Francisco. The results with 100% local control and a 4-year operating system are a dramatic 94%.

The second phase of II trails 0225 by the Radiation Oncology Group then showed that it is possible to transfer IMRT to a multi-institutional setting [66]. Three comparative randomized trials studies of IMRT and 2DRT have been applied. Chen et al. The studies confirmed a significant improvement in the therapeutic ratio by IMRT: The use of IMRT in patients with NPC demonstrated an improved terminal therapeutic ratio compared to 2DRT over a follow-up period of more than 10 years with significant improvement in OS, FFS, and L-FFS [67].

5.2 Adjuvant and neoadjuvant chemotherapy

While chemotherapy given concurrently with RT offers consistent benefits, the adjuvant chemotherapy role after alternative chemoradiotherapy is uncertain. The chemotherapy induction attempts for cases with local metastasis which include concomitant chemotherapy and radiation therapy, followed by adjuvant chemotherapy, in which an increased rate of NPC relapse in remote locations was observed in a large proportion of patients. These studies have shown the usefulness of this strategy for the OS. The administration of adjuvant chemotherapy was associated with significant toxicity, with 25-45% of the patients exhibiting high grade toxicities [68]. In addition, some research studies evaluating chemoradiotherapy protocols without adjuvant chemotherapy which provided similar results to studies using simultaneous and adjuvant chemotherapy, raising questions about the actual results and benefits of adjuvant chemotherapy for NPC control [69].

In theory, novel chemotherapy can prevent micrometastases earlier and also facilitate the mapping of RT by decreasing local metastasis, especially in large tumors. So far, phase III studies on novel adjuvant chemotherapy with post-radiation therapy alone have proven no difference in OS compared to RT [70]. An up to date meta-analysis of MAC-NPC contained data from a number of induction chemotherapy studies and showed statistically excellent results in survival without disease progression, but not in OS [71]. Increased cases with leukopenia and neutropenia rates observed during the CRT period [72]. This confirms the primary interest in the new induction/adjuvant approach, which could interfere with the delivery of chemotherapy with effective doses and/or radiation therapy during the period of CRT or increased toxicity and outweigh the potential benefits of the induction-based approach.

5.3 Treatment in advanced NPC

Although chemotherapy concurrently with radiation has resulted in many improvements with significant outcomes in NPC patients, and improve survival in locally advanced NPC over 5 years in 50-70%. A large proportion of patients have relapsed either locally or in distant sites, or both. Adding more chemotherapy drugs to available protocols is not a viable approach as CRT already exhibits significant toxicity. Instead, more research aims to identify the possibility of recurrence or relapse before treatment or at the end of the CRT assessment, who can focus on additional research methods. Second, the use of personalized target therapy in conjunction with radiation therapy or chemotherapy is assessed.

In NPC patients, the epidermal growth factor receptor (EGFR) overexpression is 80% or more and associated with lower survival results [73]. Adding of cetuximab, a monoclonal chimeric antibody in patients with squamous cell carcinoma of the head and neck against EGFR in conjunction with RT of HNSCC in locally advanced stages, which reported improvement and significant in OS in comparison to RT alone [74]. The evaluation of cetuximab in concurrent with radiation therapy in comparison to standard CRT in NPC patients has not proven to be more effective due to the association with increased rates of mucositis [75]. The combination of IMRT radiation therapy and weekly cisplatin with cetuximab was more effective in patients in advanced stages [76].

5.4 Palliative chemotherapy for metastasis and relapses NPC

Palliative chemotherapy is very important and plays role in control of disease and keep patients in good conditions as well as in extending survival of patients with NPC metastases as NPC is very sensitive to chemotherapy cancer. Standard treatment includes chemotherapy with platinum in combination with other drugs such as 5-FU with cisplatin/carboplatin and paclitaxel with gemcitabine. Patients treated for long time with platinum chemotherapy, can achieve a significant response with rates of up to 80% and an average survival rate of 12 to 18 months [77]. There is a significant correlation between higher response rates with a combination therapy regimen than monotherapy, and platinum is a good treatment, but it is not the main criterion or standard treatment. Regardless of the treatment regimen chosen for the first line, the average progression time after 7 to 10 months remains relatively constant [78, 79]; This is related to the development of platinum resistance. The response rates for a triple therapy with paclitaxel/carboplatin/ gemcitabine are impressive and close to 80%. However, the average response time is about 8 months, similar to two drug regimens [80].

5.5 Novel therapies: molecular-targeted agents

The past 10 years have seen the development of new treatments for NPC and this has been somewhat simultaneous with the development of treatment for other cancers. Little progress has been made in recent years beyond the usual cytotoxic approaches. EGFR-mediated signaling pathways inhibited by the molecular factors that lead to inhibition of cell growth and cell apoptosis which include tyrosine kinase inhibitors, for example gefitinib and monoclonal antibodies [81].

In a number of centers, Ueda and colleagues [82] investigating a combination treatment of carboplatin, paclitaxel and cetuximab in patients with metastatic or recurrent or with repeated platinum-resistant NPC showed good survival benefit, an overall response rate reach to 64 % and a median OS of 29.1 months with follow up for 30 months. The treatment with gefitinib had little response rates in metastatic and recurrent NPC treated previously with platinum-based chemotherapy. The symptomatic improvement and disease stabilization were observed in some cases [83].

Multikinase inhibitors target tyrosine kinases such as fibroblast growth factor receptor (FGFR), platelet-derived growth factor receptor (PDGFR) and vascular endothelial growth factor receptor (VEGFR) and drugs such as pazopanib (VEGFR, PDGFR, FGFR, c-KIT), sorafenib (VEGFR, PDGFR, Raf kinases), and sunitinib (PDGFR, VEGFR, C-KIT), have been evaluated in NPC [84, 85].

6. Mortality and survival

6.1 Mortality of NPC

Global mortality rates of NPCestimated 51,000 deaths in 2012 among females and males were 0.04 per 10, 000 and 0.1 per 10,000, respectively.

The mortality rate were high in Southeast Asia, East Asia, East Africa North Africa and Micronesia. Nasopharyngeal carcinoma is the native cancer of Southeast Asia and the countries with the highest mortality were Malaysia, Singapore, Indonesia, Vietnam, and Brunei [26] (**Figure 2**).

6.2 Survival patterns of NPC

Early diagnosed NPC patients respond very well to radiation, and this treatment shows promise. Radiation therapy is the strategy treatment for treating NPC. However, approximately 70% of stage III or IV NPC patients are exposed to a local and/or regional condition of distant metastases or recurrences after radiation therapy [86]. Treatment with combination of chemotherapy and radiation therapy often required for advanced NPC [87].

Studies have shown that intensity modulated radiation therapy (IMRT) often produces larger radiation dose distributions corresponding to improved tumor exposure and allows for lower doses of normal tissue for a variety of cancers that

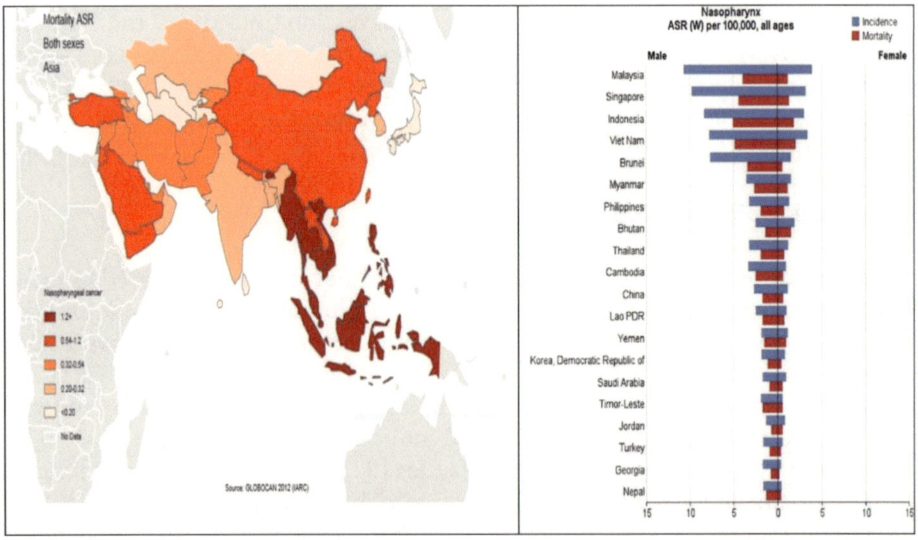

Figure 2.
Mortality rate of nasopharyngeal carcinoma in Asia in 2012 (GLOBOCAN 2012) [26].

occur in the head and neck area [88]. In addition, the prognosis of NPC associated with many factors are, including age, sex, TNM stage, histology, radiation dose, leukopenia and anemia, and the type of combined chemotherapy [89]. Therefore, minimizing the risk of late complication and distant metastasis and maximizing the local control should be the key objects in designing future treatment.

7. Conclusions

Nasopharyngeal carcinoma is a rare head and neck malignancy and the native malignancy of Southeast Asia. Nasopharyngeal carcinoma (NPC), predominantly associated with Epstein-Barr virus (EBV), is characterized by remarkable geographical and racial differences in its incidence. The incidence of NPC is generally less than 1 per 100,000 individuals; however, in southern China it is around 25 per 100,000 individuals, accounting for 18% of all cancers. Epidemiological studies over the past few decades have shown a gradual decrease in incidence and a marked decrease in NPC mortality. However, the rise in population in Asia has increased the number of deaths caused by NPCs from 45,000 in 1990 to 65,000 in 2010.

The development of image diagnostic techniques and introducing chemoradiotherapy (chemo-IMRT) followed by adjuvant chemotherapy resulted in excellent locoregional control and increased survival rates among patients with NPC.

Author details

Gamal Abdul Hamid
Faculty of Medicine and Health Sciences, University of Aden, Aden, Yemen

*Address all correspondence to: drgamal2000@yahoo.com

References

[1] MaBB, Hui EP and Chan AT: Investigational drugs for nasopharyngealcarcinoma. Expert Opin InvestigDrugs 26: 677-685, 2017.

[2] Tsao SW LK, Huang DP. Nasopharyngealcarcinoma. In: Tselis AC, Jenso n H, editors. Epsteion-Bar virus. New York: Taylor & Francis. 2006; pp. 273-295.

[3] Ferlay J, Shin H, Bray F, For man D, Mathers C, Park in D. Incidence/mortality data. GLOBOCAN 2008 v2.0. Cancer incidence and mortality worldwide: IARC Cancer Base No. 10 [Internet]. Lyon, France: International Agency for Research on Cancer, 2010

[4] Xu ZJ, Zheng RS, Zhang SW, Zou XN, Chen WQ. Nasopharyngeal carcinoma incidence and mortality in China in 2009. Chin J Cancer 2013; 32: 453-458.

[5] Chang ET, Adami HO. The enigmatic epidemiology of nasopharyngeal carcinoma. Cancer Epidemiol Biomarkers Prev 2006; 15: 1765-1777.

[6] Arnold M, Wildeman MA, Visser O, Karim-Kos HE, Middeldorp JM, Fles R, Bing Tan I, Coebergh JW. Lower mortality from nasopharyngeal cancer in The Netherlands since 1970 with differential incidence trends in histopathology. Oral Oncol 2013; 49: 237-243.

[7] Lozano, R.; Naghavi, M.; Foreman, K.; Lim, S.; Shibuya, K.; Aboyans, V.; Abraham, J.; Adair, T.; Aggarwal, R.;Ahn, S.Y.; et al. Global and regional mortality from 235 causes of death for 20 age groups in 1990 and 2010: asystematic analysis for the Global Burden of Disease Study 2010. Lancet **2012**, 380, 2095-2128.

[8] Wu, S.; Xia, B.; Han, F.; Xie, R.; Song, T.; Lu, L.; Yu,W.; Deng, X.; He, Q.; Zhao, C.; et al. Prognostic nomogramfor patients with nasopharyngeal carcinoma after intensity-modulated radiotherapy. PLoS ONE **2015**, 10,e0134491.

[9] Wu, L.; Li, C.; Pan, L. Nasopharyngeal carcinoma: A review of current updates. Exp. Ther. Med. **2018**, 15, 3687-3692.

[10] Kamran, S.C.; Riaz, N.; Lee, N. Nasopharyngeal carcinoma. Surg. Oncol. Clin. N. Am. **2015**, 24, 547-561.

[11] Zhou T, Yang DW, He YQ, et al. Associations between environmental factors and serological Epstein-Barr virus antibodies in patients with nasopharyngeal carcinoma in South China. Cancer Medicine. 2019 Aug;8(10):4852-4866. DOI: 10.1002/cam4.2348.

[12] Lee AW, Ng WT, Chan YH, et al. The battle against nasopharyngeal cancer. RadiotherOncol. 2012;104:272-278.

[13] Baujat B, Audry H, Bourhis J, et al. Chemotherapy in locally advanced nasopharyngeal carcinoma: an individual patient data meta-analysis of eight randomized trials and 1753 patients. Int J RadiatOncolBiol Phys. 2006;64:47-56.

[14] Bray F, Ferlay J, Soerjomataram I, Siegel RL, Torre LA, Jemal A. Global cancer statistics 2018: GLOBOCAN estimates of incidence and mortality worldwide for 36 cancers in 185 countries. CA Cancer J Clin. 2018;68(6):394. Epub 2018 Sep 12.

[15] Devi BC, Pisani P, Tang TS, et al. High incidence of nasopharyngeal carcinoma in native people of Sarawak, Borneo Island. Cancer Epidemiol Biomarkers Prev2004; 13:482-486

[16] Jia WH, Huang QH, Liao J, et al. Trends in incidence and mortality of

nasopharyngeal carcinomaover a 20-25 year period (1978/1983-2002) inSihui and Cangwu counties in southern China.BMC Cancer2006; 6:178

[17] Luo J, Chia KS, Chia SE, et al. Secular trends of nasopharyngeal carcinoma incidence in Singapore, Hong Kong and Los Angeles Chinese populations, 1973-1997.Eur J Epidemiol2007; 22:513-521

[18] Tse LA, Yu IT, Mang OW, et al. Incidence ratetrends of histological subtypes of nasopharyngealcarcinoma in Hong Kong.Br J Cancer2006; 95:1269-1273.

[19] Hsu C, Shen YC, Cheng CC, et al. Difference in the incidence trend of nasopharyngeal and oro-pharyngeal carcinomas in Taiwan: implication from age-period-cohort analysis.CancerEpidemiol Biomarkers Prev2006; 15:856-61.

[20] Sun LM, Epplein M, Li CI, et al. Trends in theincidence rates of nasopharyngeal carcinomaamong Chinese Americans living in Los AngelesCounty and the San Francisco metropolitan area,1992-2002.Am J Epidemiol2005; 162:1174-8.16.

[21] Yu WM, Hussain SS. Incidence of nasopharyngeal carcinoma in Chinese immigrants, compared with Chinese in China and South East Asia: review. JLaryngol Otol2009; 123:1067-74.

[22] HamdiCherif M, Serraino D, Mahnane A, et al.Time trends of cancer incidence in Setif, Algeria,1986-2010: an observational study.BMC Cancer2014; 14:637.

[23] Torre LA, Bray F, Siegel RL, et al. Global cancerstatistics, 2012.Cancer J Clin2015; 65:87-108.

[24] Y.P. Chen, A.T.C. Chan, Q.T. Le, P. Blanchard, Y. Sun, J. Ma. Nasopharyngeal carcinoma Lancet, 394 (10192) (2019), pp. 64-80

[25] A.B. Rickinson, K.W. Lo A. Lee, M. Lung, W. Ng (Eds.), Nasopharyngeal Carcinoma: A History, Nasopharyngeal Carcinoma: From Etiology to Clinical Practice Academic Press, London, United Kingdom (2019), pp. 1-16

[26] NedaMahdavifar, MahshidGhoncheh, AbdollahMohammadian-Hafshejani, BahmanKhosravi, Hamid Salehiniya. Epidemiology and Inequality in the Incidence and Mortality of Nasopharynx Cancer in Asia;Osong Public Health Res Perspect 2016 7(6), 360e372 http://dx.doi.org/10.1016/j.phrp.2016.11.002

[27] Yu MC, Yuan JM. Epidemiology of nasopharyngeal carcinoma. Semin Cancer Biol 2002 ; 12: 421-429.

[28] Jia WH, Qin HD. Non-viral environmental risk factors for nasopharyngeal carcinoma: a systematic review. Semin Cancer Biol 2012; 22: 117-126.

[29] Wang H, Seow A, Lee HP. Trends in cancer incidence among Singapore Malays: a low-risk population. Ann Acad Med Singapore 2004; 33: 57-62.

[30] Lee AW, Foo W, Mang O, Sze WM, Chappell R, Lau WH, Ko WM. Changing epidemiology of nasopharyngeal carcinoma in Hong Kong over a 20-year period (1980-99): an encouraging reduction in both incidence and mortality. Int J Cancer 2003; 103: 680-685.

[31] Shanmugaratnam K. Nasopharynx. In: Schottenfeld D, Fraumeni JF, Jr., editors. Cancer epidemiology and prevention. Philadelphia: W. B. Saunders Company 1982;pp. 536-553.

[32] JacksonC: Primarycarcinomaof thenasopharynx. atableof cases. J AmMedAssoc 37: 371-377, 1901.

[33] Zheng T, Li J, Liu X. The study of estrogen and progesterone receptor in nasopharyngeal carcinoma. Chin J Cancer Res 1996;8(1):64-66.

[34] XueWQ, QinHD, RuanHL, Shugart YY and Jia WH: Quantitative association of tobacco smoking with the risk of nasopharyngeal carcinoma: A comprehensive meta-analysis of studies conducted between1979 and 2011. Am J Epidemiol 178: 325-338, 2013.

[35] Tang M, Lautenberger JA, Gao X, Sezgin E, Hendrickson SL, Troyer JL, et al. (2012) The Principal Genetic Determinants for Nasopharyngeal Carcinoma in China Involve the *HLA* Class I Antigen Recognition Groove. PLoS Genet 8(11): e1003103. https://doi.org/10.1371/journal.pgen.1003103.

[36] Zheng YM, Tuppin P, Hubert A, Jeannel D, PanYJ, Zeng Y and de Thé G: Environmental and dietary risk factors for nasopharyngeal carcinoma: A case-control study in Zangwu County, Guangxi, China. BrJ Cancer 69: 508-514, 1994.

[37] MelbyeM, EbbesenP, LevinePH and BennikeT: Early primary infection and high Epstein-Barr virus antibody titers in Greenland Eskimosat high risk for nasopharyngeal carcinoma. Int J Cancer 34: 619-623, 1984.

[38] JeannelD, GhnassiaM, Hubert A, Sancho-Garnier H, Eschwège F, Crognier E and de-Thé G: Increased risk of nasopharyngeal carcinoma among males of French origin born in Maghreb (northAfrica). Int J Cancer 54: 536-539, 1993.

[39] HildesheimA and WangCP: Genetic predisposition factors and nasopharyngeal carcinoma risk: a review of epidemiological association studies, 2000-2011: RosettaStoneforNPC: genetics, viralinfection, and otherenvironmentalfactors. SeminCancerBiol 22: 107-116, 2012.

[40] Lung ML, Cheung AKL, Ko JMY, Lung HL, Cheng Y, Dai W. The interplay of host genetic factors and Epstein-Barr virus in the development of nasopharyngeal carcinoma. Chin J Cancer 2014; 33: 556-562.

[41] Licitra L, Bernier J, Cvitkovic E, Grandi C, Spinazzé S, Bruzzi P, Gatta G, Molinari R. Cancer of the nasopharynx. Crit Rev OncolHematol 2003; 45: 199-214

[42] Turkoz FP, Celenkoglu G, Dogu GG, KalenderME, Coskun U, Alkis N, OzkanM, Turk HM and ArslanUY: Risk factorsof nasopharyngealcarcinomainTurkey-anepidemiologicalsurveyof theAnatolianSocietyof MedicalOncology. AsianPacJ CancerPrev 12: 3017-3021, 2011.

[43] RenZF, Liu WS, QinHD, Xu YF, Yu DD, FengQS, ChenLZ, Shu XO, ZengYX and JiaWH: Effect of familyhistoryof cancersand environmentalfactorsonrisk of nasopharyngealcarcinomain Guangdong, China. CancerEpidemiol 34: 419-424, 2010.

[44] OlajosJ, FüleE, ErfánJ, KrenácsL, StelkovicsE, Francz M, Lengyel E, Al-Farhat Y and Esik O: Familialclusteringof nasopharyngealcarcinomainanon-endemicgeographicalregion. Report of twoHungariancasesand areview of theliterature. ActaOtolaryngol 125: 1008-1013, 2005.

[45] Zou J, SunQ, AkibaS, YuanY, ZhaY, TaoZ, WeiL and Sugahara T: A case-controlstudyof nasopharyngealcarcinomainthe highbackground radiationareasof Yangjiang, China. J Radiat Res 41 (Suppl): 53-62, 2000.

[46] Feng BJ, Huang W, Shugart YY, et al. Genome-wide scan for familial nasopharyngeal carcinoma reveals evidence of linkage to chromosome 4. Nat Genet. 2002;31:395e399.

[47] Li X, Fasano R, Wang E, Yao KT, Marincol a FM. HLA associations with nasopharyngeal carcinoma. CurrMol Med 2009; 9: 751-765.

[48] JiaWH, CollinsA, ZengYX, FengBJ, Yu XJ, Huang LX, Feng QS, HuangP, YaoMH and Shugart YY: Complex segregationanalysisof nasopharyngealcarcinomain Guangdong, China: Evidenceforamulti factorialmodeof inheritance(complex segregationanalysisof NPC inChina). EurJ HumGenet 13: 248-252, 2005.

[49] Yu MC, Huang TB, Henderso n BE. Diet and nasopharyngeal carcinoma: a case-control study in Guangzhou, China. Int J Cancer 1989; 43: 1077-1082.

[50] Yuan JM, Wang XL, Xiang YB, Gao YT, Ross RK, Yu MC. Preserved foods in relation to risk of nasopharyngeal carcinoma in Shanghai, China. Int J Cancer 2000; 85: 358-363.

[51] Gall icchio L, Matanosk i G, Tao XG, Chen L, Lam TK, Boy d K, Robinso n KA, Balick L, Mick elso n S, Caulfield LE, Herman JG, Guallar E, Alberg AJ. Adulthood consumption of preserved and nonpreserved vegetables and the risk of nasopharyngeal carcinoma: a systematic review. Int J Cancer 2006; 119: 1125-1135.

[52] Farrow DC, Vaughan TL, Berw ick M, Lynch CF, Swanson GM, Lyo n JL. Diet and nasopharyngeal cancer in a low-risk population. Int J Cancer 1998; 78: 675-679.

[53] Shanmugaratnam, K. Histological typing of nasopharyngeal carcinoma. In: Nasopharyngeal Carcinoma – Etiology and Control. Eds. G. De The and Y. Ito. IARC Scientific Publiction 20: 3, 1978.

[54] Vaughan TL, Shapiro JA, Burt RD, Swanso n GM, Berwick M, Lynch CF, Lyo n JL. Nasopharyngeal cancer in a low-risk population: defining risk factors by histological type. Cancer Epidemiol Biomarkers Prev 1996; 5: 587-593.

[55] Lin, T.M., Chen, K.P., Lin, C.C., Hsu, M.M., Tu, S.M., Chiang, T.C., Jung, P.F. and Hirayama, T. Retrospectives study on nasopharyngeal carcinoma. J Natl Cancer Inst 51: 1403, 1973.

[56] Cheng, Y.J., Hildesheim, A., Hsu, M.M., Chen, I.H., Brinton, L.A., Levine, P.H., Chen, C.J. and Yang, C.J. Cigarette smoking, alcohol consumption and risk of nasopharyngeal carcinoma in Taiwan. Cancer Causes Control 10: 201, 1999.

[57] Abnet CC, QiaoYL, Mark SD, DongZW, TaylorPR and Dawsey SM: Prospective study of tooth loss and incident esophageal and gastric cancers in China. Cancer Causes Control 12: 847-854, 2001.

[58] Zhiwei Liu, Ellen T. Chang, Qing Liu, et al. Oral Hygiene and Risk of Nasopharyngeal Carcinoma—A Population-Based Case–Control Study in China.Cancer Epidemiol Biomarkers Prev August 1 2016 (25) (8) 1201-1207; DOI: 10.1158/1055-9965.EPI-16-0149

[59] Meurman JH and UittamoJ: Oral micro-organisms in the etiology of cancer. ActaOdontolScand 66: 321-326, 2008

[60] Chen L, Gallicchio L, Boyd-Lindsley K, Tao XG, Robinson KA, Lam TK, Herman JG, Caulfield LE, Guallar E, Alberg AJ. Alcohol consumption and the risk of nasopharyngeal carcinoma: a systematic review. Nutr Cancer. 2009;61(1):1-15. doi: 10.1080/01635580802372633.

[61] Armstrong RW, Imrey PB , Lye MS, Armstrong MJ, Yu MC, Sani S. Nasopharyngeal carcinoma in Malaysian Chinese: occupational exposures to

particles, formaldehyde and heat. Int J Epidemiol 2000; 29: 991-998

[62] Hardell L, Johansso n B, Axelso n O. Epidemiological study of nasal and nasopharyngeal cancer and their relation to phenoxy acid or chlorophenol exposure. Am J Ind Med 1982; 3: 247-257.

[63] Rous, G.C., Walrath, J., Stayner, L.T., Kaplan, S.A., Flannery, J.T. and Blair, A. Nasopharyngeal cancer, sinonasal cancer and occupation related to formaldehyde: A case control study. J Natl Cancer Inst 76: 1221, 1987.

[64] Yu, M.C., Garabrant, D.H., Huang, T.B. and Henderson, B.E. Occupational and other non-dietary risk factors for nasopharyngeal carcinoma in Guangzhou, China. Int J Cancer 45: 1033,1990

[65] Vaughan, T.L., Stewart, P.A., Teschke, K., Lynmch, C.F., Swanson, G.M., Lyon, J.L. and Berwick, M. Occupational exposure to formaldehyde and wood dust and nasopharyngeal carcinoma. Occup Environ Med 57: 376, 2000.

[66] Lee N. ,Harris J.,Garden A.S. et al. Intensity-modulated radiation therapy with or without chemotherapy for nasopharyngeal carcinoma: radiation therapy oncology group phase II trial 0225. J ClinOncol.2009; 27: 3684-3690

[67] Chen, L., Zhang, Y., Lai, S. Z., Li, W. F., Hu, W. H., Sun, R., Liu, L. Z., Zhang, F., Peng, H., Du, X. J., Lin, A. H., Sun, Y., & Ma, J. (2019). 10-Year Results of Therapeutic Ratio by Intensity-Modulated Radiotherapy Versus Two-Dimensional Radiotherapy in Patients with Nasopharyngeal Carcinoma. *The oncologist*, *24*(1), e38–e45. https://doi.org/10.1634/theoncologist.2017-0577

[68] Lee AW, Tung SY, Chua DT, et al. Randomized trial of radiotherapy Plus concurrent–Adjuvant chemotherapy vs radiotherapy Alone for regionally Advanced Nasopharyngeal carcinoma. J Natl Cancer Inst 2010;102:1188-1198.

[69] Blanchard P, Lee A, Marguet S, et al. Chemotherapy and radiotherapy in nasopharyngeal carcinoma: an update of the MAC-NPC meta-analysis. Lancet Oncol 2015;16:645-655.

[70] Ma J, Mai HQ, Hong MH, et al. Results of a prospective randomized trial comparing neoadjuvant chemotherapy plus radiotherapy with radiotherapy alone in patients with locoregionally advanced nasopharyngeal carcinoma. J ClinOncol 2001;19:1350-1357.

[71] Hui EP, Ma BB, Leung SF, et al. Randomized phase II trial of concurrent cisplatin-radiotherapy with or without neoadjuvantdocetaxel and cisplatin in advanced nasopharyngeal carcinoma. J ClinOncol 2009;27:242-249.

[72] Tan T, Lim WT, Fong KW, et al. Concurrent Chemo-Radiation With or Without Induction Gemcitabine, Carboplatin, and Paclitaxel: A Randomized, Phase 2/3 Trial in Locally Advanced Nasopharyngeal Carcinoma. Int J RadiatOncolBiolPhys 2015;91:952-960

[73] Ma BB, Poon TC, To K, et al. Prognostic significance of tumor angiogenesis, Ki 67, p53 oncoprotein, epidermal growth factor receptor and HER2 receptor protein expression in undifferentiated nasopharyngeal carcinoma—a prospective study. Head Neck 2003;25:864-872.

[74] Bonner JA, Harari PM, Giralt J, et al. Radiotherapy plus cetuximab for locoregionally advanced head and neck cancer: 5-year survival data from a phase 3 randomised trial, and relation between cetuximab-induced rash and survival. Lancet Oncol 2010;11:21-28.

[75] Xu T, Liu Y, Dou S, et al. Weekly cetuximab concurrent with IMRT aggravated radiation-induced oral mucositis in locally advanced nasopharyngeal carcinoma: Results of a randomized phase II study. Oral Oncol 2015;51:875-879.

[76] Ma BB, Kam M, Leung S, et al. A phase II study of concurrent cetuximab–cisplatin and intensity-modulated radiotherapy in locoregionally advanced nasopharyngeal carcinoma. Ann Oncol 2012;23:1287-1292.

[77] Ma BB, Hui EP, Chan AT. Systemic approach to improving treatment outcome in nasopharyngeal carcinoma: current and future directions. Cancer Sci 2008;99:1311-1318.

[78] Ngan RK, Yiu H, Lau W, et al. Combination gemcitabine and cisplatin chemotherapy for metastatic or recurrent nasopharyngeal carcinoma: report of a phase II study. Ann Oncol 2002;13:1252-1258.

[79] Chua DT, Yiu HH, Seetalarom K, et al. Phase II trial of capecitabine plus cisplatin as first-line therapy in patients with metastatic nasopharyngeal cancer. Head Neck 2012;34:1225-1230.

[80] Leong SS, Wee J, Tay MH, et al. Paclitaxel, carboplatin, and gemcitabine in metastatic nasopharyngeal carcinoma. Cancer 2005;103:569-575.

[81] Hsu CH, Gao M, Chen CL, et al. Inhibitors of epidermoid growth factor receptor suppress cell growth and enhance chemosensitivity of nasopharyngeal cancer cells in vitro. Oncology 2005;68:538-547.

[82] Ueda Y, Enokida T, Okano S, Fujisawa T, Ito K and Tahara M (2020) Combination Treatment With Paclitaxel, Carboplatin, and Cetuximab (PCE) as First-Line Treatment in Patients With Recurrent and/or Metastatic Nasopharyngeal Carcinoma. *Front. Oncol.* 10:571304. doi: 10.3389/fonc.2020.571304

[83] Chua DT, Wei WI, Wong MP, et al. Phase II study of gefitinib for the treatment of recurrent and metastatic nasopharyngeal carcinoma. Head Neck 2008;30:863-867.

[84] Lim WT, Ng QS, Ivy P, et al. A Phase II study of pazopanib in Asian patients with recurrent/metastatic nasopharyngeal carcinoma. Clin Cancer Res 2011;17:5481-5489

[85] Xue C, Huang Y, Huang P, et al. Phase II study of sorafenib in combination with cisplatin and 5-fluorouracil to treat recurrent or metastatic nasopharyngeal carcinoma. Ann Oncol 2013;24:1055-1061

[86] Zhang L, Zhao C, Ghimire B, et al. The role of concurrent chemoradiotherapy in the treatment of locoregionally advanced nasopharyngeal carcinoma among endemic population: a meta-analysis of the phase iii randomized trials. BMC Canc. 2010;10:558.

[87] Rossi A, Molinari R, Boracchi P, et al. Adjuvant chemotherapy with vincristine, cyclophosphamide, and doxorubicin after radiotherapy in local-regional nasopharyngeal cancer: results of a 4-year multicenter randomized study. J ClinOncol. 1988;6:1401e1410.

[88] Wang J, Shi M, Hsia Y, et al. Failure patterns and survival in patients with nasopharyngeal carcinoma treated with intensity modulated radiation in Northwest China: a pilot study. RadiatOncol. 2012;7:2. https://doi.org/10.1186/1748-717X-7-2

[89] Wei WI, Sham JST. Nasopharyngeal carcinoma. Lancet. 2005;365:2041e2054.

Chapter 5

Diagnosis and Therapy of Nasopharyngeal Carcinoma

Tingting Huang, Zhe Zhang and Xiaoying Zhou

Abstract

Nasopharyngeal carcinoma (NPC) is a malignancy with unique biological and clinical characteristics. It has highly associated with Epstein–Barr virus (EBV) infection and is sensitive to radiotherapy. Due to the extreme relevance between EBV infection and incidence of NPC, testing antibodies against EBV has been applied to screening "high-risk" populations of NPC. The pathological diagnosis of nasopharyngeal biopsy is the gold standard for the diagnosis of NPC. Radiotherapy has been recognized as the first choice for NPC treatment. With the improvement of intensity-modulated radiation therapy (IMRT), the 5-year disease-specific survival rate in NPC patients at an early stage has reached 95%. However, the efficacy brought by radiotherapy has reached the bottleneck in advanced patients. Recently, the 5-year overall survival rate was increased around 60-80% in locoregionally advanced NPC patients by introducing concurrent chemoradiotherapy. In addition, molecular targeted therapy and immunotherapy have been introduced to many clinical trials. In this chapter, we mainly focus on the current early screening and diagnosis of NPC patients, and the development of therapeutic approaches.

Keywords: nasopharyngeal carcinoma, population-based screening, symptoms, diagnosis, treatment

1. Introduction

As a part of the pharynx, the nasopharynx lies behind and communicates with the nasal cavities. It is up to the cranial base, down to the soft palate plane, forward through the back of the nose to the nasal cavity, and pharynx tonsils in the backward. Behind the inferior turbinate, there is an opening of the eustachian tube, which leads through the nasopharynx to the tympanic cavity. A recess in the lateral of the pharyngeal wall extending posteriorly to the opening of the eustachian tubal torus, which is called Fossa of Rosenmüller, is the predilection site of nasopharyngeal carcinoma (NPC).

As one of the malignant head and neck cancer, NPC arises from epithelial cells within the nasopharyngeal mucosa, with a unique geographical and ethnic distribution.. Epstein–Barr virus (EBV) infection, carcinogen exposure, and genetic susceptibility contribute to the carcinogenesis of NPC. In the endemic area, more than 95% of NPC patients were EBV positive, therefore, testing antibodies against EBV or cell-free EBV DNA has been established for screening assays targeted "high-risk" populations of NPC. Nasopharyngeal endoscopy is recommended for EBV-seropositive individuals to find out NPC patients at an early stage. The common clinical symptoms of NPC were nasal congestion, bloody nose, hearing loss, and headache, but not specific at early stages. At present, the pathological diagnosis of nasopharyngeal biopsy remains the golden standard for NPC. Most undifferentiated NPC is moderately sensitive to radiation therapy, leading it the first choice for NPC treatment. Taking advantage of accurate staging systems, modern radiotherapy techniques, and concurrent chemotherapy, the locoregional control and overall survival of NPC patients have substantially improved along with the decline of treatment-induced toxicity in the past two decades. However, residual/recurrent disease and metastatic disease are still crucial challenges in managing NPC.

1.1 Epidemiology

Globally, NPC is uncommon cancer with approximately 129,000 new cases reported in 2018 and accounting for 0.7% of all cancers [1]. The incidence of NPC is relatively concentrated, about 80% of NPC occurs in Asia, and China accounts for almost half of the total [2]. For instance, the incidence rate in North America and Europe is less than 1/100,000 person-years, but greater than 20/100,000 person-years in Southern China and Southeast Asia [3, 4]. Importantly, NPC incidence is higher in males than in females, with a ratio of 2-3 [5]. The age-specific incidence of NPC is different from other types of cancer as well. The bimodal distribution of age showed two peaks between 16 and 20 and 45-60 years [3]. Besides, family aggregation is a characteristic of NPC in the endemic area which is well documented [6, 7]. Even people migrate from Southern China to non-endemic areas, the incidence remains high, suggesting that genetic inheritance is one of the main factors for NPC pathogenesis. However, the reduced incidence has been observed in second-generation migrants [8]. In addition, according to recent epidemiology studies, the global incidence of NPC is also declining gradually [9–11]. These findings indicate that lifestyle alterations are highly correlated with the pathogenesis of NPC.

1.2 Etiology

So far, the etiology of NPC is not fully clear. It is widely accepted that genetic susceptibility, EBV infection, and exposure to harmful carcinogens such as intake of salted fish and preserved food, etc., are the main pathogenic factors for NPC. The single factor mentioned above can not induce the occurrence of NPC in animal models, therefore all these factors contribute together and their interaction might be more important and worth deeply understanding [12]. Recently, poor oral hygiene has been proposed as a risk factor for NPC [13]. The composition of the oral microbiome is shown to be different between NPC patients and their population-based controls [14]. Moreover, the anaerobic metabolites of *F. nucleatum*, *n*-butyrate acid is a strong lytic-cycle inducer of EBV [15]. More potential pathogenic factors are being discovered.

In the endemic area, almost all NPC patients are associated with EBV infection and are more sensitive to radiotherapy [16]. Besides, it is difficult to achieve effective treatment by surgery in NPC patients, because the anatomy of the nasopharynx is concealed and the peripheral nerves and blood vessels, and more than 80% of patients show lymph node metastasis at the time of diagnosis [17, 18]. Therefore, radiotherapy is the first choice in the treatment of NPC. At present, the local control rate of NPC patients under radiotherapy exceeds 90%, and the 5-year survival rate is close to 80% [19, 20]. It is noteworthy that early diagnosis is a key point. The earlier diagnosis of NPC patients, the greater improvement of survival [21]. To date, distant organ metastasis remains the largest obstacle and the main factor of failure. In this chapter, we mainly introduce the early population screening of NPC in the endemic area, as well as the approaches for NPC diagnosis and treatment.

2. Population screening of NPC

As literature reported, before the clinical onset of NPC, the serological EBV antibody level has already been sustained elevated within a window of 37 months, which serves as an efficient screening biomarker [22]. At present, serological detection of EBV, testing the titers of viral capsid antigen (VCA)-IgA, early antigen (EA)-IgA, and EBV nuclear antigen 1 (EBNA1)-IgA antibodies of EBV is widely used in the mass screening of NPC in an endemic region, which is helpful for early diagnosis [23–25]. No matter using the traditional immunofluorescent/Immunoenzymatic assays or enzyme-linked immunosorbent assays (ELISA) assay, once the elevated EBV-IgA were detected in screening participants, they were defined as "high-risk" objects of NPC. Next, an indirect mirror examination in the nasopharynx and/or lymphatic palpation should be carried out. If abnormal enlargement of the lymph node in the upper neck and elevate, rough nasopharyngeal surface were observed, the objects will be concluded as suspicious NPC patients. Further fiberoptic endoscopy and biopsy are necessary for diagnosis [25]. The benefit of screening was illustrated by finding early NPC cases.

Scientists are devoted to improving the methods of detecting EBV to enhance the effectiveness of screening. For instance, collecting nasopharyngeal swabs for additional nasopharyngeal EBV DNA load analysis could effectively reduce the "high risk" population who needed follow-up examination [26]. Recently, utilizing circulating cell-free EBV DNA has been proposed for early NPC screening, with sensitivity and specificity as 97.1% and 98.6%, respectively [27].

3. Symptoms and diagnosis of NPC

Due to the concealed anatomical location of NPC, most cases show no specific symptoms at all when the disease is initiated, until they present lymph node metastasis, typically in the neck. Thus, most of the patients missed the opportunity of diagnosis at the early stages.

3.1 Symptoms of NPC

NPC usually occurs in the lateral walls, it grows either within the nasopharynx or extends outward. Being a malignant tumor, NPC can infiltrate or invade surrounding structures, for instance, the base of the skull, the palates, nasal cavity, and the oropharynx. The most common presenting symptom is cervical lymph node enlargement, followed by nasal, aural, and neurological symptoms. Among them, the most noteworthy early symptoms of NPC are the first retracted snot with blood in the morning, which is often overlooked by patients. Enlargement of NPC within the nasopharynx may cause nasal obstruction-related symptoms, such as congestion, and bleeding. A blockage of the eustachian tube may lead to unilateral tinnitus, hearing loss, and catarrhal otitis media. The brain nerve invasion or skull base bone damage by NPC are often the causes of headaches [28].

3.2 Diagnosis

The detection of NPC is based on clinical symptoms and physical examination, but a definitive diagnosis requires a biopsy of the lesion. The first choice of the diagnosis of the primary NPC is biopsy under the nasopharynx endoscope [28]. Cervical lymph node biopsy by fine-needle aspiration should only be used when the pathological finding in primary tumor biopsy is negative but remains highly suspicious of NPC. Combining with EBV encoded small RNAs (EBERs) *in situ* hybridization examination could help clinical doctors promptly identify the primary lesions [29]. To further assess the tumor size and location, a series of radiologic tests, including computed tomography (CT) scans and magnetic resonance imaging (MRI) of the head and neck are required. This provides additional but necessary information for evaluating the stage of NPC.

Currently, the staging system of NPC is the eighth edition of the International Union Against Cancer (UICC) and the American Joint Committee on Cancer (AJCC) TNM Classification, based on the tumor-node-metastasis (TNM) criteria (**Table 1**) [30]. This system is an important guideline for the treatment, as well as the basis for evaluating the treatment outcomes of patients. With the development of imaging techniques and treatment approaches for NPC patients, the TNM classification systems will be significantly refined again. Notably, monitoring plasma EBV DNA and circulating tumor cells (CTC) can further improve the prediction of prognosis [31, 32].

Primary tumor (T)	
T_X	Primary tumor cannot be assessed.
T_0	No tumor was identified, but EBV positive cervical node(s) involvement.
T_1	Nasopharynx, oropharynx, or nasal cavity without parapharyngeal extension.
T_2	Parapharyngeal extension, adjacent soft tissue involvement (medial pterygoid, lateral pterygoid, prevertebral muscles.
T_3	Bony structures (skull base, cervical vertebra) and/or paranasal sinuses
T_4	Intracranial extension, cranial nerve, hypopharynx, orbit, extensive soft tissue involvement (beyond the lateral surface of the lateral pterygoid muscle), parotid gland.
Lymph nodes (N)	
N_X	Regional lymph nodes cannot be assessed.
N_0	No regional lymph node metastasis.
N_1	Unilateral cervical, unilateral or bilateral retropharyngeal lymph nodes, above the caudal border of cricoid cartilage;≤6 cm.
N_2	Bilateral metastasis in lymph node(s), 6 cm or less in greatest dimension, above the caudal border of the cricoid cartilage.
N_3	>6 cm and/or below the caudal border of the cricoid cartilage (regardless of laterality).
Distant metastasis (M)	
M_0	No distant metastasis.
M_1	Distant metastasis.
Group staging	
I	T1N0M0
II	T1N0M0; T2N0-1 M0
III	T1-2N2M0; T3N0-2 M0
IV	IVA: T4 or N3M0; IVB: Any T Any N M1

Table 1.
The UICC/AJCC staging system for nasopharyngeal carcinoma (8th edition).

3.3 Pathological classification

Histologically, NPC cells are regarded to be squamous in origin, but with a high background of lymphoid cells. According to the world health organization (WHO), NPC was categorized into three types: nonkeratinizing carcinoma, keratinizing squamous cell carcinoma, and basaloid squamous cell carcinoma [33]. In the endemic areas, over 95% of the cases belong to the nonkeratinizing type, while less than 5% belong to the keratinizing squamous cell carcinoma type, and basaloid squamous cell carcinoma type is extremely rare. On the contrary, in nonendemic western countries like the United States, keratinizing squamous cell carcinoma accounts for more than 25% of NPC cases [34, 35].

4. Treatment of NPC

NPC is relatively sensitive to ionizing radiation, and radiation therapy (RT) is the mainstay modality of curative-intent treatment for patients with the non-disseminated disease. The 5-year disease-specific survival rate in stage I NPC is now expected to be around 95% with IMRT alone [36]. By introducing concurrent chemoradiotherapy to patients with locoregionally advanced diseases, the 5-year overall survival rate was around 60-80% recently [37]. Researchers are making exploratory effects on molecular-targeted medicine and immunotherapy in the treatment of NPC. Several encouraging results from clinical trials will be discussed below.

4.1 Radiation therapy

The ideal modality of RT should fully cover the complex-shaped gross tumor with high doses needed for eradication while providing maximum sparing for adjacent organs. Photon-based radiotherapy techniques have evolved from conventional two-dimensional (2D) radiotherapy to 3D conformal radiotherapy and intensity-modulated radiation therapy (IMRT). Charged particle therapy is gaining more and more attention in the treatment of NPC, especially the locoregionally advanced disease.

IMRT technique allows for the conform radiation dose to deliver precisely to a gross tumor and minimize the dose to adjacent normal tissues by controlling the intensity of the radiation beam. There is compelling evidence from numerous randomized controlled trials (RCTs) reporting a superiority of IMRT over conventional techniques. Over 90% 5-year locoregional control rate and 80% of overall survival rate were achieved, along with significant protection of the saliva gland and reduction of other radiation-induced complications [38–44]. Compared with 2D or 3D radiotherapy, IMRT was significantly associated with better 5-year locoregional control and overall survival [45].

Despite the rapid improvement in radiotherapy techniques, successful RT of NPC relies on precise delineation and accurate dose delivery to the gross tumor volume (GTV), clinical target volume (CTV), and critical organs at risk (OARs) [46]. Advanced imaging techniques, such as MRI, CT, 18F-fluorodeoxyglucose (18F-FDG)-positron emission tomography (PET)/CT, and fusion of images from different techniques with the planning CT images of radiotherapy, together with endoscopy and clinical examination are most commonly used for facilitating primary GTV delineation. The international guidelines and consensus have recently been propounded for the delineation of CTV and OARs, allowing improved consistency and providing helpful references in NPC radiation management [41, 47–49].

Besides, the application of automation, deep learning, and artificial intelligence has been investigated currently [50–52]. It will be an integral piece of RT to improve accuracy, consistency, and cost-efficiency while reducing labor-intensive costs soon.

4.2 Chemotherapy in non-metastatic NPC

While stage I NPC is treated by IMRT alone with little doubt, locoregionally advanced disease (stage II to stage IVB) requires the combination of chemotherapy with comprehensive consideration [53, 54] (**Table 2**). The modalities of chemotherapy include concurrent chemoradiotherapy (CRT), adjuvant chemotherapy, and induction chemotherapy, while the regimens vary between studies/centers.

For stage II NPC, the National Comprehensive Cancer Network (NCCN) guideline suggests RT plus concurrent chemotherapy ± sequential chemotherapy, whereas the EHNS-ESMO-ESTRO clinical practice guideline proposes concurrent chemoradiotherapy (**Table 2**). The controversy between the two guidelines may partly reflect the contentious evidence from numerous clinical trials based on different RT techniques [2, 55–57]. In the IMRT era, many recently retrospective studies and meta-analyses demonstrated that RT alone might be sufficient for patients with stage II disease to achieve desirable long-term outcomes and avoid increased toxicity [58–61].

There is a consensus among guidelines that concurrent chemoradiotherapy ± sequential chemotherapy may be mainstay treatment in stage III to IVB diseases with a remarkable survival benefit [2, 48]. Recently, a study based on 7,940 patients from 27 trials suggests that patients treated with induction-concurrent CRT (IMRT) gained the highest overall survival, progress-free survival, and distant metastasis-free survival [62]. To date, induction-concurrent CRT is becoming more and more important in treating locoregionally advanced NPC and adopted by many treatment centers. Several ongoing trials (NCT01536223, NCT01872962, NCT02512315, NCT 03306121, and NCT03503136) comparing induction-concurrent CRT and concurrent CRT with detailed combinations of different regimens, such as taxane, cisplatin, and 5-fluorouracil are anticipated, which results would provide further evidence for clinical practice.

Stage (8th Ed[a])	NCCN (v2.2020[b])	EHNS-ESMO-ESTRO (2012[c])
Stage I	Radiotherapy (RT) alone	RT alone
Stage II	RT plus Chemotherapy (C): Concurrent C + Adjuvant C (2A[d])	RT + C: Concurrent (I, B[e])
Stage III	or Induction C + Concurrent C (2A)	RT + C: Concurrent ± Adjuvant (I, A)
Stage IVA-B	or Concurrent C (2B)	RT + C: Concurrent ± Adjuvant (I, A) or Induction C + Concurrent C (II, B)
Stage IVC	C alone or RT + C	

[a]*Stage: American Joint Committee on Cancer (AJCC) – TNM Staging System for the Nasopharyngeal Carcinoma (8th ed. 2017).*
[b]*National Comprehensive Cancer Network (NCCN) Guidelines Version 2.2020.*
[c]*EHNS-ESMO-ESTRO Clinical Practice Guidelines (2012).*
[d]*NCCN Categories (1-3) of Evidence and consensus.*
[e]*Level of evidence (I-V) used in the EHNS-ESMO-ESTRO Clinical Practice Guidelines.*

Table 2.
Treatment strategies for different stages.

4.3 Disease surveillance, management of residual/recurrent disease

Close follow-up for NPC patients is essential in terms of disease surveillance. Despite relatively desirable treatment outcomes among solid cancers, unfortunately, about 10-20% of NPC patients will suffer from residual disease or develop recurrent disease after primary treatment, T4 disease among them is reported with up to 45% local recurrence rate [43, 63–67]. Early detection is critical given that extent of relapse determines the chance of salvage, and patients with T1-T2 recurrent disease are more likely to achieve long-term benefit [68, 69]. Initial assessment of residual disease is usually conducted at 12 weeks after the completion of RT or CRT [70, 71]. A detailed history and physical examination, nasopharyngoscopy (with/without biopsy), and radiation imaging (CT/MRI/18F-FDG-PET-CT) are highly recommended in a comprehensive response assessment. Recently, the post-treatment plasma EBV DNA is considered for monitoring for NPC in the context of locoregional failure, distant metastasis, and survival [72].

Emerging evidence suggests that aggressive salvage modalities might increase the chances of better prognosis among patients with recurrent NPC [68, 73, 74]. Neck dissection is widely recommended for isolated regional failure. Re-irradiation is considered for a tumor that recurs more than one year after the completion of primary RT. In contrast, salvage surgery is esteemed if the one recurs within one year and is resectable.

4.4 Management of metastatic disease

Patients with metastatic NPC have various clinical characteristics and outcomes. Around 10% of newly diagnosed NPC patients present with synchronous distance metastases. Unfortunately, up to 15%-30% of the non-metastatic NPC patients will experience distant failure after primarily curative treatment [2, 48]. Compelling evidence suggests these patients may achieve a median overall survival of 10-15 months by receiving palliative chemotherapy. The overall survival can be improved among those who are indicated for locoregional RT and local treatment of metastatic lesions [63, 75–81]. Thus, a personalized treatment strategy is necessary for metastatic NPC. Researchers and clinicians have made a hard effort to build up predictive models for prognosis to stratify risk groups and provide treatment strategies accurately [82–87].

Recommending by NCCN guideline, the first-line regimens of systemic therapy for NPC patients with recurrent, or unresectable, or metastatic disease are cisplatin plus gemcitabine. Other recommended regimens include the combination of cisplatin/5-fluorouracil, cisplatin or carboplatin/docetaxel or paclitaxel, carboplatin/cetuximab, gemcitabine/carboplatin, as well as the single-use of them. A recent view suggests that neither VEGFR nor EGFR targeting therapies are recommended as high priority for recurrent and/or metastatic NPC, with unimpressive response rates around 10% or less [67, 88–93]. Reported toxicities of anti-VEGF therapy and anti-EGFR therapy can be severe and life-threatening, which should not be neglected.

Remarkably, several single-arm trials evaluating immunotherapy targeted the programmed death 1/programmed death-ligand 1 (PD1/PD-L1) pathway in recurrent/metastatic NPC patients have shown promising outcomes [94–96]. In principle, NPC tumors are featured by high PD-L1 expression and abundant infiltration of non-malignant lymphocytes, suggesting the feasibility of immune checkpoint blockade therapies in NPC patients [97–100]. Some ongoing phase 3 trials investigating anti-PD-1 therapies among treatment naïve locoregionally advanced disease, recurrent, or metastatic disease, will improve clinical practice [2]. Likewise, a phase

1 trial of a recombinant vaccinia virus (MVA-EL), which encodes an EBNA1/LMP2 fusion protein designed to boost T-cell immunity to these antigens, has shown clinical efficacy in heavily pretreated NPCs [101]. Evidence from phage 2/3 RCTs on immunotherapies targeting EBV and/or PD1/PD-L1 is awaited to manage locoregional, recurrent, and metastatic NPC in the near future.

5. Conclusion

Early diagnosis and early therapy is the most effective method to improve the curative effect of NPC. It is necessary to strengthen the population-based screening of NPC in the endemic region and optimize the screening methods to elevate efficiency. Improving the treatment approach is critical as well. With the great progress in staging systems, radiotherapy techniques, and concurrent chemotherapy, the locoregional control and overall survival of NPC patients have improved substantially. Meanwhile, molecular targeted therapy and immunotherapy have gained much interest and are now being introduced to many clinical trials. Although encouraging outcomes are achieved, treatment-related toxicities, residual/recurrent disease, and metastatic disease are still crucial challenges in managing NPC, worthy of further attention and effort.

Acknowledgements

This work was supported by grants from the National Natural Science Foundation of China (81660445, 81772882), and the Natural Science Foundation of Guangxi Province (2018GXNSFBA281028).

Conflict of interest

The authors declare no conflict of interest.

Author details

Tingting Huang[1,2], Zhe Zhang[3] and Xiaoying Zhou[4*]

1 Department of Medical Epidemiology and Biostatistics, Karolinska Institutet, Stockholm, Sweden

2 Department of Radiation Oncology, First Affiliated Hospital of Guangxi Medical University, Nanning, China

3 Department of Otolaryngology-Head and Neck Surgery, First Affiliated Hospital of Guangxi Medical University, Nanning, China

4 Life Science Institute, Guangxi Medical University, Nanning, China

*Address all correspondence to: zhouxiaoying1982@foxmail.com

References

[1] Bray, F., et al., *Global cancer statistics 2018: GLOBOCAN estimates of incidence and mortality worldwide for 36 cancers in 185 countries.* CA Cancer J Clin, 2018. **68**(6): p. 394-424.

[2] Chen, Y.P., et al., *Nasopharyngeal carcinoma.* Lancet, 2019. **394**(10192): p. 64-80.

[3] Yu, M.C. and J.M. Yuan, *Epidemiology of nasopharyngeal carcinoma.* Semin Cancer Biol, 2002. **12**(6): p. 421-9.

[4] Zhang, L.F., et al., *Incidence trend of nasopharyngeal carcinoma from 1987 to 2011 in Sihui County, Guangdong Province, South China: an age-period-cohort analysis.* Chin J Cancer, 2015. **34**(8): p. 350-7.

[5] Chen, W., et al., *Cancer statistics in China, 2015.* CA Cancer J Clin, 2016. **66**(2): p. 115-32.

[6] Ko, J.Y., et al., *Familial clustering of nasopharyngeal carcinoma.* Otolaryngol Head Neck Surg, 1998. **118**(5): p. 736-7.

[7] Zeng, Y.X. and W.H. Jia, *Familial nasopharyngeal carcinoma.* Semin Cancer Biol, 2002. **12**(6): p. 443-50.

[8] Yu, W.M. and S.S. Hussain, *Incidence of nasopharyngeal carcinoma in Chinese immigrants, compared with Chinese in China and South East Asia: review.* J Laryngol Otol, 2009. **123**(10): p. 1067-74.

[9] Li, K., et al., *Time trends of nasopharyngeal carcinoma in urban Guangzhou over a 12-year period (2000-2011): declines in both incidence and mortality.* Asian Pac J Cancer Prev, 2014. **15**(22): p. 9899-903.

[10] Lee, A.W., et al., *Changing epidemiology of nasopharyngeal carcinoma in Hong Kong over a 20-year period (1980-99): an encouraging reduction in both incidence and mortality.* Int J Cancer, 2003. **103**(5): p. 680-5.

[11] Tang, L.L., et al., *Global trends in incidence and mortality of nasopharyngeal carcinoma.* Cancer Lett, 2016. **374**(1): p. 22-30.

[12] Lee, H.M., et al., *Current Perspectives on Nasopharyngeal Carcinoma.* Adv Exp Med Biol, 2019. **1164**: p. 11-34.

[13] Liu, Z., et al., *Oral Hygiene and Risk of Nasopharyngeal Carcinoma-A Population-Based Case-Control Study in China.* Cancer Epidemiol Biomarkers Prev, 2016. **25**(8): p. 1201-7.

[14] Debelius, J.W., et al., *Subspecies Niche Specialization in the Oral Microbiome Is Associated with Nasopharyngeal Carcinoma Risk.* mSystems, 2020. **5**(4).

[15] Ito, Y., M. Kishishita, and S. Yanase, *Induction of Epstein-Barr virus antigens in human lymphoblastoid P3HR-1 cells with culture fluid of Fusobacterium nucleatum.* Cancer Res, 1980. **40**(11): p. 4329-30.

[16] Young, L.S. and C.W. Dawson, *Epstein-Barr virus and nasopharyngeal carcinoma.* Chin J Cancer, 2014. **33**(12): p. 581-90.

[17] King, A.D., et al., *Neck node metastases from nasopharyngeal carcinoma: MR imaging of patterns of disease.* Head Neck, 2000. **22**(3): p. 275-81.

[18] Tomita, N., et al., *Factors associated with nodal metastasis in nasopharyngeal cancer: an approach to reduce the radiation field in selected patients.* Br J Radiol, 2011. **84**(999): p. 265-70.

[19] Sun, X.S., et al., *Future of Radiotherapy in Nasopharyngeal Carcinoma.* Br J Radiol, 2019. **92**(1102): p. 20190209.

[20] Kong, F., et al., *Long-term survival and late complications of intensity-modulated radiotherapy for recurrent nasopharyngeal carcinoma.* BMC Cancer, 2018. **18**(1): p. 1139.

[21] Liu, D.H., et al., *Survival of stage II nasopharyngeal carcinoma patients with or without concurrent chemotherapy: A propensity score matching study.* Cancer Med, 2020. **9**(4): p. 1287-1297.

[22] Ji, M.F., et al., *Sustained elevation of Epstein-Barr virus antibody levels preceding clinical onset of nasopharyngeal carcinoma.* Br J Cancer, 2007. **96**(4): p. 623-30.

[23] Zeng, Y., et al., *Serological mass survey for early detection of nasopharyngeal carcinoma in Wuzhou City, China.* Int J Cancer, 1982. **29**(2): p. 139-41.

[24] Liu, Y., et al., *Establishment of VCA and EBNA1 IgA-based combination by enzyme-linked immunosorbent assay as preferred screening method for nasopharyngeal carcinoma: a two-stage design with a preliminary performance study and a mass screening in southern China.* Int J Cancer, 2012. **131**(2): p. 406-16.

[25] Liu, Z., et al., *Two Epstein-Barr virus-related serologic antibody tests in nasopharyngeal carcinoma screening: results from the initial phase of a cluster randomized controlled trial in Southern China.* Am J Epidemiol, 2013. **177**(3): p. 242-50.

[26] Chen, Y., et al., *Nasopharyngeal Epstein-Barr Virus Load: An Efficient Supplementary Method for Population-Based Nasopharyngeal Carcinoma Screening.* PLoS One, 2015. **10**(7): p. e0132669.

[27] Chan, K.C.A., et al., *Analysis of Plasma Epstein-Barr Virus DNA to Screen for Nasopharyngeal Cancer.* N Engl J Med, 2017. **377**(6): p. 513-522.

[28] Zhou, X., et al., *The progress on genetic analysis of nasopharyngeal carcinoma.* Comp Funct Genomics, 2007: p. 57513.

[29] Zhang, Y., et al., *Diagnostic utility of immunohistochemical analysis and Epstein-Barr virus-encoded small RNAs in situ hybridisation of cell block sections obtained using fine-needle aspiration in nasopharyngeal carcinoma with lymph node metastasis.* Diagn Cytopathol, 2019. **47**(3): p. 200-205.

[30] Guo, R., et al., *The evolution of nasopharyngeal carcinoma staging.* Br J Radiol, 2019. **92**(1102): p. 20190244.

[31] Tan, L.P., et al., *Systematic comparison of plasma EBV DNA, anti-EBV antibodies and miRNA levels for early detection and prognosis of nasopharyngeal carcinoma.* Int J Cancer, 2020. **146**(8): p. 2336-2347.

[32] You, R., et al., *Relationship of circulating tumor cells and Epstein-Barr virus DNA to progression-free survival and overall survival in metastatic nasopharyngeal carcinoma patients.* Int J Cancer, 2019. **145**(10): p. 2873-2883.

[33] Tabuchi, K., et al., *Early detection of nasopharyngeal carcinoma.* Int J Otolaryngol, 2011. **2011**: p. 638058.

[34] Jeyakumar, A., et al., *Review of nasopharyngeal carcinoma.* Ear Nose Throat J, 2006. **85**(3): p. 168-70, 172-3, 184.

[35] Wei, W.I. and J.S. Sham, *Nasopharyngeal carcinoma.* Lancet, 2005. **365**(9476): p. 2041-54.

[36] Chua, D.T., et al., *Treatment outcome after radiotherapy alone for patients with Stage I-II nasopharyngeal carcinoma.* Cancer, 2003. **98**(1): p. 74-80.

[37] Kong, M., Y.J. Lim, and Y. Kim, *Concurrent Chemoradiotherapy for Loco-regionally Advanced Nasopharyngeal*

Carcinoma: Treatment Outcomes and Prognostic Factors. Asian Pac J Cancer Prev, 2018. **19**(6): p. 1591-1599.

[38] Kam, M.K., et al., *Prospective randomized study of intensity-modulated radiotherapy on salivary gland function in early-stage nasopharyngeal carcinoma patients.* J Clin Oncol, 2007. **25**(31): p. 4873-9.

[39] Pow, E.H., et al., *Xerostomia and quality of life after intensity-modulated radiotherapy vs. conventional radiotherapy for early-stage nasopharyngeal carcinoma: initial report on a randomized controlled clinical trial.* Int J Radiat Oncol Biol Phys, 2006. **66**(4): p. 981-91.

[40] Fang, F.M., et al., *Quality of life and survival outcome for patients with nasopharyngeal carcinoma receiving three-dimensional conformal radiotherapy vs. intensity-modulated radiotherapy-a longitudinal study.* Int J Radiat Oncol Biol Phys, 2008. **72**(2): p. 356-64.

[41] Lee, N., et al., *Intensity-modulated radiation therapy with or without chemotherapy for nasopharyngeal carcinoma: radiation therapy oncology group phase II trial 0225.* J Clin Oncol, 2009. **27**(22): p. 3684-90.

[42] Wong, F.C., et al., *Whole-field simultaneous integrated-boost intensity-modulated radiotherapy for patients with nasopharyngeal carcinoma.* Int J Radiat Oncol Biol Phys, 2010. **76**(1): p. 138-45.

[43] Sun, X., et al., *Long-term outcomes of intensity-modulated radiotherapy for 868 patients with nasopharyngeal carcinoma: an analysis of survival and treatment toxicities.* Radiother Oncol, 2014. **110**(3): p. 398-403.

[44] Peng, G., et al., *A prospective, randomized study comparing outcomes and toxicities of intensity-modulated radiotherapy vs. conventional two-dimensional radiotherapy for the treatment of nasopharyngeal carcinoma.* Radiother Oncol, 2012. **104**(3): p. 286-93.

[45] Zhang, B., et al., *Intensity-modulated radiation therapy versus 2D-RT or 3D-CRT for the treatment of nasopharyngeal carcinoma: A systematic review and meta-analysis.* Oral Oncol, 2015. **51**(11): p. 1041-1046.

[46] Wu, H.T., et al., *Analysis of the Differentially Expressed Genes Induced by Cisplatin Resistance in Oral Squamous Cell Carcinomas and Their Interaction.* Front Genet, 2019. **10**: p. 1328.

[47] Sun, Y., et al., *Recommendation for a contouring method and atlas of organs at risk in nasopharyngeal carcinoma patients receiving intensity-modulated radiotherapy.* Radiother Oncol, 2014. **110**(3): p. 390-7.

[48] Lee, A.W., et al., *Management of Nasopharyngeal Carcinoma: Current Practice and Future Perspective.* J Clin Oncol, 2015. **33**(29): p. 3356-64.

[49] Lee, A.W., et al., *International guideline for the delineation of the clinical target volumes (CTV) for nasopharyngeal carcinoma.* Radiother Oncol, 2018. **126**(1): p. 25-36.

[50] Cardenas, C.E., et al., *Deep Learning Algorithm for Auto-Delineation of High-Risk Oropharyngeal Clinical Target Volumes With Built-In Dice Similarity Coefficient Parameter Optimization Function.* Int J Radiat Oncol Biol Phys, 2018. **101**(2): p. 468-478.

[51] Lin, L., et al., *Deep Learning for Automated Contouring of Primary Tumor Volumes by MRI for Nasopharyngeal Carcinoma.* Radiology, 2019. **291**(3): p. 677-686.

[52] van Dijk, L.V., et al., *Improving automatic delineation for head and neck organs at risk by Deep Learning Contouring.* Radiother Oncol, 2020. **142**: p. 115-123.

[53] Chan, A.T., et al., *Nasopharyngeal cancer: EHNS-ESMO-ESTRO Clinical Practice Guidelines for diagnosis, treatment and follow-up.* Ann Oncol, 2012. **23 Suppl** 7: p. vii83-5.

[54] *National Comprehensive Cancer Network. (NCCN) Clinical Practice Guidelines in Oncology. Head and Neck Cancers. [Internet]. 2020. Available from:* https://www.nccn.org/professionals/physician_gls/pdf/head-and-neck.pdf; [Accessed 2020-09-09]

[55] Chen, Q.Y., et al., *Concurrent chemoradiotherapy vs radiotherapy alone in stage II nasopharyngeal carcinoma: phase III randomized trial.* J Natl Cancer Inst, 2011. **103**(23): p. 1761-70.

[56] Lee, A.W., et al., *Treatment results for nasopharyngeal carcinoma in the modern era: the Hong Kong experience.* Int J Radiat Oncol Biol Phys, 2005. **61**(4): p. 1107-16.

[57] Lee, A.W., et al., *Evolution of treatment for nasopharyngeal cancer--success and setback in the intensity-modulated radiotherapy era.* Radiother Oncol, 2014. **110**(3): p. 377-84.

[58] Tham, I.W., et al., *Intensity-modulated radiation therapy without concurrent chemotherapy for stage IIb nasopharyngeal cancer.* Am J Clin Oncol, 2010. **33**(3): p. 294-9.

[59] Xu, T., et al., *Omission of Chemotherapy in Early Stage Nasopharyngeal Carcinoma Treated with IMRT: A Paired Cohort Study.* Medicine (Baltimore), 2015. **94**(39): p. e1457.

[60] Xu, C., et al., *Chemoradiotherapy Versus Radiotherapy Alone in Stage II Nasopharyngeal Carcinoma: A Systemic Review and Meta-analysis of 2138 Patients.* J Cancer, 2017. **8**(2): p. 287-297.

[61] Liu, F., et al., *The role of concurrent chemotherapy for stage II nasopharyngeal carcinoma in the intensity-modulated radiotherapy era: A systematic review and meta-analysis.* PLoS One, 2018. **13**(3): p. e0194733.

[62] You, R., et al., *The Changing Therapeutic Role of Chemo-radiotherapy for Loco-regionally Advanced Nasopharyngeal Carcinoma from Two/Three-Dimensional Radiotherapy to Intensity-Modulated Radiotherapy: A Network Meta-Analysis.* Theranostics, 2017. **7**(19): p. 4825-4835.

[63] Chua, D.T., et al., *Phase II trial of capecitabine plus cisplatin as first-line therapy in patients with metastatic nasopharyngeal cancer.* Head Neck, 2012. **34**(9): p. 1225-30.

[64] Cao, C.N., et al., *Clinical outcomes and patterns of failure after intensity-modulated radiotherapy for T4 nasopharyngeal carcinoma.* Oral Oncol, 2013. **49**(2): p. 175-81.

[65] Zhang, M.X., et al., *Intensity-modulated radiotherapy prolongs the survival of patients with nasopharyngeal carcinoma compared with conventional two-dimensional radiotherapy: A 10-year experience with a large cohort and long follow-up.* Eur J Cancer, 2015. **51**(17): p. 2587-95.

[66] Mao, Y.P., et al., *Prognostic factors and failure patterns in non-metastatic nasopharyngeal carcinoma after intensity-modulated radiotherapy.* Chin J Cancer, 2016. **35**(1): p. 103.

[67] Le, Q.T., et al., *Current Treatment Landscape of Nasopharyngeal Carcinoma and Potential Trials Evaluating the Value of Immunotherapy.* J Natl Cancer Inst, 2019. **111**(7): p. 655-663.

[68] Yu, K.H., et al., *Survival outcome of patients with nasopharyngeal carcinoma with first local failure: a study by the Hong Kong Nasopharyngeal Carcinoma Study Group.* Head Neck, 2005. **27**(5): p. 397-405.

[69] ANNE W.M. LEE, M.L.L., WAI TONG NG, *Nasopharyngeal Carcinoma*. 2019, United Kingdom: Stacy Masucci. p. 396.

[70] Kwong, D.L., et al., *The time course of histologic remission after treatment of patients with nasopharyngeal carcinoma.* Cancer, 1999. **85**(7): p. 1446-53.

[71] Lin, G.W., et al., *The use of MR imaging to detect residual versus recurrent nasopharyngeal carcinoma following treatment with radiation therapy.* Eur J Radiol, 2013. **82**(12): p. 2240-6.

[72] Chan, A.T.C., et al., *Analysis of Plasma Epstein-Barr Virus DNA in Nasopharyngeal Cancer After Chemoradiation to Identify High-Risk Patients for Adjuvant Chemotherapy: A Randomized Controlled Trial.* J Clin Oncol, 2018: p. JCO2018777847.

[73] Lee, A.W., et al., *Retrospective analysis of patients with nasopharyngeal carcinoma treated during 1976-1985: survival after local recurrence.* Int J Radiat Oncol Biol Phys, 1993. **26**(5): p. 773-82.

[74] Teo, P.M., et al., *How successful is high-dose (> or = 60 Gy) reirradiation using mainly external beams in salvaging local failures of nasopharyngeal carcinoma?* Int J Radiat Oncol Biol Phys, 1998. **40**(4): p. 897-913.

[75] Tan, E.H., et al., *Phase II trial of a paclitaxel and carboplatin combination in Asian patients with metastatic nasopharyngeal carcinoma.* Ann Oncol, 1999. **10**(2): p. 235-7.

[76] Ngan, R.K., et al., *Combination gemcitabine and cisplatin chemotherapy for metastatic or recurrent nasopharyngeal carcinoma: report of a phase II study.* Ann Oncol, 2002. **13**(8): p. 1252-8.

[77] Lee, A.W., et al., *The battle against nasopharyngeal cancer.* Radiother Oncol, 2012. **104**(3): p. 272-8.

[78] Chan, O.S. and R.K. Ngan, *Individualized treatment in stage IVC nasopharyngeal carcinoma.* Oral Oncol, 2014. **50**(9): p. 791-7.

[79] Zeng, L., et al., *Retrospective analysis of 234 nasopharyngeal carcinoma patients with distant metastasis at initial diagnosis: therapeutic approaches and prognostic factors.* PLoS One, 2014. **9**(9): p. e108070.

[80] Zou, X., et al., *Establishment and validation of M1 stage subdivisions for de novo metastatic nasopharyngeal carcinoma to better predict prognosis and guide treatment.* Eur J Cancer, 2017. **77**: p. 117-126.

[81] Sun, X.S., et al., *Identifying optimal candidates for local treatment of the primary tumor among patients with de novo metastatic nasopharyngeal carcinoma: a retrospective cohort study based on Epstein-Barr virus DNA level and tumor response to palliative chemotherapy.* BMC Cancer, 2019. **19**(1): p. 92.

[82] Ong, Y.K., et al., *Design of a prognostic index score for metastatic nasopharyngeal carcinoma.* Eur J Cancer, 2003. **39**(11): p. 1535-41.

[83] Toh, C.K., et al., *Validation of a new prognostic index score for disseminated nasopharyngeal carcinoma.* Br J Cancer, 2005. **92**(8): p. 1382-7.

[84] Jin, Y., et al., *To build a prognostic score model containing indispensible tumour markers for metastatic nasopharyngeal carcinoma in an epidemic area.* Eur J Cancer, 2012. **48**(6): p. 882-8.

[85] Jiang, R., et al., *Development of a ten-signature classifier using a support vector machine integrated approach to subdivide the M1 stage into M1a and M1b stages of nasopharyngeal carcinoma with synchronous metastases to better predict patients' survival.* Oncotarget, 2016. **7**(3): p. 3645-57.

[86] Zeng, Z., et al., *A nomogram for predicting survival of nasopharyngeal carcinoma patients with metachronous metastasis.* Medicine (Baltimore), 2016. **95**(27): p. e4026.

[87] Chee, J., et al., *Prognostic stratification of patients with metastatic nasopharyngeal carcinoma using a clinical and biochemical scoring system.* J Cancer Res Clin Oncol, 2017. **143**(12): p. 2563-2570.

[88] Chan, A.T., et al., *Multicenter, phase II study of cetuximab in combination with carboplatin in patients with recurrent or metastatic nasopharyngeal carcinoma.* J Clin Oncol, 2005. **23**(15): p. 3568-76.

[89] Chua, D.T., et al., *Phase II study of gefitinib for the treatment of recurrent and metastatic nasopharyngeal carcinoma.* Head Neck, 2008. **30**(7): p. 863-7.

[90] Hui, E.P., et al., *Hemorrhagic complications in a phase II study of sunitinib in patients of nasopharyngeal carcinoma who has previously received high-dose radiation.* Ann Oncol, 2011. **22**(6): p. 1280-1287.

[91] You, B., et al., *A Phase II trial of erlotinib as maintenance treatment after gemcitabine plus platinum-based chemotherapy in patients with recurrent and/or metastatic nasopharyngeal carcinoma.* Am J Clin Oncol, 2012. **35**(3): p. 255-60.

[92] Lim, W.T., et al., *A Phase II study of pazopanib in Asian patients with recurrent/metastatic nasopharyngeal carcinoma.* Clin Cancer Res, 2011. **17**(16): p. 5481-9.

[93] Xue, C., et al., *Phase II study of sorafenib in combination with cisplatin and 5-fluorouracil to treat recurrent or metastatic nasopharyngeal carcinoma.* Ann Oncol, 2013. **24**(4): p. 1055-61.

[94] Hsu, C., et al., *Safety and Antitumor Activity of Pembrolizumab in Patients With Programmed Death-Ligand 1-Positive Nasopharyngeal Carcinoma: Results of the KEYNOTE-028 Study.* J Clin Oncol, 2017. **35**(36): p. 4050-4056.

[95] Ma, B.B.Y., et al., *Antitumor Activity of Nivolumab in Recurrent and Metastatic Nasopharyngeal Carcinoma: An International, Multicenter Study of the Mayo Clinic Phase 2 Consortium (NCI-9742).* J Clin Oncol, 2018. **36**(14): p. 1412-1418.

[96] Fang, W., et al., *Camrelizumab (SHR-1210) alone or in combination with gemcitabine plus cisplatin for nasopharyngeal carcinoma: results from two single-arm, phase 1 trials.* Lancet Oncol, 2018. **19**(10): p. 1338-1350.

[97] Lee, V.H., et al., *Correlation of PD-L1 Expression of Tumor Cells with Survival Outcomes after Radical Intensity-Modulated Radiation Therapy for Non-Metastatic Nasopharyngeal Carcinoma.* PLoS One, 2016. **11**(6): p. e0157969.

[98] Zhu, Q., et al., *Tumor cells PD-L1 expression as a favorable prognosis factor in nasopharyngeal carcinoma patients with pre-existing intratumor-infiltrating lymphocytes.* Oncoimmunology, 2017. **6**(5): p. e1312240.

[99] Larbcharoensub, N., et al., *Characterization of PD-L1 and PD-1 Expression and CD8+ Tumor-infiltrating Lymphocyte in Epstein-Barr Virus-associated Nasopharyngeal Carcinoma.* Am J Clin Oncol, 2018. **41**(12): p. 1204-1210.

[100] Wang, Y.Q., et al., *Prognostic significance of tumor-infiltrating lymphocytes in nondisseminated nasopharyngeal carcinoma: A large-scale cohort study.* Int J Cancer, 2018. **142**(12): p. 2558-2566.

[101] Hui, E.P., et al., *Phase I trial of recombinant modified vaccinia ankara encoding Epstein-Barr viral tumor antigens in nasopharyngeal carcinoma patients.* Cancer Res, 2013. **73**(6): p. 1676-88.

Chapter 6

Chemotherapy in Nasopharyngeal Carcinoma

Lekha Madhavan Nair, Rejnish Ravi Kumar, Malu Rafi, Farida Nazeer, Kainickal Cessal Thommachan and Kunnambath Ramadas

Abstract

Nasopharyngeal carcinoma is a unique disease entity among head and neck cancers due to its epidemiology and clinical behavior. Non-keratinizing or undifferentiated carcinoma is the most common histological type in endemic areas. Radiotherapy is the treatment for early-stage disease. With the widespread use of IMRT, loco-regional control has improved significantly in locally advanced diseases. But distant metastasis continues to be the most common pattern of failure. To address this issue, chemotherapy has been incorporated into radiotherapy in various settings; as concurrent, induction, and adjuvant. The initial trials of concurrent chemotherapy incorporated adjuvant chemotherapy also and the magnitude of benefit contributed by each treatment was not clear. Later trials proved that adjuvant chemotherapy was not beneficial. Induction chemotherapy when added to concurrent chemoradiation resulted in improvement in Failure Free Survival, Overall Survival, and Distant Metastasis Free Survival. Thus, induction chemotherapy followed by concurrent chemoradiation became the standard of care for locally advanced disease (stage III and IVA). The role of chemotherapy in stage II disease is still evolving. Metastatic nasopharyngeal carcinoma is treated by platinum doublet chemotherapy, Cisplatin-gemcitabine is the standard regimen.

Keywords: Nasopharyngeal carcinoma, locally advanced, metastatic, concurrent chemotherapy, induction chemotherapy, adjuvant chemotherapy

1. Introduction

Nasopharyngeal carcinoma (NPC) is unique from other head and neck cancers due to its difference in epidemiology, etiology and propensity for distant metastasis. It is endemic in Southern China, South East Asia, North Africa, and Artic region. Non-keratinizing or undifferentiated carcinoma is the most common histological type in endemic areas. Radiotherapy is the backbone of treatment owing to the complex anatomical location and high radiosensitivity. Higher local control and survival are reported for early-stage disease with radiotherapy alone [1]. But around 70% of patients present with locoregionally advanced disease and outcomes with radiotherapy alone are poor [2]. Many strategies have been tried to improve outcomes in locoregionally advanced NPC; the incorporation of chemotherapy and the use of modern radiotherapy techniques. IMRT when compared with two-dimensional radiotherapy showed significantly better locoregional control and survival with a lower incidence of radiation- induced toxicities [3, 4]. IMRT is mainly aimed at reducing the toxicities in the early stages whereas it improves loco-regional control (LRC) in advanced stages. After the widespread use of IMRT, distant metastasis remains the predominant pattern of failure. Hence chemotherapy was added to radiotherapy in various settings; as concurrent, induction, and adjuvant. Patients with metastatic disease are treated by palliative chemotherapy or palliative radiotherapy.

2. Evolution of chemoradiation in NPC

Stage I disease is treated by radical radiotherapy. Locally advanced disease (stage III and IVA) was treated by radiotherapy till the early '90s. Chemo-radiation was first studied in the landmark intergroup trial by Al Saraaf et al [5]. This trial compared chemoradiation followed by adjuvant chemotherapy versus radiotherapy (RT) alone in stage III and IV NPC (N = 147). The radiotherapy dose was 70Gy, delivered by conformal technique. There was a significant improvement in PFS and OS with the addition of chemotherapy. The 3-year PFS rate was 69% versus 24% (P < .001) and the 3-year OS was 78% versus 47% (P = .005) in the chemoradiation and radiotherapy arms respectively. But this trial was conducted in a non-endemic area and 22% of patients had keratinizing SCC. Hence the results could not be extrapolated to endemic areas.

Four randomized trials were conducted in a similar fashion in the endemic population, one each from Singapore and China and two from Hongkong. Wee et al randomized patients (N = 221) with stage T3-4NxM0 or TxN2-3 M0 NPC with WHO type II or III histology to radiotherapy alone or chemoradiotherapy followed by adjuvant chemotherapy [6]. Patients on chemoradiotherapy received concurrent cisplatin (25 mg/m2 on days 1 to 4) on weeks 1, 4, and 7 of RT and adjuvant cisplatin (20 mg/m2 on days 1 to 4) and fluorouracil (1,000 mg/m2 on days 1 to 4) every 4 weeks (weeks 11, 15, and 19) for three cycles after completion of RT. RT dose was 70Gy in 7 weeks by conventional technique. The 3-year survival rate was 65% and 80% for RT alone and CCRT, respectively (HR 0.51 (95% CI, 0.31 to 0.81; P = .0061). There was a 17% decrease in cumulative incidence of distant metastasis in the chemotherapy arm (p = 0029).

Two parallel RCTs from Hongkong namely NPC 9901 and NPC 9902 were done for advanced regional disease and advanced local disease respectively in the endemic population [7, 8]. In NPC 9901, patients with nonkeratinizing/undifferentiated NPC staged T1–4N2-3 M0 were randomized to chemo-RT followed by adjuvant chemotherapy or RT alone (N = 348). There was a significant improvement in LRC and failure free survival (FFS) but at the expense of significantly higher rates of acute and late toxicities. The update also showed significant improvement in 5 year FFS (67% vs 55%, P = .014) and PFS (62% vs 53%, P = .035) in favor of chemotherapy [9]. There was an increase in acute toxicities (CRT vs RT: 83% vs 53%; P < .001), but late toxicities were not different. OS did not show any benefit, probably due to the increased rates of noncancer death in the chemotherapy arm. NPC 9902 included Stage T3-4N0-1M0, nonkeratinizing or undifferentiated carcinoma of the nasopharynx (N = 189). There were 4 arms; RT with conventional fractionation alone, RT with accelerated fractionation alone, RT with conventional fractionation + concurrent /adjuvant chemotherapy (CF + C), and RT with accelerated fractionation + concurrent/ adjuvant chemotherapy (AF- + C). There was a significant improvement in FFS in the AF + C compared to the CF arm (94% vs. 70% at 3 years, p = 0.008), but the difference was not significant between the AF arm and the CF + C. There was no significant difference in OS between the 4 arms.

Acute toxicities were significantly more in both the chemo-RT arms. The late toxicity was more in the AF + C arm compared to the CF arm($p = 0.05$).

Another prospective trial with a similar design was conducted in the endemic population of China by Chen et al [10]. RT dose was 70Gy in 7 weeks by conventional technique. The chemotherapy arm received concurrent cisplatin (40 mg/m2 on Day 1) weekly during RT, followed by cisplatin (80 mg/m2 on Day 1) and fluorouracil (800 mg/m2 on Days 1–5) every 4 weeks (Weeks 5, 9, and 13) for three cycles after completion of RT. The 2 year overall survival rate (89.8% vs. 79.7%, $p = 0.003$), failure-free survival rate (84.6% vs. 72.5%, $p = 0.001$), distant failure-free survival rate (86.5% vs. 78.7%, $p = 0.024$), and locoregional failure-free survival rate (98.0% vs. 91.9%, $p = 0.007$) was better in the chemotherapy arm. But acute toxicities were more in the chemotherapy arm (62.6% vs. 32%, $p = 0.000$).

Different trials used different concurrent cisplatin schedules. A randomized phase 3 trial was conducted by Liang et al to identify the ideal concurrent regimen. Weekly cisplatin 40 mg/m2 was shown to have efficacy similar to 3 weekly cisplatin 100 mg/m2 but at the expense of increased hematological toxicities [11].

The chemoradiation trials showed improvement in failure-free survival and distant metastasis-free survival with the addition of chemotherapy at the expense of increased acute toxicities. But overall survival benefit was not consistent among trials. A meta-analysis of 7 randomized trials done in endemic population by Zhang et al showed significantly better 5 years OS in favor of the CCRT treatment groups with a relative risk (RR) of 0.74 [0.62–0.89]. Locoregional recurrence (RR of 0.67,95% CI, 0.49 to 0.91) and distant metastasis (RR of 0.71;95% CI, 0.58 to 0.88) was significantly lower in the chemo-RT arm [12].

A meta-analysis with ten RCTs was done by Langendijk et al (4 neoadjuvant trials, 3 concurrent +/−adjuvant trials, and 2 adjuvant trials) to identify the additional benefit of chemotherapy when added to radiation [13]. There was an absolute survival benefit of 4% at 5 years with chemotherapy. Among the three chemotherapy timings, concomitant chemotherapy was associated with an absolute survival benefit of 20% at 5 years (HR of 0.48 (95% CI, 0.32 to 0.72). There was a significant reduction in locoregional recurrences with the addition of chemotherapy. The RR for locoregional recurrence was 0.47 ($p < 0.0001$) with concomitant chemotherapy and 0.74 ($p = 0.005$) with induction chemotherapy. But there was no benefit with adjuvant chemotherapy for locoregional control. The addition of chemotherapy demonstrated significant benefit in reducing distant metastasis also($p < 0.001$).

The MAC NPC collaborative group meta-analysis included trials 8 trials that used chemotherapy in induction, concurrent or adjuvant setting [14]. There was an absolute survival benefit of 6% at 5 years with the addition of chemotherapy to RT which corresponds to an 18% reduction in the HR of death (HR 0.82; $p = 0.006$). The concomitant schedule showed more benefit (HR = 0.60) than induction (HR = 0.99) and adjuvant (HR = 0.97) regimens. There was an absolute EFS benefit of 10% at 5 years with the addition of chemotherapy. Chemotherapy decreased the risk of locoregional failure (p 0.003; HR, 0.76) and distant failure ($p = 0.001$; HR, 0.72) irrespective of the timing of chemotherapy. Chemotherapy was more efficient against WHO type 1 disease than against WHO type 2 or 3 diseases ($p = 0.003$ for OS and $p = 0.0001$ for EFS). The survival outcomes were favoring the chemotherapy arms even after excluding WHO type 1 patients ($p = 0.03$).

The updated MAC NPC meta-analysis included 19 trials and with a median follow-up of 7.7 years [15]. There was an absolute survival benefit of 6.3% at 5 years by the addition of chemotherapy to radiotherapy. The addition of chemotherapy resulted in significant improvement in PFS, LRC, distant control, and cancer mortality. The outcome was analyzed separately for concurrent chemotherapy with or without adjuvant chemotherapy. The benefit of chemotherapy was dependent on the timing of chemotherapy. HR was 0·65 (0·56–0·76) for concomitant plus adjuvant chemotherapy, and 0·80 (0·70–0·93) for concomitant with out adjuvant chemotherapy. There was no significant benefit with induction chemotherapy alone or adjuvant chemotherapy alone.

A meta-analysis of 28 RCTs on the association of chemoradiotherapy regimens and survival done by Zhang et al showed that concurrent chemoradiotherapy (CCRT) was significantly associated with improved OS, PFS, DMFS, and LRFS compared with radiotherapy. The addition of induction chemotherapy resulted in improvement in OS ([HR 0.84; 95%CI 0.74–0.95), PFS (HR 0.73; 95% CI, 0.64–0.84), DMFS (HR, 0.67; 95% CI, 0.59–0.78), and LRFS (HR, 0.74; 95% CI, 0.64–0.85). The addition of adjuvant chemotherapy was not associated with survival benefits [16].

3. Role of adjuvant chemotherapy after concurrent chemoradiation

The above-mentioned five chemoradiation trials used adjuvant chemotherapy also. Hence the benefit of adjuvant chemotherapy when added to chemoradiation is not clear. Moreover, with the advancements in radiation techniques, the local control has increased significantly and distant metastasis remains the common mode of failure. This prompted investigators to test the value of adjuvant chemotherapy when added to chemoradiation. Chen et al randomized stage III and IV nonmetastatic non-keratinizing NPC patients to concurrent chemoradiotherapy plus adjuvant chemotherapy versus concurrent chemoradiotherapy alone. Cisplatin 40 mg/m2 weekly was used as the concurrent regimen. Adjuvant chemotherapy consisted of 3 cycles of cisplatin 80 mg/m on day 1 and 5FU 800 mg/m^2 per day on days 1–5. After a median follow-up of 37·8 months, the 2 year FFS was 86% in the adjuvant chemotherapy group compared to 84% in the CCRT group($p = .13$). There was no significant difference in Overall survival, Distant failure-free survival, and loco-regional failure-free survival [17]. The update also showed similar results [18]. The outcomes in the two arms were similar irrespective of the radiotherapy technique (2D vs 3Dvs IMRT). All three cycles of adjuvant chemotherapy were completed by only 63% of patients in the adjuvant arm.

Adjuvant chemotherapy after concurrent chemoradiation is associated with significant toxicities and poor compliance without any survival advantage. There is no evidence to recommend routine use of adjuvant chemotherapy in locally advanced NPC.

4. Adjuvant chemotherapy-risk adjusted treatment

EBV is related to NPC in endemic areas. EBV DNA load has been correlated with the prognosis of NPC in many studies [19, 20]. Hong Kong 0502 trial included patients with detectable plasma EBV DNA after curative radiotherapy. Patients were randomized to adjuvant chemotherapy with cisplatin-gemcitabine or observation [20]. After a median follow-up of 6.6 years, there was no significant difference in the 5-year relapse-free survival (RFS) rate between the two arms (49.3% versus 54.7%; HR 1.09, $P = 0.75$).

5. Induction chemotherapy in NPC

Concurrent chemo-RT with advanced radiotherapy techniques have increased the locoregional control in locally advanced NPC. But distant metastasis continued

Author (year)	Control	Intervention	Median follow up	DFS/FFS (Intervention vs. control arm in %)	OS	DMFS
Yang et al [22] (2019) N = 476	CCRT (cisplatin 80 mg/m^2)	CDDP+5FU infusion X 2 cycles →CCRT	82.6 months	5 year DFS 73.4 vs. 63.1 P = 0.007	5 year OS 80.8 vs. 76.8 P = 0.040	5 year DMFS 82.8 vs. 73.1 P = 0.014
Li et al [24] (2019) N = 480	CCRT (Cisplatin 100 mg/m^2)	Docetaxel 60 mg/m^2 D1, cisplatin 60 mg/m2D1,5FU 600 mg/m^2 D1–5 X 3 cycles→CCRT	71.5 months	5 year FFS 77.4 vs. 66.4 P = 0.019	5 year OS 85.6vs 77.7 P = 0.042	5 year DMFS 88vs 79.8 P = 0.030
Zhang et al. [25] (2019) N = 480	CCRT (cisplatin 100 mg/m^2)	Cisplatin 80 mg/m^2 D1, gemcitabine 1 g/m^2 D1, D8 X 3 cycles→ CCRT	42.7 months	3 year Recurrence Free Survival 85.3 vs. 76.5 P = 0.001	3 year OS 94.6 vs. 90.3 HR 0.43(0.24–0.77)	3 year DMFS 91.1 VS 84.4 HR 0.43(0.25–0.73)
Frikha et al [26] (2018) N = 83	CCRT Weekly cisplatin 40 mg/m^2	Docetaxel 75 mg/m^2, cisplatin 75 mg/m^2,5Fu 750 mg/m^2 D 1–5 X 3 cycles → CCRT	43.1 months	3 year PFS 73.9 vs. 57.2 P = 0.042	3 year OS 86.3 vs. 68.9 P = 0.059	3 year DMFS HR 0.53 P = 0.18
Hong et al. [27] (2018) N = 479	CCRT (cisplatin 80 mg/m^2)	MEPFL regimen (mitomycin 8 mg/m^2 D1, Epirubicin 60 mg/m^2 D1, Cispaltin 60 mg/m^2 D1,5FU 450 mg/m^2 D8. caLV 30 mg/m^2 D8) X3 cycles→CCRT	72 months	5 year DFS 61 vs. 50 P = 0.0264	5 year OS 72 vs. 68 P = 0.624	5 year DMFS 76 vs. 71 P = 0.28
Tan et al. [28] (2015) N = 180	CCRT (cisplatin (40 mg/m^2 weekly)	Paclitaxel 70 mg/m^2, carboplatin AUC(2.5),Gemcitabine 1 g/m^2 D1,D8X 3 cycles→ CCRT	3.2 years	3 year DFS 74.9 vs. 67.4 P = 0.362	3 year OS 94.3 vs. 92.3 P = 0.494	3 year DMFS 83.8 vs. 79.9 P = 0.547
Jin et al. [29] (2019) N = 276	Cisplatin 100 mg/m^2 D1,5FU 800 mg/m^2 D1–5→CCRT (cisplatin 80 mg/m2)	Docetaxel 75 mg/m2 D1, Cisplatin 75 mg/m2 D1,5FU 600 mg/m2 D1–4 X 3 cycles→ CCRT	36 months	3 year PFS 84.5 vs. 77.9 P = 0.380	3 year OS 91.1vs 91.1 P = 0.082	—

(CCRT- Concurrent Chemoradiotherapy, OS-Overall Survival, DFS-Disease Free Survival, FFS- Failure Free survival, DMFS- Distant Metastasis Free Survival, HR-Hazard Ratio)

Table 1.
Phase 3 trials of induction chemotherapy in locally advanced nasopharyngeal carcinoma.

to be a major problem and hence adjuvant chemotherapy was tried. But it failed to show benefit and the compliance to chemotherapy after chemoradiation was poor. Induction chemotherapy was tried to decrease the rates of distant metastasis, to increase survival, and to reduce radiotherapy toxicities by decreasing treatment volumes.

Six randomized trials on induction chemotherapy have been published; three from China, one each from Europe, Taiwan, and Singapore. These trials used different induction regimens, radiotherapy techniques, and dosage schedules. The three Chinese trials showed improvement in DFS, OS, and DMFS with the addition of induction chemotherapy [21–25]. But GORTEC, Taiwan, and Singapore trials did not show any advantage in terms of DMFS or OS [26–28]. All these trials reported significantly higher rates of acute toxicities with induction chemotherapy. Jin et al tested TPF against PF as induction therapy in locally advanced NPC and reported similar outcomes with better tolerance and compliance in the PF arm [29]. The details of induction chemotherapy trials are given in **Table 1**.

Three meta-analyses of induction chemotherapy have been published. Tan et al included 6 RCTs and five observational studies with 2802 patients. Induction chemotherapy was associated with significantly improved PFS (HR 0.69, P = 0.0003) and OS (HR 0.77, P = 0.03,) at the expense of increased toxicities. There was a statistically significant 37% reduction in the hazard for the development of distant metastases (HR 0.63, P = 0.001) in favor of induction chemotherapy [30]. Individual patient data pooled analysis of 4 randomized trials from endemic areas by Chen et al reported an absolute benefit of 9.3% in 5 year PFS with the addition of induction chemotherapy to CCRT (P = 0.0009). Induction chemotherapy also improved OS (HR = 0.75; p = 0.04) and reduced distant failure (HR0.68; P = 0.008) [31]. Meta-analysis of 8 randomized trials with 2384 patients by Mane et al reported a significant benefit in OS (HR 0.68, P = 0.001) and PFS (HR 0.657, P < 0.001) with the addition of induction chemotherapy to CCRT, but acute toxicities were more with induction chemotherapy [32].

Induction chemotherapy before chemoradiation is associated with improvement in PFS, OS, and DMFS. TPF did not show any advantage over PF and the optimal induction regimens are cisplatin-infusion 5FU and cisplatin-gemcitabine.

6. Chemotherapy in stage II NPC

Radical radiotherapy is the treatment for stage I disease. Stage III and IVA are managed by induction chemotherapy followed by chemoradiation or chemoradiotherapy with or without adjuvant chemotherapy. But the treatment of stage II disease is controversial. Stage II is a heterogeneous group with T2N0M0, T1N1M0, and T2N1M0disease. A phase 3 trial done by Chen et al in the conventional RT era randomized stage II patients into RT or CCRT [33]. Chemo-RT resulted in better 5 year OS, PFS and Distant metastasis-free survival at the expense of increased acute toxicities. IMRT resulted in improvement in OS by reducing local and regional recurrence with decreased toxicities and better quality of life compared to 2D RT. The benefit of concurrent chemotherapy in the IMRT era is doubtful. Many comparative studies were done to study the effect of the addition of chemotherapy to IMRT. But most of the studies are retrospective in nature. A randomized phase 2 trial by Huang et al showed no significant difference in OS, LFFS, RFFS, DFS, and DMFS after a median follow-up of 75 months. There was a detrimental effect on bone marrow function with chemo-RT [34]. Two retrospective studies from endemic areas showed no improvement in survival with the addition of chemotherapy to IMRT [35, 36]. Propensity score matching analysis in intermediate-risk NPC by Zhang et al showed no survival benefit (OS, FFS) by adding concurrent chemotherapy to IMRT [37]. Two meta-analyses of stage 2 trials have been published. Xu et al included 2D and IMRT studies [38]. CRT had significantly higher OS (HR 0.67, P = 0.04) and LRRFS (HR = 0.61, P = 0.0003) compared to RT alone, but there was no difference in DMFS. Acute toxicities were more in the chemo-RT arm. Subgroup analysis showed that IMRT alone achieved equivalent OS(P = 0.14), LRRFS(P-0.06) and DMFS(P = 0.89) compared to CRT. Liu et al published a meta-analysis of seven trials that compared IMRT alone with IMRT plus concurrent chemotherapy [39]. There was no benefit with the addition of chemotherapy to IMRT in terms of OS, PFS, DMFS, or LRRFS. Moreover CCRT was associated with increased rates of grade 3–4 leukopenia.

The benefit of adding chemotherapy to intensity-modulated radiotherapy in stage II disease is doubtful and is still under investigation.

7. Chemotherapy in metastatic NPC

Being a chemosensitive tumor, chemotherapy is the mainstay of treatment for metastatic NPC. Single-agent chemotherapy was used previously. Standard chemotherapy agents used now are platinum doublets with gemcitabine, 5FU, or paclitaxel [40, 41]. Higher response rates are associated with combination regimens than monotherapy. Cisplatin-5FU continuous infusion regimen resulted in a response rate of 55–65% [42]. Paclitaxel when added to carboplatin resulted in response rates as high as 75% [43]. A Randomized phase 3 trial from China compared Cisplatin gemcitabine (GP) with cisplatin 5FU(FP) in recurrent and metastatic NPC [44]. Gemcitabine plus cisplatin prolonged progression-free survival in patients with recurrent or metastatic NPC. The updated results showed an improvement in OS with Cisplatin -gemcitabine regimen (HR 0.723 (95% CI, 0.578 to 0.904; P = .004). The median OS was 22.1 months with GP versus 18.6 months with FP [45]. Triplet regimens tried in metastatic settings resulted in higher response rates and increased median OS, but with increased toxicities [46]. There is no head-on comparison with the standard doublets and triplet regimens are not recommended for first-line therapy.

These patients eventually progress on platinum-based chemotherapy due to the development of platinum resistance. The selection of second line treatment depends on the chemotherapy agent used in first line. The common second-line agents are 5-FU (including capecitabine), taxanes (paclitaxel, docetaxel), irinotecan, vinorelbine, and gemcitabine [47–50] The response rates are inferior compared to the first-line agents.

8. Future directions

The role of adjuvant chemotherapy according to risk-adapted approach is evolving. Two trials of adjuvant chemotherapy according to post-treatment plasma EBV DNA measurements (NRG-HN001- NCT02135042 and NCT02363400) are underway [51, 52]. The benefit of concurrent chemotherapy in stage II NPC is not clear. NCT02610010, NCT02116231, and NCT02633202 are ongoing randomized phase2/3 trials evaluating the same [53–55]. There is no proven role for targeted therapy or immunotherapy in locally advanced or metastatic NPC [56, 57]. A phase 3 trial (NCT02633176) comparing cisplatin, docetaxel plus cetuximab with cisplatin and docetaxel induction chemotherapy followed by concurrent chemoradiation in previously untreated metastatic NPC is underway [58]. PD-1 antibody Camrelizumab is being compared with best supportive care after Chemoradiotherapy in Locoregionally Advanced NPC in a phase 3 trial [59]. Camrelizumab in combination with chemotherapy is tested against chemotherapy alone in recurrent and metastatic NPC in another randomized phase 3 trial [60].

9. Conclusion

Stage I NPC is treated by radical radiotherapy. Stage II disease is treated by IMRT alone or concurrent chemoradiation. Stage III and stage IVA disease are treated by induction chemotherapy followed by concurrent chemoradiation or concurrent chemoradiation +/−adjuvant radiotherapy. Metastatic NPC is usually treated by chemotherapy using platinum doublets, cisplatin-gemcitabine is the standard regimen.

Conflict of interest

The authors declare no conflict of interest.

Author details

Lekha Madhavan Nair, Rejnish Ravi Kumar, Malu Rafi, Farida Nazeer, Kainickal Cessal Thommachan* and Kunnambath Ramadas
Department of Radiation Oncology, Regional Cancer Centre, Thiruvananthapuram, Kerala, India

*Address all correspondence to: drcessalthomas@gmail.com

References

[1] Lee AWM, Ng WT, Chan LLK, Hung WM, Chan CCC, Sze HCK, et al. Evolution of treatment for nasopharyngeal cancer - success and setback in the intensity-modulated radiotherapy era. Radiotherapy and Oncology [Internet]. 2014;110(3): 377-384. Available from: http://dx.doi.org/10.1016/j.radonc.2014.02.003

[2] Bhattacharyya T, Babu G, Kainickal CT. Current Role of Chemotherapy in Nonmetastatic Nasopharyngeal Cancer. Journal of Oncology. vol. 2018, Article ID 3725837, 7 pages, 2018. https://doi.org/10.1155/2018/3725837.

[3] Peng G, Wang T, Yang KY, Zhang S, Zhang T, Li Q, et al. A prospective, randomized study comparing outcomes and toxicities of intensity-modulated radiotherapy vs. conventional two-dimensional radiotherapy for the treatment of nasopharyngeal carcinoma. Radiotherapy and Oncology. 2012;104(3):286-293.

[4] Du T, Xiao J, Qiu Z, Wu K. The effectiveness of intensity-modulated radiation therapy versus 2D-RT for the treatment of nasopharyngeal carcinoma: A systematic review and meta-analysis. PLoS ONE. 2019;14(7):1-14.

[5] Al-sarraf BM, Leblanc M, Giri PGS, Fu KK, Cooper J, Vuong T, et al. Randomized intergroup study 0099. Society. 1998;16(4):1310-1317.

[6] Wee J, Tan EH, Tai BC, Wong HB, Leong SS, Tan T, et al. Randomized trial of radiotherapy versus concurrent chemoradiotherapy followed by adjuvant chemotherapy in patients with American joint committee on cancer/ International Union against Cancer stage III and IV nasopharyngeal cancer of the endemic variety. Journal of Clinical Oncology. 2005;23(27): 6730-6738.

[7] Lee AWM, Lau WH, Tung SY, Chua DTT, Chappell R, Xu L, et al. Preliminary results of a randomized study on therapeutic gain by concurrent chemotherapy for regionally-advanced nasopharyngeal carcinoma: NPC-9901 trial by the Hong Kong nasopharyngeal cancer study group. Journal of Clinical Oncology. 2005;23(28):6966-6975.

[8] Lee AWM, Tung SY, Chan ATC, Chappell R, Fu YT, Lu TX, et al. Preliminary results of a randomized study (NPC-9902 trial) on therapeutic gain by concurrent chemotherapy and/ or accelerated fractionation for locally advanced nasopharyngeal carcinoma. International Journal of Radiation Oncology Biology Physics. 2006;66(1): 142-151.

[9] Lee AWM, Tung SY, Chua DTT, Ngan RKC, Chappell R, Tung R, et al. Randomized trial of radiotherapy plus concurrent-adjuvant chemotherapy vs radiotherapy alone for regionally advanced nasopharyngeal carcinoma. Journal of the National Cancer Institute. 2010;102(15):1188-1198.

[10] Chen Y, Liu MZ, Liang SB, Zong JF, Mao YP, Tang LL, et al. Preliminary results of a prospective randomized trial comparing concurrent Chemoradiotherapy plus adjuvant chemotherapy with radiotherapy alone in patients with Locoregionally advanced nasopharyngeal carcinoma in endemic regions of China. International Journal of Radiation Oncology Biology Physics. 2008;71(5):1356-1364.

[11] Liang H, Xia W-X, Lv X, Sun R, Zeng Q, Li S-W, et al. Concurrent chemoradiotherapy with 3-weekly versus weekly cisplatin in patients with locoregionally advanced nasopharyngeal carcinoma: A phase 3 multicentre randomised controlled trial (ChiCTR-TRC-12001979). Journal of Clinical Oncology. 2017 May 20;35(15_suppl):6006-6006.

[12] Zhang L, Zhao C, Ghimire B, Hong MH, Liu Q, Zhang Y, et al. The role of concurrent chemoradiotherapy in the treatment of locoregionally advanced nasopharyngeal carcinoma among endemic population: A meta-analysis of the phase iii randomized trials. BMC Cancer. 2010;10.

[13] Langendijk JA, Leemans CR, Buter J, Berkhof J, Slotman BJ. The additional value of chemotherapy to radiotherapy in locally advanced nasopharyngeal carcinoma: A meta-analysis of the published literature. Journal of Clinical Oncology. 2004;22(22):4604-4612.

[14] Baujat B, Audry H, Bourhis J, Chan ATC, Onat H, Chua DTT, et al. Chemotherapy in locally advanced nasopharyngeal carcinoma: An individual patient data meta-analysis of eight randomized trials and 1753 patients. International Journal of Radiation Oncology Biology Physics. 2006;64(1):47-56.

[15] Blanchard P, Lee A, Marguet S, Leclercq J, Ng WT, Ma J, et al. Chemotherapy and radiotherapy in nasopharyngeal carcinoma: An update of the MAC-NPC meta-analysis. The Lancet Oncology [Internet]. 2015;16(6):645-655. Available from: http://dx.doi.org/10.1016/S1470-2045(15)70126-9

[16] Zhang B, Li MM, Chen WH, Zhao JF, Chen WQ, Dong YH, et al. Association of Chemoradiotherapy Regimens and Survival among patients with nasopharyngeal carcinoma: A systematic review and meta-analysis. JAMA Network Open. 2019;1-20.

[17] Chen L, Hu CS, Chen XZ, Hu GQ, Cheng Z Bin, Sun Y, et al. concurrent chemoradiotherapy plus adjuvant chemotherapy versus concurrent chemoradiotherapy alone in patients with locoregionally advanced nasopharyngeal carcinoma: A phase 3 multicentre randomised controlled trial. The Lancet Oncology. 2012;13(2): 163-171.

[18] Chen L, Hu CS, Chen XZ, Hu GQ, Cheng Z Bin, Sun Y, et al. adjuvant chemotherapy in patients with locoregionally advanced nasopharyngeal carcinoma: Long-term results of a phase 3 multicentre randomised controlled trial. European Journal of Cancer. 2017;75(December 2016):150-158.

[19] Leung SF, Zee B, Ma BB, Hui EP, Mo F, Lai M, et al. Plasma Epstein-Barr viral deoxyribonucleic acid quantitation complements tumor-node-metastasis staging prognostication in nasopharyngeal carcinoma. Journal of Clinical Oncology. 2006;24(34): 5414-5418.

[20] Hui EP, Ma BBY, Chan KCA, Chan CML, Wong CSC, To KF, et al. Clinical utility of plasma Epstein-Barr virus DNA and ERCC1 single nucleotide polymorphism in nasopharyngeal carcinoma. Cancer. 2015;121(16): 2720-2729.

[21] Cao SM, Yang Q, Guo L, Mai HQ, Mo HY, Cao KJ, et al. Neoadjuvant chemotherapy followed by concurrent chemoradiotherapy versus concurrent chemoradiotherapy alone in locoregionally advanced naso pharyngeal carcinoma: A phase III multicentre randomised controlled trial. European Journal of Cancer [Internet]. 2017;75:14-23. Available from: http://dx.doi.org/10.1016/j.ejca.2016.12.039

[22] Yang Q, Cao SM, Guo L, Hua YJ, Huang PY, Zhang XL, et al. Induction chemotherapy followed by concurrent chemoradiotherapy versus concurrent chemoradiotherapy alone in locoregionally advanced nasopharyngeal carcinoma: Long-term results of a phase III multicentre randomised controlled trial. European journal of cancer [internet].

2019;119:87-96. Available from: https://doi.org/10.1016/j.ejca.2019.07.007

[23] Sun Y, Li WF, Chen NY, Zhang N, Hu GQ, Xie FY, et al. Induction chemotherapy plus concurrent chemoradiotherapy versus concurrent chemoradiotherapy alone in locoregionally advanced nasopharyngeal carcinoma: A phase 3, multicentre, randomised controlled trial. The Lancet Oncology [Internet]. 2016;17(11):1509-1520. Available from: http://dx.doi.org/10.1016/S1470-2045(16)30410-7

[24] Li WF, Chen NY, Zhang N, Hu GQ, Xie FY, Sun Y, et al. Concurrent chemoradiotherapy with/without induction chemotherapy in locoregionally advanced nasopharyngeal carcinoma: Long-term results of phase 3 randomized controlled trial. International Journal of Cancer. 2019;145(1):295-305.

[25] Zhang Y, Chen L, Hu G-Q, Zhang N, Zhu X-D, Yang K-Y, et al. Gemcitabine and cisplatin induction chemotherapy in nasopharyngeal carcinoma. New England Journal of Medicine. 2019; 381(12):1124-1135.

[26] Frikha M, Auperin A, Tao Y, Elloumi F, Toumi N, Blanchard P, et al. A randomized trial of induction docetaxel-cisplatin- 5FU followed by concomitant cisplatin-RT versus concomitant cisplatin-RT in nasopharyngeal carcinoma (GORTEC 2006-02). Annals of Oncology. 2018;29(3):731-736.

[27] Hong RL, Hsiao CF, Ting LL, Ko JY, Wang CW, Chang JTC, et al. Final results of a randomized phase III trial of induction chemotherapy followed by concurrent chemoradiotherapy versus concurrent chemoradiotherapy alone in patients with stage IVA and IVB nasopharyngeal carcinoma-Taiwan cooperative oncology group (TCOG). Annals of Oncology. 2018;29(9):1972-1979.

[28] Tan T, Lim WT, Fong KW, Cheah SL, Soong YL, Ang MK, et al. Concurrent chemo-radiation with or without induction gemcitabine, carboplatin, and paclitaxel: A randomized, phase 2/3 trial in locally advanced nasopharyngeal carcinoma. International Journal of Radiation Oncology Biology Physics [Internet]. 2015;91(5):952-960. Available from: http://dx.doi.org/10.1016/j.ijrobp.2015.01.002

[29] Jin T, Qin W Feng, Jiang F, Jin Q feng, Wei Q chun, Jia Y shi, et al. cisplatin and fluorouracil induction chemotherapy with or without docetaxel in Locoregionally advanced nasopharyngeal carcinoma. Translational oncology [internet]. 2019;12(4):633-9. Available from: https://doi.org/10.1016/j.tranon.2019.01.002

[30] Tan TH, Soon YY, Cheo T, Ho F, Wong LC, Tey J, et al. Induction chemotherapy for locally advanced nasopharyngeal carcinoma treated with concurrent chemoradiation: A systematic review and meta-analysis. Radiotherapy and Oncology. 2018;129(1):10-17.

[31] Chen YP, Tang LL, Yang Q, Poh SS, Hui EP, Chan ATC, et al. Induction chemotherapy plus concurrent chemoradiotherapy in endemic nasopharyngeal carcinoma: Individual patient data pooled analysis of four randomized trials. Clinical Cancer Research. 2018;24(8):1824-1833.

[32] Mané M, Benkhaled S, Dragan T, Paesmans M, Beauvois S, Lalami Y, et al. Meta-analysis on induction chemotherapy in locally advanced nasopharyngeal carcinoma. Oncologist. 2021;26(1):e130–e141.

[33] Chen QY, Wen YF, Guo L, Liu H, Huang PY, Mo HY, et al. Concurrent

chemoradiotherapy vs radiotherapy alone in stage ii nasopharyngeal carcinoma: Phase iii randomized trial. Journal of the National Cancer Institute. 2011;103(23):1761-1770.

[34] Huang X, Chen X, Zhao C, Wang J, Wang K, Wang L, et al. Adding concurrent chemotherapy to intensity-modulated radiotherapy does not improve treatment outcomes for stage II nasopharyngeal carcinoma: A phase 2 multicenter clinical trial. Frontiers in Oncology. 2020;10(August):1-7.

[35] Su Z, Mao YP, Tang J, Lan XW, OuYang PY, Xie FY. Long-term outcomes of concurrent chemoradiotherapy versus radiotherapy alone in stage II nasopharyngeal carcinoma treated with IMRT: A retrospective study. Tumor Biology. 2016;37(4):4429-4438.

[36] Xu T, Shen C, Zhu G, Hu C. Omission of chemotherapy in early stage nasopharyngeal carcinoma treated with IMRT a paired cohort study. Medicine (United States). 2015;94(39):e1457.

[37] Zhang F, Zhang Y, Li WF, Liu X, Guo R, Sun Y, et al. Efficacy of concurrent chemotherapy for intermediate risk NPC in the intensity-modulated radiotherapy era: A propensity-matched analysis. Scientific Reports. 2015;5(74):1-11.

[38] Xu C, Zhang LH, Chen YP, Liu X, Zhou GQ, Lin AH, et al. Chemoradiotherapy versus radiotherapy alone in stage II nasopharyngeal carcinoma: A systemic review and meta-analysis of 2138 patients. Journal of Cancer. 2017;8(2):287-297.

[39] Liu F, Jin T, Liu L, Xiang Z, Yan R, Yang H. The role of concurrent chemotherapy for stage II nasopharyngeal carcinoma in the intensity-modulated radiotherapy era: A systematic review and meta-analysis. PLoS ONE [Internet]. 2018 Mar 1 [cited 2021 May 13];13(3). Available from: https://pubmed.ncbi.nlm.nih.gov/29566078/

[40] Ma BBY, Chan ATC. Recent perspectives in the role of chemotherapy in the management of advanced nasopharyngeal carcinoma. Cancer. 2005;103(1):22-31.

[41] Lee AWM, Ma BBY, Ng WT, Chan ATC. Management of nasopharyngeal carcinoma: Current practice and future perspective. Journal of Clinical Oncology. 2015;33(29): 3356-3364.

[42] Au E, Ang PT. A phase II trial of 5-fluorouracil and cisplatinum in recurrent or metastatic nasopharyngeal carcinoma. Annals of Oncology. 1994;5(1):87-89.

[43] Tan EH, Khoo KS, Wee J, Fong KW, Lee KS, Lee KM, et al. Phase II trial of a paclitaxel and carboplatin combination in Asian patients with metastatic nasopharyngeal carcinoma. Annals of Oncology. 1999;10(2):235-237.

[44] Zhang L, Huang Y, Hong S, Yang Y, Yu G, Jia J, et al. Gemcitabine plus cisplatin versus fluorouracil plus cisplatin in recurrent or metastatic nasopharyngeal carcinoma: A multicentre, randomised, open-label, phase 3 trial. The Lancet [Internet]. 2016;388(10054):1883-1892. Available from: http://dx.doi.org/10.1016/S0140-6736(16)31388-5.

[45] Hong S, Huang Y, Yang Y, Yu G, Jia J, Peng J, et al. GEM20110714: Final overall survival results of the phase III study of first-line gemcitabine plus cisplatin versus fluorouracil plus cisplatin in recurrent or metastatic nasopharyngeal carcinoma. Journal of Clinical Oncology. 2020 May 20;38 (15_suppl):6521-6521.

[46] Leong SS, Wee J, Tay MH, Toh CK, Tan SB, Thng CH, et al. Paclitaxel,

carboplatin, and gemcitabine in metastatic nasopharyngeal carcinoma: A phase II trial using a triplet combination. Cancer. 2005;103(3): 569-575.

[47] Chua DTT, Sham JST, Au GKH. A phase II study of capecitabine in patients with recurrent and metastatic nasopharyngeal carcinoma pretreated with platinum-based chemotherapy. Oral Oncology. 2003;39(4):361-366.

[48] Poon D, Chowbay B, Cheung YB, Leong SS, Tan EH. Phase II study of irinotecan (CPT-11) as salvage therapy for advanced nasopharyngeal carcinoma. Cancer. 2005;103(3): 576-581.

[49] Wang CC, Chang JY, Liu TW, Lin CY, Yu YC, Hong RL. Phase II study of gemcitabine plus vinorelbine in the treatment of cisplatin-resistant nasopharyngeal carcinoma. Head and Neck. 2006;28(1):74-80.

[50] Foo KF, Tan EH, Leong SS, Wee JTS, Tan T, Fong KW, et al. Gemcitabine in metastatic nasopharyngeal carcinoma of the undifferentiated type. Annals of Oncology. 2002;13(1):150-156.

[51] Nancy Lee. Randomized Phase II and Phase III Studies of Individualized Treatment for Nasopharyngeal Carcinoma Based on Biomarker Epstein Barr Virus (EBV) Deoxyribonucleic Acid (DNA). https://clinicaltrials.gov/ct2/show/NCT02135042. Accessed on May 16,2021.

[52] Jin-Ching Lin. Phase III Randomized Trial of Immediate Adjuvant Chemotherapy or Delayed Salvage Chemotherapy in Nasopharyngeal Carcinoma Patients With Post-radiation Detectable Plasma EBV DNA. https://clinicaltrials.gov/ct2/show/NCT02363400. Accessed on May 16,2021.

[53] Fang-Yun Xie. Intensity-modulated Radiotherapy With or Without Concurrent Chemotherapy for Stage II Nasopharyngeal Carcinoma: a Phase 3 Non-inferior Multicenter Randomized Controlled Trial. https://clinicaltrials.gov/ct2/show/NCT02610010. Accessed on May 16,2021.

[54] Song Qu. Phase II Study Comparing Intensity Modulated Radiotherapy (IMRT) in Combination With Concurrent Chemotherapy and IMRT Alone for Stage II Nasopharyngeal Carcinoma. https://clinicaltrials.gov/ct2/show/NCT02116231. Accessed on May16,2021.

[55] Lei Chen. Prospective Non-inferior Clinical Trial Comparing Concurrent Chemoradiotherapy or Radiotherapy Alone in Patients With Intermediate Risk Nasopharyngeal Carcinoma in Intensity-modulated Radiotherapy Era. https://clinicaltrials.gov/ct2/show/NCT02633202. Accessed on May16,2021.

[56] Chen X, Liang R, Zhu X. Anti-EGFR therapies in nasopharyngeal carcinoma. Biomedicine and pharmacotherapy [internet]. 2020;131(July):110649. Available from: https://doi.org/10.1016/j.biopha.2020.110649

[57] Jain A, Chia WK, Toh HC. Immunotherapy for nasopharyngeal cancer-a review. Chinese Clinical Oncology. 2016;5(2):1-10.

[58] Tongyu Lin. Phase III Randomized Trial of Cisplatin Plus Docetaxel Versus Cetuximab, Cisplatin, and Docetaxel Induction Chemotherapy Followed by Concurrent Chemoradiation in Previously Untreated Patients Metastatic Nasopharyngeal Carcinoma. https://clinicaltrials.gov/ct2/show/NCT02633176. Accessed on May16,2021.

[59] Jun Ma. Camrelizumab (PD-1 Antibody) Compared With Best Supportive Care After Chemo radiotherapy in Locoregionally Advanced Nasopharyngeal Carcinoma:

a Multi-center, Randomised Controlled, Phase 3 Trial. (NPaCific). https://clinicaltrials.gov/ct2/show/NCT03427827. Accessed on May16,2021.

[60] Li Zhang. A Phase III, Randomized, Double-Blind, Multi-center Study to Investigate the Efficacy and Safety of Camrelizumab+Gemcitabine+Cisplatin Versus Placebo+Gemcitabine+Cisplatin in Subjects With Recurrent/Metastatic Nasopharyngeal Carcinoma. https://clinicaltrials.gov/ct2/show/NCT03707509. Accessed on May 16,2021.

Chapter 7

Hypopharyngeal Cancer: Staging, Diagnosis, and Therapy

Yi Huang, Yushan Liang and Weilin Zhao

Abstract

Hypopharyngeal carcinoma is uncommon in all head and neck cancers. With a synergistic reaction of each, tobacco consumption and alcohol abuse contribute to the tumorigenesis. The aerodigestive tract epithelium exposure to similar risks causing multiple cancers. Thus, a pan-endoscopic screening offers a practical approach for evaluating second primary esophageal cancer. The common symptoms of hypopharyngeal carcinoma were globus pharyngeus, sore throat, dysphagia, otalgia, neck mass, hoarseness, and dyspnoea. However, approximately 75–80% of patients are initial diagnosed with advanced-stage. Although improvements in therapy, the prognosis is still lacking. In early-stage patients, primary surgical resection and radiotherapy achieved similar survival and locoregional control rates. T1–T2 malignancies with N0–N1 can usually be treated with radiation alone, open surgery, or transoral surgery. In some people, after primary surgery or transoral approaches is often required adjuvant radiotherapy. However, most cases have been in the advanced-stage when screened. Individual therapy programs should be chosen carefully to achieve a balance between swallowing-voice rehabilitation and organ preservation in advanced-stage ones. Meanwhile, reasonable reconstruction of intraoperative defect is essential for a surgeon who seeks satisfied postoperative outcomes. Considerable treatment (surgery or non-surgery) remains the key point of improving the survival rate.

Keywords: hypopharyngeal carcinoma, etiology, staging, diagnosis, treatment

1. Introduction

Hypopharyngeal carcinoma is relatively rare in all head and neck cancers (approximately 3–5%) [1, 2]. The overall worldwide age-standardized incidence rates occur at a rate of 0.8 per 100,000 (1.4 in men and 0.3 in women) in hypopharyngeal cancer [3]. Bangladesh had the highest incidence with 4.8 per 100,000 [4]. In the past four decades, the incidence of hypopharyngeal cancer has declined smoothly in America, in part due to decreasing intake of tobacco [5–7]. Overall, it is five times greater in males than in females [8] and mainly occurs in the aged 50 to 70 years [5, 9]. However, this tumor rarely occurs at young ages [10].

Epidemiologic studies showed a series of potential environmental risk factors for hypopharyngeal carcinoma development. Tobacco consumption (> 90% of patients) and alcohol abuse (> 70% of patients) are the two well-established risk factors for hypopharyngeal squamous cell carcinoma [11–13]. Heinz Maier et al. reported a time-response correlation between tobacco intake and hypopharyngeal cancer. Besides, the amount of alcohol consumption is also related to cancer development. Compared to non-smokers, it increased the risk by 9.5-fold (adjusted for alcohol consumption) for the long-term smoker (40–60 tobacco years). Also, alcohol drinkers increased the risk of this cancer that was up to 125.2-fold (adjusted for tobacco consumption) for alcoholics (> 100 g/day) [13]. Moreover, there is a synergistic carcinogenic effect between tobacco use and alcohol abuse [14]. Quitting smoking and refrain from drinking may reduce the risks of hypopharyngeal cancer.

Other risk factors, such as nutritional factors, diet, Plummer-Vinson syndrome, gastroesophageal reflux disease [15], and chronic infectious diseases have been reported to increase the risk of hypopharyngeal tumor. An inadequate caloric intake may lead to cancer cachexia, associated with a poor prognosis for hypopharyngeal carcinoma [16]. Plummer-Vinson syndrome is responsible for post-cricoid carcinoma, characterized by dysphagia and iron deficiency anemia [17, 18]. It has been reported that oncogenic viral infection has a close relationship with head and neck cancers. The human papillomavirus (HPV) is involved in the malignant transformation of oropharyngeal carcinoma [7]. Epstein–Barr virus (EBV) infection is relevant to nasopharyngeal carcinoma (NPC) tumorigenesis [19]. Nevertheless, HPV and EBV infection in hypopharyngeal cancer are rare [20–22]. To date, the possible role of HPV in tumorigenesis of hypopharyngeal cancer is still controversial, EBV as well [23, 24].

In hypopharyngeal cancer, most histological types are squamous cell carcinoma (SCC) (up to 95%). That is usually represented poorly differentiated [25]. Adenocarcinoma is less frequent than in hypopharyngeal malignancies, accounted for around 5%. Other rare malignant tumors: papillary (exophytic) squamous cell carcinoma, verrucous carcinoma, and lymphoepithelial-like carcinoma, have been reported. However, the non-epithelial neoplasms that may arise in the hypopharynx include mucosal malignant melanoma, synovial sarcoma, fibrosarcoma, and liposarcoma, are not included [26]. Both histologic confirmations and histopathologic grading of squamous carcinoma should be recorded in hypopharyngeal cancers.

2. Symptoms and diagnosis

2.1 Relevant anatomy of hypopharynx

There are three parts to the pharynx: nasopharynx, oropharynx, and hypopharynx. As part of the pharynx, the hypopharynx is located behind the entire length of the larynx. It extends from the plane of the epiglottis to the lower border of the cricoid cartilage. Moreover, the pharynx is further classified into three regions (**Figure 1**): (1) the piriform sinuses, (2) the posterior pharyngeal wall, and (3) the post-cricoid area.

The pyriform sinus, a bilateral area, is bounded by the aryepiglottic fold and laterally by the esophagus's upper end. The posterior pharyngeal wall is bounded from the superior level of the epiglottis to the lower border of the cricoid cartilage and from the vertex of one pyriform sinus to the other. The post-cricoid region lies on the arytenoid cartilages' level and connecting to the plane of the inferior border of the cricoid cartilage.

In general, hypopharyngeal cancer occurs most in the piriform sinuses in 60–85% of patients, followed by the posterior pharyngeal wall up to 10–20% and rarely in the post-cricoid area in 5–15% of patients (**Figure 2**) [9, 27]. Also, during these three hypopharyngeal subsites, the tumor of the pyriform sinus and the posterior pharyngeal wall is mainly in males, while post-cricoid carcinoma is more often occurs in females [5, 9].

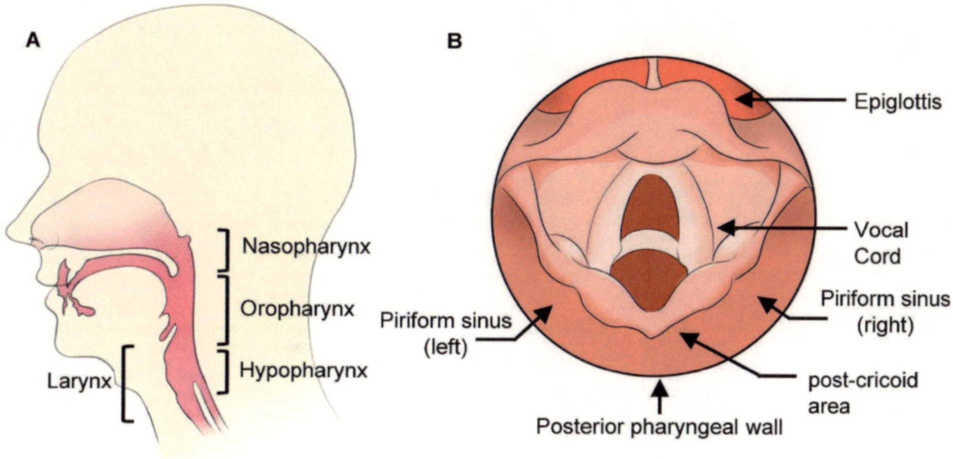

Figure 1.
Anatomical subsites of hypopharynx. (A) The pharynx includes three parts: The nasopharynx, oropharynx, and hypopharynx. (B) The hypopharynx is situated posterior to the larynx. It is further subdivided into the pyriform sinuses (left and right), posterior pharyngeal wall, and post-cricoid area.

2.2 Symptoms and signs of hypopharyngeal carcinoma

Early in hypopharyngeal cancer is not easy to be found due to the asymptomatic for an extended period. Something sticking or irritative sensation in the throat could be the early symptoms. If the tumor increases to a considerable size, sore throat, increasing dysphagia, and referred otalgia on swallowing may be present. Besides, progressive dysphagia frequently leads to significant weight loss.

A neck mass is now recognized as the typical clinical manifestation of hypopharyngeal carcinoma. There are a rich lymphatic network and vascular anatomy in the neck, allowing tumors to easily metastasize to the cervical nodal. Clinically, more than half of patients have enlarged cervical nodes at initial presentation because of the vibrant lymph nodes network in the pharynx [28]. The neck metastases rate is higher (> 75% of patients) in pyriform sinus cancers, as compared with the neck metastases rate in the posterior pharyngeal wall and post-cricoid cancers [29, 30]. Lymphatics from pyriform sinuses usually result in levels II-III and retropharyngeal node metastasis. And the posterior pharyngeal wall lymphatic metastasis area is more occurred to level II lymph node metastasis. In contrast, lymph node metastasis of the post-cricoid region prefers to levels IV-VI metastasis [31–33].

The larynx functions mainly in airway protection and respiration, which is in front of the hypopharynx. The hypopharynx configuration may allow tumor invasion or involvement of these adjacent organs, for instance, the larynx. When the throat symptoms appear, the tumor is considered significant in particular hoarseness, invading the larynx. Furthermore, some of the patients may present aggressive laryngeal invasion with life-threatening airway obstruction.

2.3 Second primary cancer

Patients with hypopharyngeal cancer have an exceptionally high risk of diagnosing a synchronous or metachronous second primary cancer, which may be associated with the prognosis's deterioration [34]. One possible mechanism causing second primary cancer in hypopharyngeal cancer is the phenomenon of "field cancerization" [35]. Anatomically, the cervical esophagus is originated at the upper esophageal sphincter, contiguous with the post-cricoid region

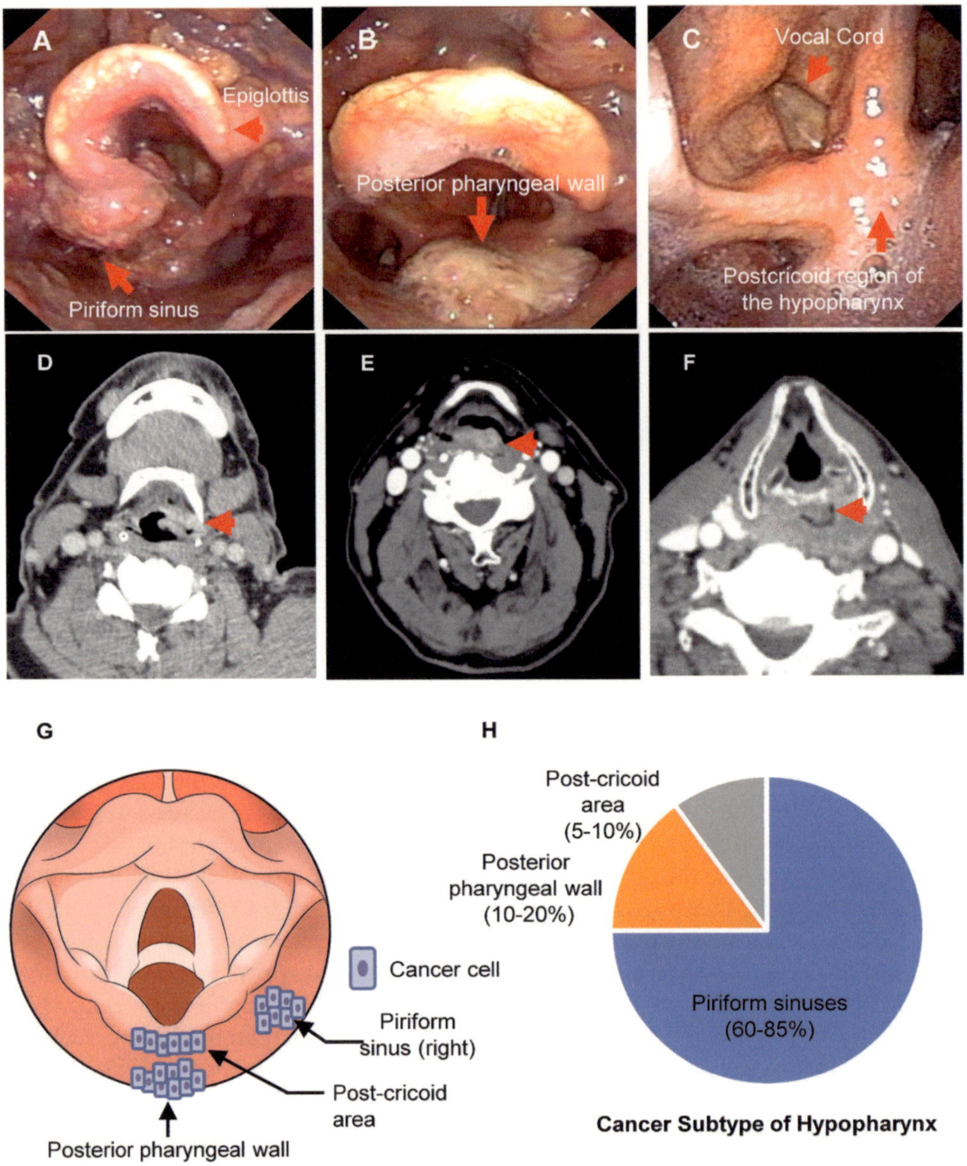

Figure 2.
Typical subtypes of hypopharyngeal carcinoma. (A, D) The pyriform sinus carcinoma (left) (red arrow) involving the left side of aryepiglottic fold in endoscopy (A) and (D) CT scan. (B, E) The posterior pharyngeal wall carcinoma (red arrow) in endoscopy (B) and (E) CT scan. (C, F) The hypopharyngeal carcinoma (red arrow) arising from the post-cricoid region in endoscopy (C) and (F) CT scan. (G) The patterns of hypopharyngeal carcinoma. (H) The percentages of hypopharyngeal carcinoma in three subtypes.

and behind the lower border of the cricoid cartilage. The aerodigestive tract mucosa, including hypopharynx and esophagus epithelium, is the squamous epithelium. During the carcinogenesis process, both hypopharynx epithelium and esophagus epithelium are exposed to similar environmental risk factors resulting in multiple cancers in the aerodigestive tract [35–37]. Tobacco use and alcohol abuse are considered as the significant risks contributing to field cancerization.

In head and neck cancers, the overall incidence of the synchronous second primary cancer was estimated to be 12% [38]. However, hypopharyngeal cancer has a high incidence of second primary cancer. The commonest sites in

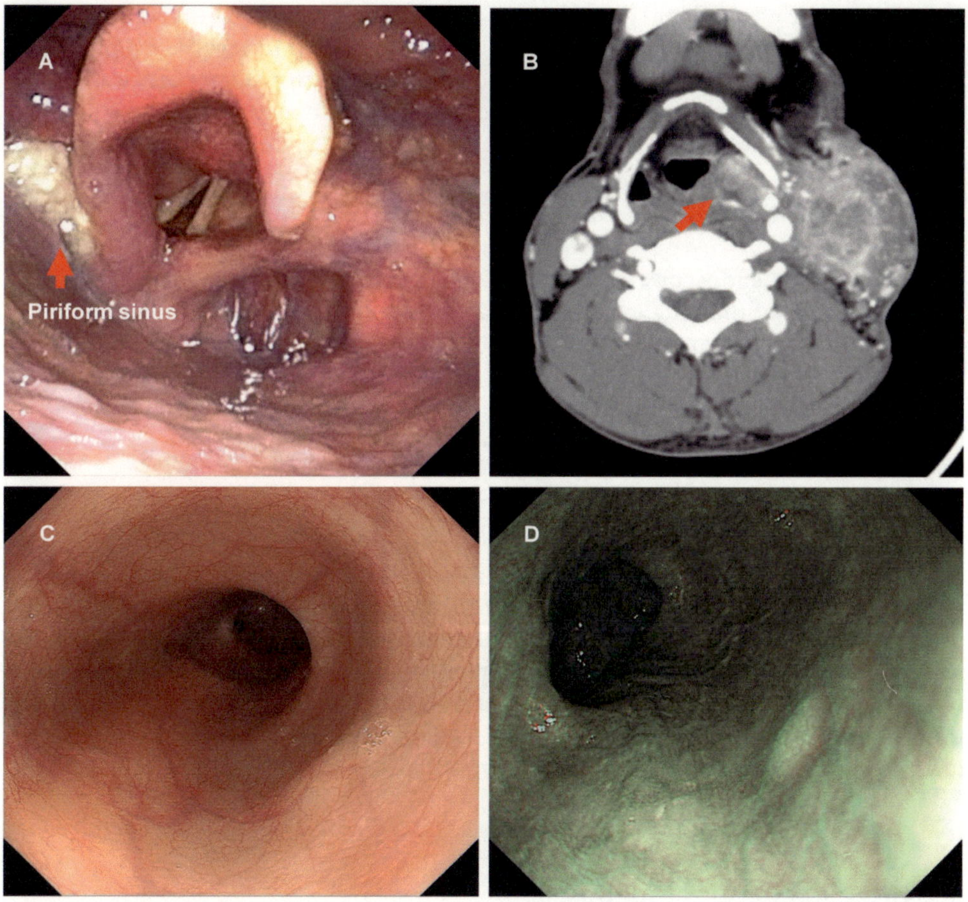

Figure 3.
The second primary cancer in hypopharyngeal cancer. (A, B) Hypopharyngeal cancer involving pyriform sinus (red arrow) by endoscopy and CT scan, respectively. (C, D) Second primary esophageal cancer of hypopharyngeal cancer, imaged with (C) white light endoscopy; (D) narrow-band imaging.

the second primary cancer [39] were the esophagus (27%) and lung (6.34%) [40–42]. Therefore, patients with hypopharyngeal carcinoma are suggested to undergo regular surveillance endoscopy (**Figure 3**) and chest CT scan to detect a second malignancy. Precancerous lesions or neoplasm are the targets of surveillance endoscopy. In case of suspected neoplasm, an endoscopic biopsy can be done to diagnose second primary esophageal cancer. The use of narrow-band imaging (NBI) shows high accuracy to screen early esophageal lesions, Lugol chromoendoscopy (LCE) endoscopy as well [43]. Most of the second primary cancer followed the hypopharyngeal cancer diagnosis within one year [34, 40].

2.4 Diagnostics of Hypopharyngeal carcinoma

2.4.1 History and physical examination

To assess the patient's condition, a thorough history of presenting symptoms must be obtained. It also is crucial to document and quantification of tobacco or alcohol use history. And then, a complete head and neck examination should be performed. Neoplasm and its extent can often be seen on indirect or laryngoscopy tests. While the post-cricoid growths may difficult to diagnose on the laryngoscopy. The pooling of secretions in the pyriform sinus is indicated to cervical esophageal involvement. Both sides of the neck should be examined to evaluate cervical lymph nodes, and the level, number, size, and mobility of palpable lymph nodes should be carefully documented.

2.4.2 Endoscopic evaluation and pathology diagnosis

In early cases, endoscopy of the laryngopharynx is best performed in the patient under suspicion of malignancy. The panendoscopy can evaluate the entire scope of cancer and find a synchronous primary at any other site. A biopsy can be done under general anesthesia with endoscopes. It is essential for histological typing. Since lymphonodi cervical metastasis often occurs as the first symptom, a fine-needle aspiration (FNA) in the neck is recommended.

2.4.3 Imaging studies

Nowadays, the application of imaging measurement offers an efficient approach for evaluating the tumor extent, lymph nodal staging, potential laryngeal impingement, and cartilage involvement. A CT enhanced scan of the laryngopharynx and neck is exceptionally worthy in evaluating laryngeal cartilage invasion. At the same time, MRI is better for the soft-tissue extension. They are complementary examinations of each other and reveal the tumor invasive range. Due to the distant metastasis (approximately 6% of patients) in hypopharyngeal cancer, a chest CT scan or PET/CT is also recommended [44].

3. Cancer staging and prognosis

The newly updated TNM classification system (8th edition), an anatomic-based classification, was published in 2017 by The American Joint Committee on Cancer (AJCC). This cancer stage classification aims to provide information for the clinical trial, cancer control activity, therapy selection, and outcome. Compared to the previous version, the new vision reflects a better understanding of cancer therapy and research design. Here we showed an overview of modifications in cancers of pharynx: (1) the revision of TNM classifications in nasopharyngeal cancer; (2) the division of pharyngeal malignancies into HPV-related (p16+) oropharyngeal cancer, oropharynx (p16-) and hypopharynx cancer, and nasopharyngeal cancer; (3) the extranodal extension (ENE) is formulated into the N category for non-viral related head and neck cancer for the first time [45]. Besides, the TNM staging of hypopharyngeal cancer is delineated in **Figures 4** and 5.

Generally, the cancer of hypopharynx has an abysmal prognosis in all head and neck cancers. Numerous patients (75–80%) are advanced-stage ones (stage III/IV) when initially diagnosed [46, 47]. About 60–75% of patients with cervical lymph node metastasis (N1–3) were detected [46, 47].

A population-based study reported that the five-year overall survival (OS) rate increased from 37.5% (1973–1989) to 41.3% (1990–2003) [9]. Also, Henry T. Hoffman, etc., showed the five-year disease-specific survival segregated into clinical stages increased: 63.1% (stage I), 67.6% (stage II), 41.8% (stage III), and 22% (stage IV), respectively [48]. Although the treatments have improved, the tumor

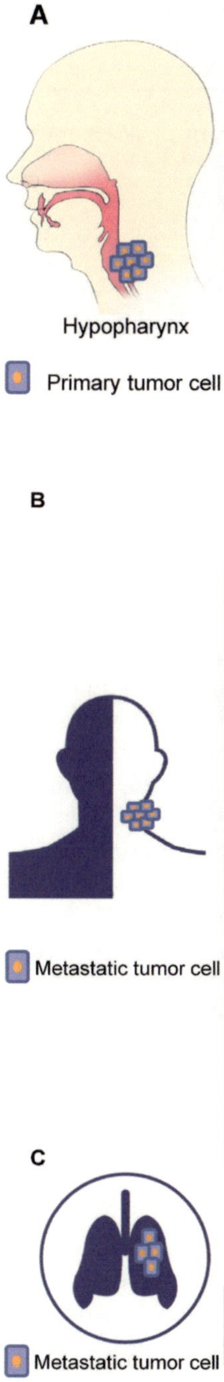

Primary Tumor (T)

Tx Primary tumor cannot be assessed

Tis Carcinoma in situ

T1 Tumor limited to one subsite of hypopharynx and/or 2 cm or smaller in greatest dimension

T2 Tumor invades more than one subsite of hypopharynx or an adjacent site, or measures larger than 2 cm but not larger than 4 cm in greatest dimension without fixation of hemilarynx

T3 Tumor larger than 4 cm in greatest dimension or with fixation of hemilarynx or extension to esophageal mucosa

T4 Moderately advanced and very advanced local disease

T4a Moderately advanced local disease

Tumor invades thyroid/cricoid cartilage, hyoid bone, thyroid gland, esophageal muscle or central compartment soft tissue

T4b Very advanced local disease

Tumor invades prevertebral fascia, encases carotid artery, or involves mediastinal structures

Regional Lymph Nodes (N)

Nx Regional lymph nodes cannot be assessed

N0 No regional lymph node metastasis

N1 Metastasis in a single ipsilateral lymph node, 3 cm or smaller in greatest dimension and ENE(−)

N2 Metastasis in a single ipsilateral lymph node, 3 cm or smaller in greatest dimension and ENE(+); or larger than 3 cm but not larger than 6 cm in greatest dimension and ENE(−); or metastases in multiple ipsilateral lymph nodes, none larger than 6 cm in greatest dimension and ENE(−); or in bilateral or contralateral lymph node(s), none larger than 6 cm in greatest dimension and ENE(−)

N2a Metastasis in single ipsilateral node 3 cm or smaller in greatest dimension and ENE(+); or a single ipsilateral node larger than 3 cm but not larger than 6 cm in greatest dimension and ENE(−)

N2b Metastases in multiple ipsilateral nodes, none larger than 6 cm in greatest dimension and ENE(−)

N2c Metastases in bilateral or contralateral lymph node(s), none larger than 6 cm in greatest dimension and ENE(−)

N3 Metastasis in a lymph node larger than 6 cm in greatest dimension and ENE(−); or in a single ipsilateral node larger than 3 cm in greatest dimension and ENE(+); or multiple ipsilateral, contralateral or bilateral nodes, any with ENE(+); or a single contralateral node of any size and ENE(+)

N3a Metastasis in a lymph node larger than 6 cm in greatest dimension and ENE(−))

N3b Metastasis in a single ipsilateral node larger than 3 cm in greatest dimension and ENE(+); or multiple ipsilateral, contralateral or bilateral nodes, any with ENE(+) or a single contralateral node of any size and ENE(+)

Distant Metastasis (M)

M0 No distant metastasis

M1 Distant metastasis

Figure 4.
TNM classification of hypopharyngeal cancer. The TNM staging system is the common language for classifying the extent of spread of cancer. Here we reveal the newest edition in hypopharyngeal carcinoma.

recurrence within one year and half of first recurrences with distance metastases [1]. Unfortunately, about 50% of the untreated cancer patients surviving within four months after the initial diagnosis, and less than 20% of patients surviving more than one year [49, 50].

		No	N1	N2	N3	M1
Tis	0					
T1		I	III	IVA	IVB	IVC
T2		II	III	IVA	IVB	IVC
T3		III	III	IVA	IVB	IVC
T4a		IVA	IVA	IVA	IVB	IVC
T4b		IVB	IVB	IVB	IVB	IVC

Figure 5.
Prognostic stage of hypopharyngeal cancer.

4. Treatment

Different treatment strategies, surgery, and nonoperative treatment were adopted according to the scope of the tumor. However, the existing literature has limitations due to the shortage of multicenter large sample randomized controlled tests. In the setting of unbalanced development in economic, academic, and medical conditions in different regions, remain in the effect of treatment, it is difficult to unify the mode of diagnosis and treatment, and the differences are present in curative effects. The general principle is to improve the postoperative life quality for patients on the premise of ensuring that the tumor is removed completely. Treatment selection requires optimizing swallowing and speaking functions to prevent a long-term aspiration and tracheostomy/G- tube dependence and acquire a balance between disease cure and anatomical preservation of tissue [19, 51].

In addition to taking effective measures to accurately determine the scope and clinical stage of the tumor, multidisciplinary treatment (MDT) should also run through the whole process of tumor diagnosis, treatment, and rehabilitation to gain optimal rehabilitation effect.

4.1 Early-stage tumor (T1/T2 with N0/N1)

4.1.1 Primary radiotherapy or open surgical procedures

Refinement in technology has improved radiation oncology across the past 20 years. The newer "more precise" techniques, such as intensity-modulated radiotherapy, compared with standard therapy, ameliorate locoregional control of hypopharyngeal carcinoma [52–54]. These techniques extend the concentration of dose to the primary tumor and concomitantly lower collateral injuries to normal tissues [53]. The results of the retrospective analysis showed the similarity between the long-term survival prognosis of primary radiotherapy and laryngectomy [55–57]. However, prospective evidence is limited for the similarity between locoregional control and survival rates [46, 58, 59]. Postradiation local control rate was achieved in 68–90% of patients with T1 tumors and approximately 75% cases in T2 lesions [58, 60–62]. The goal of radiation with concurrent chemotherapy is to acquire speaking and swallowing functional of invaded area and laryngeal preservation rates for five years above 70% [52, 63, 64]. Radical radiation-related injuries to the neck tissues need to be taken seriously, including substantial acute and late

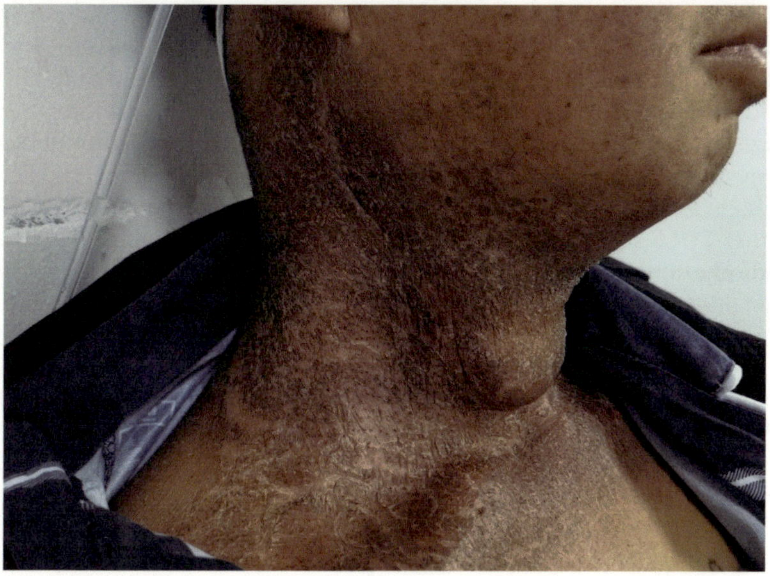

Figure 6.
Radiotherapy toxicity of neck.

toxicity (**Figure 6**). Although a majority of acute toxicities are temporary (such as radiation-related dermatitis usually alleviated within 6–12 weeks of treatment), permanent xerostomia at least partly is present invariably. Post-radiotherapy complications such as aspiration and chronic dysphagia may also occur in some cases, depending on the permanent feeding tube. The incidence is growing associated with intensive protocols (e.g., concurrent chemoradiotherapy). Therefore, effective quality assurance mechanisms and appropriate expertise are needed to be established to limit treatment-related toxicity and optimize results.

The skin injury often occurs during radiotherapy, including red swollen of skin, painful blisters, and pigmentation.

Open surgery is also an available approach for early-stage lesions compared with radiotherapy [65]. The posterior pharynx tumors can be excised through the transhyoid approach [66, 67]. Meanwhile, reservation of the internal branch of the superior laryngeal nerve is necessary. The transhyoid approach is critical for the disease that cannot be exposed transorally, especially in advanced tumors [51]. The more noticeable problem is that the postoperative T1T2 diseases with high-risk factors (e.g., positive margins, positive lymph nodes, extracapsular tumor extension) and locally advanced tumors should perform radiotherapy [68].

4.1.2 Transoral approaches

For T1/T2 tumor, minimally invasive surgery with reducing morbidity has become a surgical option for patients. In addition to open surgery, a variety of transoral surgical techniques/instrumentation, such as laser, plasma, oral robot surgery, and so on, setting primary tumor resection as a rising feasible option, with preserving laryngeal function [69, 70]. Transoral surgery (TORS/TLM) are considered as promising alternatives with better functional consequence compared with open surgery. It presents fewer complications than open surgery with nasogastric tube dependence down from 31–3% within 1 year [71]. Supporters of surgery pose that the transoral method rise the laryngeal conservation rate by over 70% through lots of single-institution series [72, 73].

Over the past few decades, with growing prevalence in a transoral path for getting into the upper aerodigestive tract, especially transoral laser surgery (TOLS), which initially was used for cancer of the larynx, gradually spread to the hypopharyngeal tumor [72–76]. Local control and cancer-free survival rates via radiotherapy and open surgery inT1/T2 diseases have been achieved through transoral routes, especially in early-stage lesions [72, 77–80]. The procedural complications of TOLS include fistula, granulation tissue formation, and fatal bleeding. [77–80]. But, in other TOLS series reported, 83% of patients were received adjuvant treatment (radiotherapy or concurrent chemoradiotherapy) after TOLS according to pathologic outcomes [77–80]. In T3, T4 cases, because of the limitation of detailed data about the use of TOLS for these lesions, the potential effects (if any) of TOLS remains poorly explained [78, 79]. Transoral robotic surgery has been considered a valid treatment for early hypopharyngeal carcinoma [81–83]. Meanwhile, it is also regarded as more appropriate for early cases without adjuvant treatment [81].

The complete resection of the tumor should be taken as the premise, with the corresponding bilateral neck dissection, combining with intraoperative frozen section examination to achieve radical procedures. If the postoperative pathological or histological examination indicates high-risk factors, postoperative adjuvant radiotherapy is required.

4.2 Advanced-stage tumor (T3/T4 or $\geq$ N2)

4.2.1 Non-surgical management

For the need of larynx-preservation, non-surgical treatments are considered as valid notions involved when appropriate [84]. At present, the non-operative treatment of larynx reservation is mainly combined with radiotherapy and chemotherapy (such as simultaneous radiotherapy and chemotherapy, induction chemotherapy sequential radiotherapy). Targeted therapy and immunotherapy are still being explored. The advanced patients involved postoperative adjuvant radiotherapy acquired improvement of local control, cancer-free survival rate, and overall survival [60, 85–88].

For stage IV malignancy, chemotherapy (induction therapy or concomitant therapy) heightens therapeutic efficacy, which is better in locoregional control and survival rates than radiation alone and combination therapies (surgery + radiation [84, 89–92]. A randomized trial including 202 cases indicated that chemotherapy group (induction chemotherapy +radiotherapy) achieve almost same disease survival as immediate surgery, with13.1% (the chemotherapy group) versus 13.8% (the surgery group) in a 10-year overall survival rate and with 8.5% versus 10.8% in10-year progression-free survival rates [93]. For optimizing chemotherapeutic effectiveness, organ-preservation strategies have to be abandoned in some advanced diseases in order to optimize chemotherapeutic effectiveness [94]. Pretreatment organ dysfunction, e.g., status vocal cord fixation and tracheostomy dependence, are related to posttreatment poor functional outcomes [95].

When considering organ-preservation strategy, the therapeutics must be implemented not only for saving of the anatomical units but also the return of upper aerodigestive function [96–98]. Meanwhile, the advanced patients with extensive invasion of surrounding tissue and serious decline of pharynx and larynx function present low pathologic complete response by non-operative treatment. The opinions of various disciplines should be integrated into decision-making. The American Society of Clinical Oncology (ASCO) guidelines recommend total laryngectomy for T3/T4patients with heavy tumor load and poor laryngeal function before induction chemotherapy [99].

4.2.2 Surgery

Surgery remains the preferred treatment for advanced-stage hypopharyngeal cancers [100]. Kinds of surgical manners are achieved in locally advanced cancers. Considering the possibility of aspiration after laryngeal preservation surgery, assessment of preoperative lung function is necessary. The cut margins (inferior or esophageal margin) must be extended carefully for safe boundaries. [25, 101, 102]. We should pay more attention to the extent of surgical margins, especially the inferior margin of the tumor (nearly to the esophageal part). Wide margins surgically are often considering in the skip disease and submucosal positive pathology. But researches have shown that patients did not benefit from extended edges (3–5 cm) compared with traditional (1–1.5 cm) incisal edges [103].

Partial pharyngectomy integrated with a partial laryngectomy, e.g.: vertical hemilaryngectomy, supraglottic laryngectomy, or supracricoid laryngectomy etc. is utilized in a series of hypopharyngeal cancers for hypopharyngeal cancers with small to medium lesions [104–107]. Laccourreye et share their extensive experience with the methods described above in their researches, including 135 cases with pyriform fossa lesions [104, 105]. The patients were executed supracricoid hemilaryngopharyngectomy combined with postoperative induction chemotherapy (IC) (96%). Five-year actuarial survival rates were assessed at 46.7%, with tracheostomy tubes removed in all patients (average = 9 days), and a 91.9% recovering oral intake (gastrostomy-free) at one year [105]. The conservation of competing cricoarytenoid units is important to achieve good functional outcomes. The unit comprises a single arytenoid, cricoid cartilage, ipsilateral recurrent/superior laryngeal nerves, and ipsilateral intrinsic laryngeal muscles. At least a single company should be reserved to obtain suitable swallowing function and upper respiratory function [108].

Due to roughly 10% of lesions invade the thyroid parenchyma directly, the cases with macroscopic cancer extension outside the larynx should be performed thyroid lobectomy or total thyroidectomy. In salvage treatments, considering thyroid vessel damages in response to radiation, preoperative hypothyroidism screening (routine pre- and post-operative thyroid hormone screening) is often necessary [109, 110]. In a prospective study including 137 laryngeal/hypopharyngeal patients, the incidence of hypothyroidism after treatment for laryngeal or hypopharyngeal tumors is 47.7%, especially after combination treatment [110]. Hypoparathyroidism is an important consideration in treatment, so the reservation or reimplantation of parathyroid glands must be noted during cricopharyngeal resection and/or paratracheal + mediastinal lymph node dissection [103].

4.2.3 Reconstruction

Laryngopharyngeal defect reconstruction is also an important approach for the surgeon to optimize surgery. The reconstruction presents a certain advantage in reducing the incidence of postoperative complications such as pharyngeal fistula, fatal bleeding, or infection. Meanwhile, it shows satisfactory outcomes in rehabilitating functions of speaking, swallowing, and breathing. The methods include local issue, regional flap or more vascularized free tissue transfer (**Figure 7**). Regional flaps contain the submental island flap, the supraclavicular island flap, the deltopectoral flap, the pectoralis, myocutaneous flap or latissimus dorsi myocutaneous flaps. Vascularized free tissue transfer methods include radial forearm free flap, anterolateral thigh free flap. In partial pharyngectomy with a partial laryngectomy, the small defects are repaired by local closure, and the larger defects (> 3 cm in size), regional flaps, and free tissue transfer are recommended. For partial pharyngeal defects

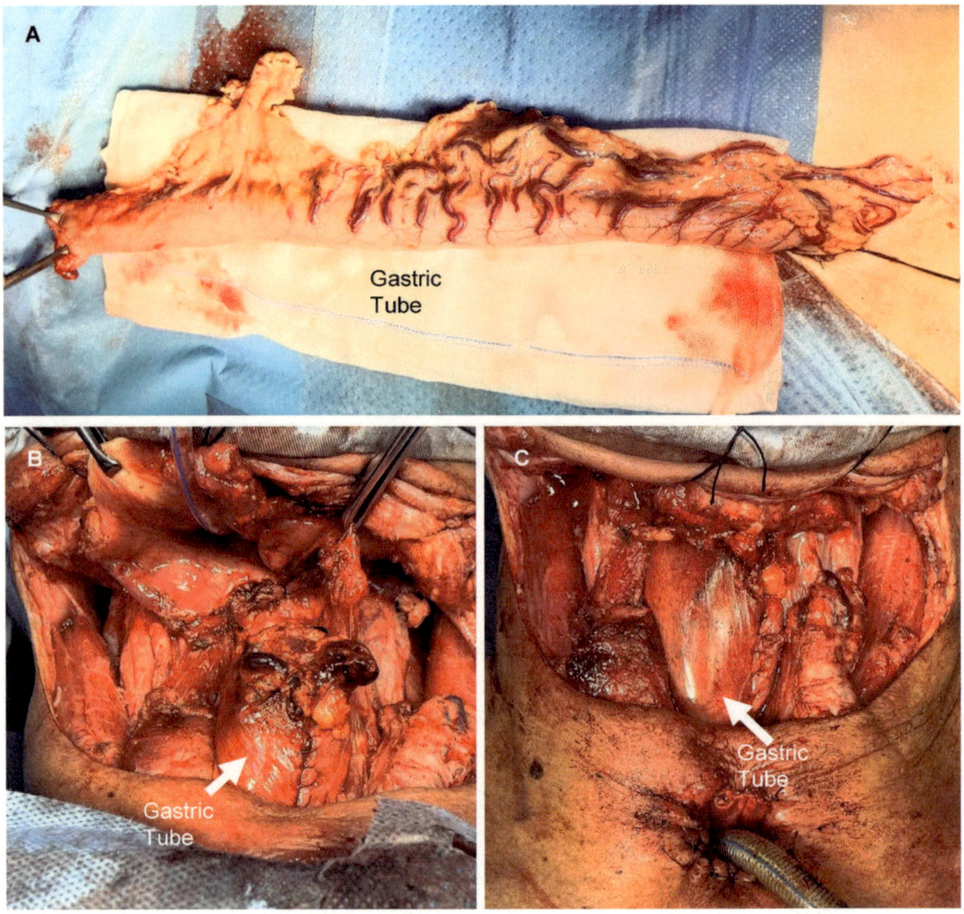

Figure 7.
Surgical reconstruction of hypopharyngeal cancer involving the larynx and esophageal. (A) The tubular gastric reconstruction was applied to repair the esophagus by video-assisted thoracoscopic surgery (VATS). (B, C) Inset of the gastric tube into the operative cavity of total laryngopharyngectomy.

with a total laryngectomy, despite other options, such as primary closure, primary closure with bolster flap, and regional tissue transfer, free tissue transfer has become one of the most utilized reconstructive selections. The major advantages of free tissue transfer are donor-site tissue, healthy tissue to repair circumferential defects. It is reconstructed in a tubular shape to provide a good swallowing tract and low incidence by avoiding entrance to other body cavities for total laryngopharyngectomy defects is usually rebuilt by the approaches such as enteric flap transposition, gastric pull-up, colonic Interposition, or jejunal free flap.

4.3 Nodal metastases in neck

Almost all patients with hypopharyngeal carcinoma have a high incidence of lymph node metastasis in the neck [30, 111]. Pyriform fossa cancer has the highest cervical metastasis rate (> 75%), while the lymph node metastasis rate of the posterior pharyngeal wall and posterior ring carcinoma is currently between 30% and 60% [29, 30, 111, 112]. For clinically negative (cN0) neck, the high-risk lymph node group must be included in the scope of dissection. Bilateral neck dissection should be considered with the tumor across the midline and tumors located in the posterior pharyngeal wall, medial Pyriform wall, or posterior annular region [96, 111]. In the cN0 cases, most of the lymph nodes with positive pathological examination were located in levels II and III of the lateral neck [46, 111, 113, 114]. Thus levels II to IV should be taken into consideration for elective neck dissection in the CN+ patients, despite the low incidence of metastases at levels I and V, the cutting of levels I through V is incorporated into an overall neck dissection for reducing relapses in a node. The internal jugular vein (IJV), sternocleidomastoid muscle, and accessory nerve are recommended to be preserved and attacked directly by cancer.

Paratracheal (level VI) and retropharyngeal nodes must be brought to attention because of The risk of tumor invasion [46, 115]. Paratracheal positive nodes (level VI) are frequently involved by tumors located in the pyriform apex or post-cricoid area [111, 116–119]. A series of reports by Chung et al. poses a 27.9% occult metastasis rate in IV nodes with a much worse prognosis (26% vs. 55% 5-year disease-specific survival) [119]. So paratracheal node dissection should be strongly involved in this crowd both for the thoroughness of removing all tumor and strict disease staging. The retropharyngeal nodal disease is common in lateral pyriform and posterior pharyngeal, existing in 40% of advanced patients [120]. Retropharyngeal nodes should be taken into adjuvant radiotherapy in the setting of unremovable surgically. In advanced stages, these positive nodes clinically/radiographically may be an indication for non-surgical treatment [120].

5. Surveillance, and recurrent

Due to most tumors relapse within two years after initiate treatment, rigorous surveillance should be followed three months after treatment until two years and every six months for 3–5 years to screen early local recurrence and second primary tumors [121–123]. A favorable scanning should involve a combination of history, physical, endoscope, images (CT, MRI, PET/CT), and biopsy [124]. For suspicion cases, repeated biopsies are necessary for positive results. PET/CT has been demonstrated to be more accurate than CT/MRI for screening false-positive results [125, 126]. Surgery is considered an optimal option for recurrent cases (especially small recurrent). For unresectable recurrence or metastatic, re-irradiation or re-irradiation+chemo is one selection with improving median survival. Meanwhile, related toxicities cannot be ignored, with complications range from 9 to 32% in adjuvant chemotherapy cases [127, 128]. Therefore, the multidisciplinary team must seek a balance between the serious toxic reactions and the rescue therapy while paying attention to the progress of the disease in the long term.

There are not many options available for recurrent and metastasis, so it is urgent to develop new targeted agents in this population. The innovative drugs may be proved as another promising avenue for recurrence and metastasis. A variety of molecular targeting drugs are developed in the exploratory stage. These drugs have anti-cancer affection on aberrantly expressed intracellular proteins. In recent years, immunotherapy has been proved to ameliorate overall survival over standard, single-agent therapy for platinum-refractory cases [129, 130]. Anti-programmed cell death 1 (PD-1) therapies were assessed as a treatment for platinum-refractory recurrent and/or metastatic head and neck squamous cell carcinoma (HNSCC). Meanwhile, a small number of patients with the PD-1 approach acquire lower toxic effects than traditional therapies. Immunotherapy brings hope to this subtype of treat-limited patients [130, 131].

6. Conclusion

The primary type of hypopharyngeal cancer is squamous cell carcinoma, with a poor prognosis. Approximately up to a third of patients are diagnosed with second primary esophageal cancer. The infrequent incidence of hypopharyngeal cancer limits the extensive clinical trial application. Early-stage disease achieved successful tumor management after treatment (radiation alone or surgery resection). However, despite the improvements of therapy, measures alone may not be sufficient to preserve the laryngeal function in advanced-stage ones. Formulating an accurate and useful treatment plan depends on a comprehensive assessment of the patient's general condition and tumor staging before treatment. To explore a functional tumor remission and improve survival outcomes, researchers are seeking a balance between swallowing-voice rehabilitation and organ preservation. Also, the treatment requires cooperation involved specialized expertise and a multi-disciplinary team to benefit patients. Future directions will focus on refining surgery to afford functional organ preservation and radiotherapy techniques. Furthermore, it is important to regard to influence patient outcomes; there also needs to be more emphasis on non-surgery therapy's toxicity.

Acknowledgements

This work was supported by grants from the Youth Program of Guangxi Natural Science Foundation of China (2018GXNSFBA281158) and High-level Talent Introduction Plan of the First Affiliated Hospital of Guangxi Medical University (the fifth level).

Conflict of interest

The authors declare no conflict of interest.

Author details

Yi Huang, Yushan Liang and Weilin Zhao*
Department of Otolaryngology-Head and Neck Surgery, First Affiliated Hospital of Guangxi Medical University, Nanning, China

*Address all correspondence to: zhaoweilin6392@hotmail.com

References

[1] Hall, S.F., et al., The natural history of patients with squamous cell carcinoma of the hypopharynx. Laryngoscope, 2008. **118**(8): p. 1362-1371. DOI: 10.1097/MLG.0b013e318173dc4a

[2] Silver, C.E., et al., Current trends in initial management of laryngeal cancer: the declining use of open surgery. Eur Arch Otorhinolaryngol, 2009. **266**(9): p. 1333-1352. DOI: 10.1007/s00405-009-1028-2

[3] Ferlay, J., et al., Cancer incidence and mortality worldwide: sources, methods and major patterns in GLOBOCAN 2012. Int J Cancer, 2015. **136**(5): p. E359–E386. DOI: 10.1002/ijc.29210

[4] Shield, K.D., et al., The global incidence of lip, oral cavity, and pharyngeal cancers by subsite in 2012. CA Cancer J Clin, 2017. **67**(1): p. 51-64. DOI: 10.3322/caac.21384

[5] Kuo, P., et al., Hypopharyngeal cancer incidence, treatment, and survival: temporal trends in the United States. Laryngoscope, 2014. **124**(9): p. 2064-9. DOI: 10.1002/lary.24651

[6] Global Burden of Disease Cancer, C., et al., Global, Regional, and National Cancer Incidence, Mortality, Years of Life Lost, Years Lived With Disability, and Disability-Adjusted Life-years for 32 Cancer Groups, 1990 to 2015: A Systematic Analysis for the Global Burden of Disease Study. JAMA Oncol, 2017. **3**(4): p. 524-548. DOI: 10.1001/jamaoncol.2016.5688

[7] Chow, L.Q.M., Head and Neck Cancer. N Engl J Med, 2020. **382**(1): p. 60-72. DOI: 10.1056/NEJMra1715715

[8] Canto, M.T. and S.S. Devesa, Oral cavity and pharynx cancer incidence rates in the United States, 1975-1998. Oral Oncol, 2002. **38**(6): p. 610-617. DOI: 10.1016/s1368-8375(01)00109-9

[9] Newman, J.R., et al., Survival trends in hypopharyngeal cancer: a population-based review. Laryngoscope, 2015. **125**(3): p. 624-629. DOI: 10.1002/lary.24915

[10] Siddiqui, F., et al., Squamous carcinoma of the larynx and hypopharynx in children: a distinct clinical entity? Med Pediatr Oncol, 2003. **40**(5): p. 322-324. DOI: 10.1002/mpo.10291

[11] Avincsal, M.O., et al., Impact of alcohol dehydrogenase-aldehyde dehydrogenase polymorphism on clinical outcome in patients with hypopharyngeal cancer. Head Neck, 2018. **40**(4): p. 770-777. DOI: 10.1002/hed.25050

[12] Maier, H., et al., Chronic alcohol consumption--the key risk factor for pharyngeal cancer. Otolaryngol Head Neck Surg, 1994. **110**(2): p. 168-173. DOI: 10.1177/019459989411000205

[13] Blot, W.J., et al., Smoking and drinking in relation to oral and pharyngeal cancer. Cancer Res, 1988. **48**(11): p. 3282-3287.

[14] Choi, S.Y. and H. Kahyo, Effect of cigarette smoking and alcohol consumption in the aetiology of cancer of the oral cavity, pharynx and larynx. Int J Epidemiol, 1991. **20**(4): p. 878-885. DOI: 10.1093/ije/20.4.878

[15] El-Serag, H.B., et al., Gastroesophageal reflux disease is a risk factor for laryngeal and pharyngeal cancer. Am J Gastroenterol, 2001. **96**(7): p. 2013-2018. DOI: 10.1111/j.1572-0241.2001.03934.x

[16] Couch, M.E., et al., Cancer cachexia update in head and neck cancer: Pathophysiology and treatment. Head Neck, 2015. **37**(7): p. 1057-1072. DOI: 10.1002/hed.23696

[17] Anderson, S.R. and J.T. Sinacori, Plummer-Vinson syndrome heralded by postcricoid carcinoma. Am J Otolaryngol, 2007. **28**(1): p. 22-24. DOI: 10.1016/j.amjoto.2006.06.004

[18] Wahlberg, P.C., et al., Carcinoma of the hypopharynx: analysis of incidence and survival in Sweden over a 30-year period. Head Neck, 1998. **20**(8): p. 714-719. DOI: 10.1002/(sici)1097-0347(199812)20:8<714::aid-hed9>3.0.co;2-2

[19] Lee, H.M., et al., Current Perspectives on Nasopharyngeal Carcinoma. Adv Exp Med Biol, 2019. **1164**: p. 11-34. DOI: 10.1007/978-3-030-22254-3_2

[20] Pongsapich, W., et al., Prevalence of HPV infection in hypopharyngeal and laryngeal squamous cell carcinoma at Thailand's largest tertiary referral center. Infect Agent Cancer, 2017. **12**: p. 58. DOI: 10.1186/s13027-017-0167-0

[21] Dalianis, T., et al., Human papillomavirus DNA and p16(INK4a) expression in hypopharyngeal cancer and in relation to clinical outcome, in Stockholm, Sweden. Oral Oncol, 2015. **51**(9): p. 857-861. DOI: 10.1016/j.oraloncology.2015.06.002

[22] Goldenberg, D., et al., Epstein-Barr virus in head and neck cancer assessed by quantitative polymerase chain reaction. Laryngoscope, 2004. **114**(6): p. 1027-1031. DOI: 10.1097/00005537-200406000-00013

[23] Ndiaye, C., et al., HPV DNA, E6/E7 mRNA, and p16INK4a detection in head and neck cancers: a systematic review and meta-analysis. Lancet Oncol, 2014. **15**(12): p. 1319-1331. DOI: 10.1016/S1470-2045(14)70471-1

[24] Zhou, L., et al., Evaluation of Epstein-Barr Virus infection in hypopharyngeal carcinomas from 37 Japanese patients. Mod Pathol, 1998. **11**(6): p. 509-512.

[25] Helliwell, T.R., acp Best Practice No 169. Evidence based pathology: squamous carcinoma of the hypopharynx. J Clin Pathol, 2003. **56**(2): p. 81-85. DOI: 10.1136/jcp.56.2.81

[26] Amin, M.B., American Joint Committee on Cancer., and American Cancer Society., *AJCC cancer staging manual*. Eight edition / editor-in-chief, Mahul B. Amin, MD, FCAP ; editors, Stephen B. Edge, MD, FACS and 16 others ; Donna M. Gress, RHIT, CTR - Technical editor ; Laura R. Meyer, CAPM - Managing editor. ed. 2017, Chicago IL: American Joint Committee on Cancer, Springer. xvii, 1024 pages.

[27] Sarradin, V., et al., [WHO classification of head and neck tumours 2017: Main novelties and update of diagnostic methods]. Bull Cancer, 2018. **105**(6): p. 596-602. DOI: 10.1016/j.bulcan.2018.04.004

[28] Uzcudun, A.E., et al., Clinical features of pharyngeal cancer: a retrospective study of 258 consecutive patients. J Laryngol Otol, 2001. **115**(2): p. 112-118. DOI: 10.1258/0022215011907703

[29] Spector, G.J., Distant metastases from laryngeal and hypopharyngeal cancer. ORL J Otorhinolaryngol Relat Spec, 2001. **63**(4): p. 224-228. DOI: 10.1159/000055746

[30] Newkirk, K.A., et al., Planned neck dissection for advanced primary head and neck malignancy treated with organ preservation therapy: disease control and survival outcomes. Head Neck, 2001. **23**(2): p. 73-79. DOI: 10.1002/1097-0347(200102)23:2<73::aid-hed1001>3.0.co;2-6

[31] Chung, E.J., et al., Pattern of cervical lymph node metastasis in medial wall pyriform sinus carcinoma. Laryngoscope, 2014. **124**(4): p. 882-887. DOI: 10.1002/lary.24299

[32] Kim, S.Y., et al., Clinicopathological factors influencing the outcomes of surgical treatment in patients with T4a hypopharyngeal cancer. BMC Cancer, 2017. **17**(1): p. 904. DOI: 10.1186/s12885-017-3880-6

[33] Kotwall, C., et al., Metastatic patterns in squamous cell cancer of the head and neck. Am J Surg, 1987. **154**(4): p. 439-442. DOI: 10.1016/0002-9610(89)90020-2

[34] Lee, D.H., et al., Second cancer incidence, risk factor, and specific mortality in head and neck squamous cell carcinoma. Otolaryngol Head Neck Surg, 2013. **149**(4): p. 579-586. DOI: 10.1177/0194599813496373

[35] Strong, M.S., J. Incze, and C.W. Vaughan, Field cancerization in the aerodigestive tract--its etiology, manifestation, and significance. J Otolaryngol, 1984. **13**(1): p. 1-6.

[36] Chang, C.C., et al., Influence of residential environment and lifestyle on multiple primary malignancies in Taiwan. Asian Pac J Cancer Prev, 2015. **16**(8): p. 3533-3538. DOI: 10.7314/apjcp.2015.16.8.3533

[37] Katada, C., et al., Alcohol Consumption and Multiple Dysplastic Lesions Increase Risk of Squamous Cell Carcinoma in the Esophagus, Head, and Neck. Gastroenterology, 2016. **151**(5): p. 860-869 e7. DOI: 10.1053/j.gastro.2016.07.040

[38] Shaha, A.R., et al., Synchronicity, multicentricity, and metachronicity of head and neck cancer. Head Neck Surg, 1988. **10**(4): p. 225-228. DOI: 10.1002/j.1930-2398.1988.tb00003.x

[39] Liu, W.S., et al., Secondary primary cancer in patients with head and neck carcinoma: the differences among hypopharyngeal, laryngeal, and other sites of head and neck cancer. Eur J Cancer Care (Engl), 2014. **23**(1): p. 36-42. DOI: 10.1111/ecc.12084

[40] Lee, K.D., et al., The incidence and risk of developing a second primary esophageal cancer in patients with oral and pharyngeal carcinoma: a population-based study in Taiwan over a 25 year period. BMC Cancer, 2009. **9**: p. 373. DOI: 10.1186/1471-2407-9-373

[41] Lien, C.F., et al., Cortactin as a potential predictor of second esophageal neoplasia in hypopharyngeal carcinoma. Auris Nasus Larynx, 2019. **46**(2): p. 260-266. DOI: 10.1016/j.anl.2018.08.002

[42] Kotarba, E., [Surgical treatment of tumors of the external ear]. Przegl Dermatol, 1990. **77**(1): p. 61-67.

[43] Lee, C.T., et al., Narrow-band imaging with magnifying endoscopy for the screening of esophageal cancer in patients with primary head and neck cancers. Endoscopy, 2010. **42**(8): p. 613-619. DOI: 10.1055/s-0030-1255514

[44] Eckel, H.E., et al., Surgical treatment for hypopharynx carcinoma: feasibility, mortality, and results. Otolaryngol Head Neck Surg, 2001. **124**(5): p. 561-569. DOI: 10.1067/mhn.2001.115060

[45] Lydiatt, W.M., et al., Head and Neck cancers-major changes in the American Joint Committee on cancer eighth edition cancer staging manual. CA Cancer J Clin, 2017. **67**(2): p. 122-137. DOI: 10.3322/caac.21389

[46] Takes, R.P., et al., Current trends in initial management of hypopharyngeal cancer: the declining use of open surgery. Head Neck, 2012. **34**(2): p. 270-281. DOI: 10.1002/hed.21613

[47] Olzowy, B., M. Hillebrand, and U. Harreus, Frequency of bilateral cervical metastases in hypopharyngeal squamous cell carcinoma: a retrospective analysis of 203 cases after bilateral neck dissection. Eur Arch Otorhinolaryngol, 2017. **274**(11): p.

3965-3970. DOI: 10.1007/s00405-017-4724-3

[48] Hoffman, H.T., et al., Hypopharyngeal cancer patient care evaluation. Laryngoscope, 1997. **107**(8): p. 1005-1017. DOI: 10.1097/00005537-199708000-00001

[49] Kowalski, L.P. and A.L. Carvalho, Natural history of untreated head and neck cancer. Eur J Cancer, 2000. **36**(8): p. 1032-1037. DOI: 10.1016/s0959-8049(00)00054-x

[50] Choi, H.G., B. Park, and S.H. Ahn, Untreated head and neck cancer in Korea: a national cohort study. Eur Arch Otorhinolaryngol, 2017. **274**(3): p. 1643-1650. DOI: 10.1007/s00405-016-4392-8

[51] Chan, J.Y. and W.I. Wei, Current management strategy of hypopharyngeal carcinoma. Auris Nasus Larynx, 2013. **40**(1): p. 2-6. DOI: 10.1016/j.anl.2011.11.009

[52] Mok, G., et al., Outcomes of intensity-modulated radiotherapy versus conventional radiotherapy for hypopharyngeal cancer. Head Neck, 2015. **37**(5): p. 655-661. DOI: 10.1002/hed.23649

[53] Lin, A., et al., Quality of life after parotid-sparing IMRT for head-and-neck cancer: a prospective longitudinal study. Int J Radiat Oncol Biol Phys, 2003. **57**(1): p. 61-70. DOI: 10.1016/s0360-3016(03)00361-4

[54] Eisbruch, A., et al., Recurrences near base of skull after IMRT for head-and-neck cancer: implications for target delineation in high neck and for parotid gland sparing. Int J Radiat Oncol Biol Phys, 2004. **59**(1): p. 28-42. DOI: 10.1016/j.ijrobp.2003.10.032

[55] Pracy, P., et al., Hypopharyngeal cancer: United Kingdom National Multidisciplinary Guidelines. J Laryngol Otol, 2016. **130**(S2): p. S104-S110. DOI: 10.1017/S0022215116000529

[56] Martin, A., et al., Organ preserving transoral laser microsurgery for cancer of the hypopharynx. Laryngoscope, 2008. **118**(3): p. 398-402. DOI: 10.1097/MLG.0b013e31815aeda3

[57] Rabbani, A., et al., Definitive radiotherapy for T1-T2 squamous cell carcinoma of pyriform sinus. Int J Radiat Oncol Biol Phys, 2008. **72**(2): p. 351-355. DOI: 10.1016/j.ijrobp.2008.01.003

[58] Garden, A.S., et al., Early squamous cell carcinoma of the hypopharynx: outcomes of treatment with radiation alone to the primary disease. Head Neck, 1996. **18**(4): p. 317-322. DOI: 10.1002/(SICI)1097-0347(199607/08)18:4<317::AID-HED2>3.0.CO;2-0

[59] Amdur, R.J., et al., Organ preservation with radiotherapy for T1-T2 carcinoma of the pyriform sinus. Head Neck, 2001. **23**(5): p. 353-362. DOI: 10.1002/hed.1044

[60] Amdur, R.J., et al., Postoperative irradiation for squamous cell carcinoma of the head and neck: an analysis of treatment results and complications. Int J Radiat Oncol Biol Phys, 1989. **16**(1): p. 25-36. DOI: 10.1016/0360-3016(89)90006-0

[61] Fein, D.A., et al., Pharyngeal wall carcinoma treated with radiotherapy: impact of treatment technique and fractionation. Int J Radiat Oncol Biol Phys, 1993. **26**(5): p. 751-757. DOI: 10.1016/0360-3016(93)90488-h

[62] Mendenhall, W.M., et al., Squamous cell carcinoma of the pyriform sinus treated with surgery and/or radiotherapy. Head Neck Surg, 1987. **10**(2): p. 88-92. DOI: 10.1002/hed.2890100205

[63] Nakamura, K., et al., Multi-institutional analysis of early squamous cell carcinoma of the hypopharynx treated with radical radiotherapy. Int J Radiat Oncol Biol Phys, 2006. **65**(4): p. 1045-1050. DOI: 10.1016/j.ijrobp.2006.02.001

[64] Edson, M.A., et al., Outcomes for hypopharyngeal carcinoma treated with organ-preservation therapy. Head Neck, 2016. **38 Suppl 1**: p. E2091–E2099. DOI: 10.1002/hed.24387

[65] Wei, W.I., The dilemma of treating hypopharyngeal carcinoma: more or less: Hayes Martin Lecture. Arch Otolaryngol Head Neck Surg, 2002. **128**(3): p. 229-232. DOI: 10.1001/archotol.128.3.229

[66] Julieron, M., et al., Surgical management of posterior pharyngeal wall carcinomas: functional and oncologic results. Head Neck, 2001. **23**(2): p. 80-86. DOI: 10.1002/1097-0347(200102)23:2<80::aid-hed1002>3.0.co;2-3

[67] Spiro, R.H., et al., Squamous carcinoma of the posterior pharyngeal wall. Am J Surg, 1990. **160**(4): p. 420-423. DOI: 10.1016/s0002-9610(05)80557-4

[68] Cooper, J.S., et al., Postoperative concurrent radiotherapy and chemotherapy for high-risk squamous-cell carcinoma of the head and neck. N Engl J Med, 2004. **350**(19): p. 1937-1944. DOI: 10.1056/NEJMoa032646

[69] Park, Y.M., et al., The long-term oncological and functional outcomes of transoral robotic surgery in patients with hypopharyngeal cancer. Oral Oncol, 2017. **71**: p. 138-143. DOI: 10.1016/j.oraloncology.2017.06.016

[70] Weiss, B.G., et al., Transoral laser microsurgery for treatment for hypopharyngeal cancer in 211 patients. Head Neck, 2017. **39**(8): p. 1631-1638. DOI: 10.1002/hed.24814

[71] White, H., et al., Salvage surgery for recurrent cancers of the oropharynx: comparing TORS with standard open surgical approaches. JAMA Otolaryngol Head Neck Surg, 2013. **139**(8): p. 773-8. DOI: 10.1001/jamaoto.2013.3866

[72] Steiner, W., et al., Organ preservation by transoral laser microsurgery in piriform sinus carcinoma. Otolaryngol Head Neck Surg, 2001. **124**(1): p. 58-67. DOI: 10.1067/mhn.2001.111597

[73] Vilaseca, I., et al., CO2 laser surgery: a larynx preservation alternative for selected hypopharyngeal carcinomas. Head Neck, 2004. **26**(11): p. 953-959. DOI: 10.1002/hed.20074

[74] Werner, J.A., Transoral resection of laryngeal and hypopharyngeal cancer is an established surgical procedure. Eur Arch Otorhinolaryngol, 2015. **272**(1): p. 1-2. DOI: 10.1007/s00405-014-3359-x

[75] Bernal-Sprekelsen, M., I. Vilaseca-Gonzalez, and J.L. Blanch-Alejandro, Predictive values for aspiration after endoscopic laser resections of malignant tumors of the hypopharynx and larynx. Head Neck, 2004. **26**(2): p. 103-110. DOI: 10.1002/hed.10363

[76] Imanishi, Y., et al., Clinical outcomes of transoral videolaryngoscopic surgery for hypopharyngeal and supraglottic cancer. BMC Cancer, 2017. **17**(1): p. 445. DOI: 10.1186/s12885-017-3396-0

[77] Rudert, H.H. and S. Hoft, Transoral carbon-dioxide laser resection of hypopharyngeal carcinoma. Eur Arch Otorhinolaryngol, 2003. **260**(4): p. 198-206. DOI: 10.1007/s00405-002-0520-8

[78] Suarez, C., et al., Laser surgery for early to moderately advanced glottic, supraglottic, and hypopharyngeal cancers. Head Neck, 2012. **34**(7): p. 1028-1035. DOI: 10.1002/hed.21766

[79] Vilaseca, I., J.L. Blanch, and M. Bernal-Sprekelsen, Transoral laser surgery for hypopharyngeal carcinomas. Curr Opin Otolaryngol Head Neck Surg, 2012. **20**(2): p. 97-102. DOI: 10.1097/MOO.0b013e32834fa8fe

[80] Karatzanis, A.D., et al., T1 and T2 hypopharyngeal cancer treatment with laser microsurgery. J Surg Oncol, 2010. **102**(1): p. 27-33. DOI: 10.1002/jso.21550

[81] Lorincz, B.B., et al., Feasibility and safety of transoral robotic surgery (TORS) for early hypopharyngeal cancer: a subset analysis of the Hamburg University TORS-trial. Eur Arch Otorhinolaryngol, 2015. **272**(10): p. 2993-2998. DOI: 10.1007/s00405-014-3259-0

[82] Lorincz, B.B., N. Jowett, and R. Knecht, Decision management in transoral robotic surgery: Indications, individual patient selection, and role in the multidisciplinary treatment for head and neck cancer from a European perspective. Head Neck, 2016. **38 Suppl 1**: p. E2190–E2196. DOI: 10.1002/hed.24059

[83] Park, Y.M., et al., Feasiblity of transoral robotic hypopharyngectomy for early-stage hypopharyngeal carcinoma. Oral Oncol, 2010. **46**(8): p. 597-602. DOI: 10.1016/j.oraloncology.2010.05.003

[84] Lagha, A., et al., Larynx preservation: what is the best non-surgical strategy? Crit Rev Oncol Hematol, 2013. **88**(2): p. 447-458. DOI: 10.1016/j.critrevonc.2013.05.005

[85] Peters, L.J., et al., Evaluation of the dose for postoperative radiation therapy of head and neck cancer: first report of a prospective randomized trial. Int J Radiat Oncol Biol Phys, 1993. **26**(1): p. 3-11. DOI: 10.1016/0360-3016(93)90167-t

[86] Vikram, B., et al., Failure at the primary site following multimodality treatment in advanced head and neck cancer. Head Neck Surg, 1984. **6**(3): p. 720-3. DOI: 10.1002/hed.2890060303

[87] Frank, J.L., et al., Postoperative radiotherapy improves survival in squamous cell carcinoma of the hypopharynx. Am J Surg, 1994. **168**(5): p. 476-480. DOI: 10.1016/s0002-9610(05)80105-9

[88] Tupchong, L., et al., Randomized study of preoperative versus postoperative radiation therapy in advanced head and neck carcinoma: long-term follow-up of RTOG study 73-03. Int J Radiat Oncol Biol Phys, 1991. **20**(1): p. 21-28. DOI: 10.1016/0360-3016(91)90133-o

[89] Bourhis, J., et al., Concomitant chemoradiotherapy versus acceleration of radiotherapy with or without concomitant chemotherapy in locally advanced head and neck carcinoma (GORTEC 99-02): an open-label phase 3 randomised trial. Lancet Oncol, 2012. **13**(2): p. 145-153. DOI: 10.1016/S1470-2045(11)70346-1

[90] Rosenthal, D.I. and K.K. Ang, Altered radiation therapy fractionation, chemoradiation, and patient selection for the treatment of head and neck squamous carcinoma. Semin Radiat Oncol, 2004. **14**(2): p. 153-166. DOI: 10.1053/j.semradonc.2004.01.001

[91] Pignon, J.P., et al., Meta-analysis of chemotherapy in head and neck cancer (MACH-NC): an update on 93 randomised trials and 17,346 patients. Radiother Oncol, 2009. **92**(1): p. 4-14. DOI: 10.1016/j.radonc.2009.04.014

[92] Cohen, E.E., M.W. Lingen, and E.E. Vokes, The expanding role of systemic therapy in head and neck cancer. J Clin Oncol, 2004. **22**(9): p. 1743-1752. DOI: 10.1200/JCO.2004.06.147

[93] Lefebvre, J.L., et al., Laryngeal preservation with induction

chemotherapy for hypopharyngeal squamous cell carcinoma: 10-year results of EORTC trial 24891. Ann Oncol, 2012. **23**(10): p. 2708-2714. DOI: 10.1093/annonc/mds065

[94] Rosenthal, D.I. and A.I. Blanco, Head and neck squamous cell carcinoma: optimizing the therapeutic index. Expert Rev Anticancer Ther, 2005. **5**(3): p. 501-514. DOI: 10.1586/14737140.5.3.501

[95] Staton, J., et al., Factors predictive of poor functional outcome after chemoradiation for advanced laryngeal cancer. Otolaryngol Head Neck Surg, 2002. **127**(1): p. 43-47. DOI: 10.1067/mhn.2002.124473

[96] Gourin, C.G. and D.J. Terris, Carcinoma of the hypopharynx. Surg Oncol Clin N Am, 2004. **13**(1): p. 81-98. DOI: 10.1016/S1055-3207(03)00122-4

[97] Eisbruch, A., et al., Objective assessment of swallowing dysfunction and aspiration after radiation concurrent with chemotherapy for head-and-neck cancer. Int J Radiat Oncol Biol Phys, 2002. **53**(1): p. 23-28. DOI: 10.1016/s0360-3016(02)02712-8

[98] Vokes, E.E., et al., Concomitant chemoradiotherapy as primary therapy for locoregionally advanced head and neck cancer. J Clin Oncol, 2000. **18**(8): p. 1652-1661. DOI: 10.1200/JCO.2000.18.8.1652

[99] Forastiere, A.A., N. Ismaila, and G.T. Wolf, Use of Larynx-Preservation Strategies in the Treatment of Laryngeal Cancer: American Society of Clinical Oncology Clinical Practice Guideline Update Summary. J Oncol Pract, 2018. **14**(2): p. 123-128. DOI: 10.1200/JOP.2017.027912

[100] Pfister, D.G., et al., Head and Neck Cancers, Version 2.2020, NCCN Clinical Practice Guidelines in Oncology. J Natl Compr Canc Netw, 2020. **18**(7): p. 873-898. DOI: 10.6004/jnccn.2020.0031

[101] Joshi, P., et al., Thyroid gland involvement in carcinoma of the hypopharynx. J Laryngol Otol, 2014. **128**(1): p. 64-67. DOI: 10.1017/S0022215113003277

[102] Kraus, D.H., et al., Salvage laryngectomy for unsuccessful larynx preservation therapy. Ann Otol Rhinol Laryngol, 1995. **104**(12): p. 936-941. DOI: 10.1177/000348949510401204

[103] Clark, J.R., et al., Primary and salvage (hypo)pharyngectomy: Analysis and outcome. Head Neck, 2006. **28**(8): p. 671-677. DOI: 10.1002/hed.20428

[104] Laccourreye, O., et al., Supracricoid hemilaryngopharyngectomy in selected pyriform sinus carcinoma staged as T2. Laryngoscope, 1993. **103**(12): p. 1373-1379. DOI: 10.1288/00005537-199312000-00010

[105] Laccourreye, O., et al., Supracricoid hemilaryngopharyngectomy in patients with invasive squamous cell carcinoma of the pyriform sinus. Part I: Technique, complications, and long-term functional outcome. Ann Otol Rhinol Laryngol, 2005. **114**(1 Pt 1): p. 25-34. DOI: 10.1177/000348940511400106

[106] Chevalier, D., et al., Supraglottic hemilaryngopharyngectomy plus radiation for the treatment of early lateral margin and pyriform sinus carcinoma. Head Neck, 1997. **19**(1): p. 1-5. DOI: 10.1002/(sici)1097-0347(199701)19:1<1::aid-hed1>3.0.co;2-a

[107] Lecanu, J.B., et al., Conservative surgery in T3-T4 pharyngolaryngeal squamous cell carcinoma: an alternative to radiation therapy and to total laryngectomy for good responders to induction chemotherapy. Laryngoscope, 2000. **110**(3 Pt 1): p. 412-416. DOI: 10.1097/00005537-200003000-00015

[108] Chawla, S. and A.S. Carney, Organ preservation surgery for laryngeal

cancer. Head Neck Oncol, 2009. **1**: p. 12. DOI: 10.1186/1758-3284-1-12

[109] Thorp, M.A., et al., Parathyroid and thyroid function five years after treatment of laryngeal and hypopharyngeal carcinoma. Clin Otolaryngol Allied Sci, 1999. **24**(2): p. 104-108. DOI: 10.1046/j.1365-2273.1999.00214.x

[110] Lo Galbo, A.M., et al., A prospective longitudinal study on endocrine dysfunction following treatment of laryngeal or hypopharyngeal carcinoma. Oral Oncol, 2013. **49**(9): p. 950-955. DOI: 10.1016/j.oraloncology.2013.03.450

[111] Buckley, J.G. and K. MacLennan, Cervical node metastases in laryngeal and hypopharyngeal cancer: a prospective analysis of prevalence and distribution. Head Neck, 2000. **22**(4): p. 380-385. DOI: 10.1002/1097-0347(200007)22:4<380::aid-hed11>3.0.co;2-e

[112] Lefebvre, J.L., et al., Lymph node invasion in hypopharynx and lateral epilarynx carcinoma: a prognostic factor. Head Neck Surg, 1987. **10**(1): p. 14-18. DOI: 10.1002/hed.2890100104

[113] Candela, F.C., K. Kothari, and J.P. Shah, Patterns of cervical node metastases from squamous carcinoma of the oropharynx and hypopharynx. Head Neck, 1990. **12**(3): p. 197-203. DOI: 10.1002/hed.2880120302

[114] Wu, A.J., et al., Radiotherapy after surgical resection for head and neck mucosal melanoma. Am J Clin Oncol, 2010. **33**(3): p. 281-285. DOI: 10.1097/COC.0b013e3181a879f5

[115] de Mones, E., et al., Initial staging of squamous cell carcinoma of the oral cavity, larynx and pharynx (excluding nasopharynx). Part 2: Remote extension assessment and exploration for secondary synchronous locations outside of the upper aerodigestive tract. 2012 SFORL guidelines. Eur Ann Otorhinolaryngol Head Neck Dis, 2013. **130**(2): p. 107-112. DOI: 10.1016/j.anorl.2012.09.003

[116] Timon, C.V., M. Toner, and B.J. Conlon, Paratracheal lymph node involvement in advanced cancer of the larynx, hypopharynx, and cervical esophagus. Laryngoscope, 2003. **113**(9): p. 1595-9. DOI: 10.1097/00005537-200309000-00035

[117] Martins, A.S., Neck and mediastinal node dissection in pharyngolaryngoesophageal tumors. Head Neck, 2001. **23**(9): p. 772-9. DOI: 10.1002/hed.1110

[118] Clayman, G.L., et al., Laryngeal preservation for advanced laryngeal and hypopharyngeal cancers. Arch Otolaryngol Head Neck Surg, 1995. **121**(2): p. 219-223. DOI: 10.1001/archotol.1995.01890020081015

[119] Chung, E.J., et al., Pattern of lymph node metastasis in hypopharyngeal squamous cell carcinoma and indications for level VI lymph node dissection. Head Neck, 2016. **38** Suppl 1: p. E1969–E1973. DOI: 10.1002/hed.24361

[120] Hasegawa, Y. and H. Matsuura, Retropharyngeal node dissection in cancer of the oropharynx and hypopharynx. Head Neck, 1994. **16**(2): p. 173-180. DOI: 10.1002/hed.2880160212

[121] Kirchner, J.A., Pyriform sinus cancer: a clinical and laboratory study. Ann Otol Rhinol Laryngol, 1975. **84**(6): p. 793-803. DOI: 10.1177/000348947508400611

[122] Terhaard, C.H., et al., F-18-fluoro-deoxy-glucose positron-emission tomography scanning in detection of local recurrence after radiotherapy for laryngeal/ pharyngeal cancer. Head Neck, 2001. **23**(11): p. 933-941. DOI: 10.1002/hed.1135

[123] Ho, C.M., et al., Squamous cell carcinoma of the hypopharynx--analysis of treatment results. Head Neck, 1993. **15**(5): p. 405-412. DOI: 10.1002/hed.2880150507

[124] Lowe, V.J., et al., Surveillance for recurrent head and neck cancer using positron emission tomography. J Clin Oncol, 2000. **18**(3): p. 651-658. DOI: 10.1200/JCO.2000.18.3.651

[125] Conessa, C., et al., FDG-PET scan in local follow-up of irradiated head and neck squamous cell carcinomas. Ann Otol Rhinol Laryngol, 2004. **113**(8): p. 628-635. DOI: 10.1177/000348940411300806

[126] Bataini, J.P., et al., Significance and therapeutic implications of tumor regression following radiotherapy in patients treated for squamous cell carcinoma of the oropharynx and pharyngolarynx. Head Neck, 1990. **12**(1): p. 41-49. DOI: 10.1002/hed.2880120106

[127] Chmura, S.J., M.T. Milano, and D.J. Haraf, Reirradiation of recurrent head and neck cancers with curative intent. Semin Oncol, 2004. **31**(6): p. 816-821. DOI: 10.1053/j.seminoncol.2004.09.003

[128] Creak, A.L., K. Harrington, and C. Nutting, Treatment of recurrent head and neck cancer: re-irradiation or chemotherapy? Clin Oncol (R Coll Radiol), 2005. **17**(3): p. 138-147. DOI: 10.1016/j.clon.2004.10.008

[129] Leemans, C.R., P.J.F. Snijders, and R.H. Brakenhoff, The molecular landscape of head and neck cancer. Nat Rev Cancer, 2018. **18**(5): p. 269-282. DOI: 10.1038/nrc.2018.11

[130] Ferris, R.L., et al., Nivolumab for Recurrent Squamous-Cell Carcinoma of the Head and Neck. N Engl J Med, 2016. **375**(19): p. 1856-1867. DOI: 10.1056/NEJMoa1602252

[131] Cramer, J.D., et al., The changing therapeutic landscape of head and neck cancer. Nat Rev Clin Oncol, 2019. **16**(11): p. 669-683. DOI: 10.1038/s41571-019-0227-z

Chapter 8

Role of Organ Preservation in Locally Advanced Hypopharyngeal Carcinoma

Farida Nazeer, Rejnish Ravi Kumar, Malu Rafi, Lekha M. Nair, Kainickal Cessal Thommachan and Kunnambath Ramadas

Abstract

Hypopharyngeal carcinoma is relatively rare and has the worst prognosis of all head and neck cancers. Initially, surgery followed by postoperative radiation was the standard of care for locally advanced disease. In the recent years, various organ sparing approaches have evolved. There are mainly two schools of thought regarding larynx preservation in hypopharyngeal cancers which include either induction chemotherapy followed by response assessment for radical radiotherapy or concurrent chemoradiation. An ongoing trial is comparing the effectiveness between these two established approaches. The role of anti-EGFR therapy and immunotherapy is still being evaluated. Despite all the advancements in treatment, hypopharyngeal cancers are still associated with poor treatment outcomes.

Keywords: organ preservation, hypopharyngeal cancer, locally advanced, induction chemotherapy, concurrent chemoradiation

1. Introduction

Hypopharyngeal carcinoma accounts for about 3% of all head and neck cancers [1]. Anatomically, the subsites include the piriform sinus, the posterior pharyngeal wall, and the post-cricoid region up to the esophageal inlet. Mostly squamous cell carcinoma of the hypopharynx presents as a locally advanced disease which is constituted by Stage III and IVa. Initially, surgery followed by postoperative radiotherapy was the most common treatment modality for these patients. The exploration of organ preservation approaches has opened a new area of research in hypopharyngeal and laryngeal tumors. The role of definitive radiotherapy (RT) was explored since the beginning of the twentieth century. Later, the role of chemotherapy either as induction or concurrent in addition to RT was also investigated. Despite all these available approaches, hypopharyngeal carcinomas still have the worst prognosis of all head and neck cancers with a reported 5-year overall survival rate of about 30–35% [2, 3]. About 50% of patients develop local recurrence within the first year itself and the majority develop distant metastasis too [3].

IntechOpen

2. Locally advanced carcinoma hypopharynx

Laryngeal preservation can be explained as the maintenance of the function of the larynx which excludes laryngectomy, long-term tracheostomy, and long-term feeding tube. The definition of larynx preservation was made more accurate in 2009 by a group of experts who defined the term laryngoesophageal dysfunction free survival (LEDFS) which comprised local failure, salvage laryngectomy, tracheostomy or feeding tube at 2 years or thereafter [4]. Major studies of laryngeal preservation were done in laryngeal carcinoma. The promising results of these studies have paved a way to adopt the same modalities in hypopharyngeal cancers also. Even before the publishing of any Phase 3 trials in organ preservation approaches, in a population-based review of hypopharyngeal cancers by Newman et al. [2], it was observed that there is a trend towards using radical radiotherapy than surgery since 1990.Thereafter chemotherapy has been incorporated along with radiation in various combinations in the management. The organ preservation strategies can be either nonsurgical or surgical. The various nonsurgical laryngeal preservation approaches in locally advanced hypopharyngeal squamous cell carcinoma include induction chemotherapy (IC) followed by radical radiotherapy (RT); concurrent chemoradiation (CCRT); IC followed by CCRT and use of anti EFFR or monoclonal antibodies along with RT.

2.1 Induction chemotherapy followed by radical radiotherapy

There was a paradigm shift in the management of locally advanced laryngeal cancers with the publishing of the Veterans Affairs Laryngeal Cancer Study Group (VALCSG) [5] which studied the role of induction chemotherapy (IC) followed by radiotherapy (RT) versus surgery followed by RT in Stage III and IV laryngeal cancers. This landmark trial has established IC followed by RT to be the preferred organ preservation approach in locally advanced laryngeal cancers [6]. This trial initiated many studies in organ preservation in hypopharyngeal cancers as well.

The earliest Phase 3 randomized trial that studied the role of organ preservation in hypopharyngeal cancers was the EORTC 24891 trial [7] which included 194 patients who were randomized to receive either IC (Cisplatin 100 mg/m2 Day 1 and 5Fluorouracil[5-FU] 1000 mg/m2 infusion over 5 days) for 2–3 cycles followed by RT (N = 100) for patients with a complete response or surgical resection followed by postoperative RT (PORT) (N = 94). The 3-year overall survival (OS) for the IC arm was superior to the surgical arm (57% vs. 43%) but the 5-year OS rates were similar (30% with IC Vs 35% with surgery). The trend for disease-free survival (DFS) was similar to OS with the rates at 3 and 5-years being 43% and 25% for the IC arm versus 32% and 27% for the surgical arm, respectively. The laryngectomy free survival at 3 and 5 years in the IC arm were 28% and 17% respectively. It was also seen that the 3 and 5-year rates of retaining a functional larynx in induction chemotherapy arm were 42% and 35%, respectively. The 10-year update showed that the OS rate at 10 years was 13.8% (surgery arm) and 13.1% (IC arm) and the PFS rates were 8.5% and 10.8%, respectively. The 5- and 10-year rates of survival with preserved larynx were 21.9% and 8.7% respectively, thus confirming the role of IC followed by RT in the larynx preservation approach [8]. Thus, this trial validated the role of IC followed by RT in responders to chemotherapy as an alternative to laryngectomy for locally advanced hypopharyngeal cancers without compromising on survival or disease control.

The EORTC 24954 Phase 3 randomized control trial was done to assess the feasibility of delivering more cycles of chemotherapy [9]. This study compared alternative chemotherapy with RT versus IC followed by RT in patients with laryngeal and hypopharyngeal tumors. This trial included 450 patients who were randomized to either 2 cycles of IC (Cisplatin and 5-FU) followed by additional 2 cycles in responders followed by radiotherapy (70Gy total) or alternating arm of 4 cycles of chemotherapy (cisplatin and 5-FU) alternating with RT 20Gy during the three 2 -week intervals between chemotherapy cycles (total 60Gy). Salvage surgery followed by PORT was offered to patients who did not respond to IC. The 3-year and 5-year rates of survival with a functional larynx were similar in both arms. Acute toxic effects were statistically significantly high in the sequential arm. But in this trial, the radiotherapy doses used were different (median dose for the IC arm was 71.5 Gy and for the alternating arm was 62.8Gy). The 10-year follow-up of the study also showed that the survival with functional larynx and overall survival were similar in both arms (18.7% and 33.6% in IC arm versus 18.3% and 31.6% in alternating arm) [10]. It was also observed there was a small trend for higher larynx preservation and better laryngeal function in the alternating arm. The late toxicities were similar in both arms and there was better tolerance of treatment in the alternating arm which may be explained by the lower doses of chemotherapy and radiotherapy doses in the investigational arm. Though this alternating chemotherapy and radiotherapy has been validated in the literature, this regimen has not been routinely practiced which may be due to the technical difficulty of institutions in delivering such alternating schedules.

In this background, studies investigated the benefit of addition of Docetaxel to IC along with Cisplatin and 5FU (TPF) in laryngeal and hypopharyngeal tumors. The superiority of 3 drug IC with the addition of a taxane to Cisplatin and 5 FU in terms of OS and PFS for advanced- stage head and neck cancers has been established by the TAX 323 [11] and TAX 324 trials [12]. To evaluate the same in locally advanced laryngeal or hypopharyngeal cancers, the GORTEC 2000–2001 trial was conducted [13]. This included 220 patients who were eligible for a total laryngectomy. The randomization was between IC with TPF (docetaxel at 75 mg/m2 on day 1, cisplatin at 75 mg/m2on day 1, and 5-FU at a dose of 750 mg/m2 continuous infusion over 5 days) Vs PF (cisplatin 100 mg/m2 on day 1 and 5-FU given at a dose of 1,000 mg/m2 continuous infusion over 5 days). Three cycles of IC chemotherapy were given in each arm and the responders (complete response at the primary site or partial response and recovered normal larynx mobility) received radical RT while non-responders underwent total laryngectomy and postoperative RT. The 3-year laryngeal preservation rate was 70.3% (TPF) vs. 57.5%(PF). The overall response was statistically higher in the TPF arm when compared to the PF arm (80.0% vs. 59.2%, P = .002). The acute toxicities to chemotherapy were variable in both arms with the TPF arm having more grade 2 alopecia, grade 4 neutropenia, and febrile neutropenia, while the PF arm had more grade 3 and 4 stomatitis, thrombocytopenia, and grade 4 creatinine elevation. The long-term efficacy and safety of the trial with a median follow-up of 105 months showed that the 5-year and 10-year larynx preservation rates were 74.0% vs. 58.1% and 70.3% vs. 46.5% (P = .01) in the TPF vs. PF arm, respectively [14]. Fewer grade 3–4 late toxicities were higher in the TPF arm when compared with the PF arm. (9.3% vs. 17.1%, P = .038).

Thus, IC with TPF was found to be superior to PF with respect to laryngeal preservation rates in locally advanced laryngeal and hypopharyngeal cancers hence being a reasonable organ preservation approach albeit the toxicity of chemotherapy.

The major difference between the EORTC 24954 trial and GORTEC 2000–2001 trial was that radical radiotherapy was given to only complete responders to chemotherapy in the EORTC study while RT was given to patients with complete response in primary site or partial response with recovered normal mobility of larynx in the latter study.

Moreover, in the subsite analysis of MACH-NC, induction chemotherapy has shown a 5-year absolute benefit of 5.3% in OS and 3.3% in event-free survival (EFS) in hypopharyngeal cancers [15].

2.2 Concurrent chemotherapy

The role of concurrent chemotherapy along with RT in head and neck squamous cell carcinoma was established in the large MACH-NC meta-analysis and its updates [15–19]. The addition of chemotherapy concurrently to radiotherapy had shown improved survival for all tumor sites with an absolute 5-year OS benefit of 3.9% in the subset analysis of hypopharyngeal cancers. Thus, concurrent chemoradiation is another potential strategy that can be practiced for the organ preservation approach.

The role of CCRT in organ preservation for laryngeal cancers was established in RTOG 91–11 and its update and the study had shown a higher 10-year laryngeal preservation rate in CCRT arm over IC followed by RT when compared to RT alone [20, 21]. This study was only for laryngeal cancers and did not include patients with primary in the hypopharynx. Concurrent chemoradiation in hypopharyngeal cancers was studied in a phase 3 randomized trial by Prades et al. [22]. This trial included 81 patients with T3N0 pyriform sinus tumors only and the randomization arms were either CCRT with Cisplatin or IC with Cisplatin and 5-FU followed by response assessment for RT. The 2-year laryngeal preservation rates were 68% in the IC and 92% in the CCRT arm ($p = 0.016$) and the two-year event-free survival rates were 36% (IC arm) and 41% (CCRT arm) respectively without any difference in overall survival (47% vs. 51%). Even though this trial showed that CCRT is superior to IC followed by RT in responders, it included only a specific subset of patients and the sample size was also less.

To conclude, there are two schools of thought in the organ preservation approach in hypopharyngeal cancers which include either induction chemotherapy followed by response assessment or concurrent chemoradiation. These two approaches are being compared in the ongoing Phase 3 French trial (GORTEC 2014–2103-SALTORL) which randomizes patients with laryngeal and hypopharyngeal cancers into IC with TPF followed by RT vs. CCRT with Cisplatin [23].

2.3 Induction chemotherapy followed by chemoradiation

No trials have evaluated the role of induction chemotherapy followed by chemoradiation in hypopharyngeal cancers alone. Various studies have shown that IC with 3 drugs is not superior to CCRT alone in head and neck squamous cell carcinoma and the meta-analysis by Budach et al. also showed that induction chemotherapy with TPF before CCRT did not improve OS and PFS in locally advanced head and neck cancers compared to chemoradiation [24–27].

2.4 Role of anti-EGFR therapy

Anti-EGFR therapy has been tried in different combinations in the management of various head and neck squamous cell carcinomas. Various trials have compared RT alone vs. RT plus anti-EGFR [28, 29]; CCRT vs. CCRT plus anti-EGFR [30–32]; RT with Cetuximab vs. CCRT with Cetuximab [33]; CCRT vs. RT plus anti-EGFR [34–36] and IC followed by RT with Cetuximab vs. CCRT [37]. But there has been no proven benefit for anti-EGFR therapy in addition to concurrent chemoradiation in terms of overall survival in head and neck cancers.

There are no Phase 3 trials that have evaluated the role of anti-EGFR therapy specifically in hypopharyngeal and laryngeal cancers. Two Phase 2 trials have investigated the role of Cetuximab in these tumors. These include the GORTEC TREMPLIN trial and the DELOS trial which had studied the role of addition of Cetuximab to RT following IC with TPF (38–40). Both studies did not prove any superiority with the addition of Cetuximab and showed an increase in adverse effects in those receiving Cetuximab. Thus, there is no proven data for the use of anti-EGFR therapy in hypopharyngeal cancers and more Phase 3 studies are required to establish its role.

2.5 Role of immunotherapy

Immunotherapy has no established role in the management of locally advanced hypopharyngeal cancers. The JAVELIN trial which included locally advanced cancers of hypopharynx, oropharynx, larynx, and oral cavity studied the role of Avelumab with concurrent chemoradiation [38]. The interim analysis did not show any significant improvement in PFS with the addition of Avelumab to CCRT.

2.6 Surgery

Various partial resection procedures that do not include a total pharyngolaryngectomy are available as organ preservation strategy. They include endoscopic transoral laser microsurgery (TLM), supracricoid partial laryngectomy, and partial pharyngectomy [39].

The ability to get a negative margin in hypopharyngeal cancers makes these procedures challenging. Transoral laser microsurgery (TLM) is a reasonable approach for the treatment of early and even moderately advanced tumors of the hypopharynx. Martin and Steiner et al. reported the results of 172 patients with hypopharyngeal cancer (Stage I-4%, Stage II-11%, Stage III-30% and Stage Iva-55%), mostly with piriform sinus tumors (87%) who underwent endoscopic TLM resections [40]. Even though this study demonstrated that TLM is a valid option to standard radical surgery or standard conservation treatment, it was seen that only 6% could be treated with TLM alone while 42% required TLM and neck dissection; 4% required TLM and adjuvant radiotherapy; and 48% needed TLM, neck dissection, and adjuvant radio- or radio chemotherapy. It was seen that 52% patients required adjuvant radio (chemo-)therapy. Another innovative approach is transoral robotic surgery (TORS). TORS has mainly been applied in the treatment of oropharyngeal carcinoma but has been tried in the treatment of hypopharyngeal and laryngeal cancers. As of now, there are only few case series showing better functional outcomes with TORS in T1-T2 hypopharyngeal tumors [41–44].

Even though various surgical approaches are available, they are mainly indicated in selected subset of patients, especially with early stage well defined lesions. It has to be noted that majority of the patients who undergo primary organ preservation surgery ultimately require adjuvant radiotherapy with or without chemotherapy. Adequate surgical expertise is also required for these procedures. Hence the role of surgery in organ preservation approach in locally advanced hypopharyngeal cancers remains questionable.

3. Hypopharyngeal cancers with cartilage destruction (T4a N0-N2 disease)

Patients with cartilage destruction are not ideal candidates for larynx preservation approaches and surgery followed by RT remains the standard of care in this subgroup. There is less likelihood of complete response with RT or CCRT and reduced success rates due to increased complications of salvage laryngectomy in these patients.

4. T4b or N3 disease

These subsets of patients are generally treated with palliation. Highly selective patients like those with low volume primary, absence of heavy nodes, good performance status, and younger age group may be considered for radical approach [45].

5. Future directions

Large-scale clinical trials are difficult in hypopharyngeal tumors due to the poor prognosis and uncommon incidence of such tumors. The future direction in the management of hypopharyngeal cancers is the use of immunotherapy [46]. The role of immune checkpoint inhibitors like Pembrolizumab and Nivolumab has shown promising results in recurrent or metastatic head and neck squamous cell carcinomas [47, 48]. New studies must be done to assess the effectiveness of these agents in larynx preservation. The expression of ERCC1 as a predictive biomarker in head and neck cancers including hypopharynx for chemotherapy response to 5-FU/cisplatin for both organ preservation and survival has been identified [49]. Validation of the various biomarkers is required to select the ideal candidates that can benefit from various treatments.

6. Conclusion

T1, T2 N1-N2 tumors are treated with concurrent chemoradiation. T3 N0-N2 can be treated either with concurrent chemoradiation or induction chemotherapy followed by reassessment for radical radiation. Patients with T4a N0-N2 (cartilage destruction) disease are treated with surgery followed by postoperative radiotherapy. The treatment for patients with T4b or N3 should be an individualized approach. The decreased treatment outcomes of hypopharyngeal cancers compared to laryngeal cancers are due to advanced stage at presentation disease, poor response to chemoradiation, and difficulty in salvage surgery. An ongoing trial is comparing the effectiveness between the two established organ preservation approaches. The definite role of surgery in organ preservation in locally advanced hypopharyngeal cancers requires further validation. There is no proven data for anti-EGFR or immune checkpoint inhibitors in the radical treatment of locally advanced hypopharyngeal cancers to date and trials are underway.

Conflict of interest

"The authors declare no conflict of interest."

Notes/thanks/other declarations

Nil.

Appendices and nomenclature

Nil.

Author details

Farida Nazeer, Rejnish Ravi Kumar, Malu Rafi, Lekha M. Nair,
Kainickal Cessal Thommachan* and Kunnambath Ramadas
Department of Radiation Oncology, Regional Cancer Centre,
Thiruvananthapuram, Kerala, India

*Address all correspondence to: drcessalthomas@gmail.com

References

[1] Chow LQM. Head and Neck Cancer. N Engl J Med. 2020; 382(1):60-72.

[2] Newman JR, Connolly TM, Illing EA, Kilgore ML, Locher JL, Carroll WR. Survival trends in hypopharyngeal cancer: a population-based review. Laryngoscope. 2015;125(3):624-9.

[3] Hall SF, Groome PA, Irish J, O'Sullivan B. The natural history of patients with squamous cell carcinoma of the hypopharynx. Laryngoscope. 2008;118(8):1362-71.

[4] Lefebvre JL, Ang KK, Larynx Preservation Consensus P. Larynx preservation clinical trial design: key issues and recommendations-a consensus panel summary. Int J Radiat Oncol Biol Phys. 2009;73(5):1293-303.

[5] Department of Veterans Affairs Laryngeal Cancer Study G, Wolf GT, Fisher SG, Hong WK, Hillman R, Spaulding M, et al. Induction chemotherapy plus radiation compared with surgery plus radiation in patients with advanced laryngeal cancer. N Engl J Med. 1991;324(24):1685-90.

[6] Bhattacharyya T, Kainickal CT. Current Status of Organ Preservation in Carcinoma Larynx. World J Oncol. 2018;9(2):39-45.

[7] Lefebvre JL, Chevalier D, Luboinski B, Kirkpatrick A, Collette L, Sahmoud *T. larynx* preservation in pyriform sinus cancer: preliminary results of a European Organization for Research and Treatment of Cancer phase III trial. EORTC Head and Neck Cancer Cooperative Group. J Natl Cancer Inst. 1996;88(13):890-9.

[8] Lefebvre JL, Andry G, Chevalier D, Luboinski B, Collette L, Traissac L, et al. Laryngeal preservation with induction chemotherapy for hypopharyngeal squamous cell carcinoma: 10-year results of EORTC trial 24891. Ann Oncol. 2012;23(10):2708-14.

[9] Lefebvre JL, Rolland F, Tesselaar M, Bardet E, Leemans CR, Geoffrois L, et al. Phase 3 randomized trial on larynx preservation comparing sequential vs alternating chemotherapy and radiotherapy. J Natl Cancer Inst. 2009;101(3):142-52.

[10] Henriques De Figueiredo B, Fortpied C, Menis J, Lefebvre JL, Barzan L, de Raucourt D, et al. Long-term update of the 24954 EORTC phase III trial on larynx preservation. Eur J Cancer. 2016;65:109-12.

[11] Vermorken JB, Remenar E, van Herpen C, Gorlia T, Mesia R, Degardin M, et al. Cisplatin, fluorouracil, and docetaxel in unresectable head and neck cancer. N Engl J Med. 2007;357(17):1695-704.

[12] Lorch JH, Goloubeva O, Haddad RI, Cullen K, Sarlis N, Tishler R, et al. Induction chemotherapy with cisplatin and fluorouracil alone or in combination with docetaxel in locally advanced squamous-cell cancer of the head and neck: long-term results of the TAX 324 randomized phase 3 trial. Lancet Oncol. 2011;12(2):153-9.

[13] Pointreau Y, Garaud P, Chapet S, Sire C, Tuchais C, Tortochaux J, et al. Randomized trial of induction chemotherapy with cisplatin and 5-fluorouracil with or without docetaxel for larynx preservation. J Natl Cancer Inst. 2009;101(7):498-506.

[14] Janoray G, Pointreau Y, Garaud P, Chapet S, Alfonsi M, Sire C, et al. Long-term Results of a Multicenter Randomized Phase III Trial of Induction Chemotherapy With Cisplatin, 5-fluorouracil, +/− Docetaxel for Larynx Preservation. J Natl Cancer Inst. 2016;108(4).

[15] Lacas B, Carmel A, Landais C, Wong SJ, Licitra L, Tobias JS, et al. Meta-analysis of chemotherapy in head and neck cancer (MACH-NC): An update on 107 randomized trials and 19,805 patients, on behalf of MACH-NC Group. Radiother Oncol. 2021;156:281-93.

[16] Pignon JP, Bourhis J, Domenge C, Designe L. Chemotherapy added to locoregional treatment for head and neck squamous-cell carcinoma: three meta-analyses of updated individual data. MACH-NC Collaborative Group. Meta-Analysis of Chemotherapy on Head and Neck Cancer. Lancet. 2000;355(9208):949-55.

[17] Bourhis J, Amand C, Pignon J-P. Update of MACH-NC (Meta-Analysis of Chemotherapy in Head & Neck Cancer) database focused on concomitant chemoradiotherapy. Journal of Clinical Oncology. 2004;22(14_suppl):5505-.

[18] Pignon JP, le Maitre A, Maillard E, Bourhis J, Group M-NC. Meta-analysis of chemotherapy in head and neck cancer (MACH-NC): an update on 93 randomized trials and 17,346 patients. Radiother Oncol. 2009;92(1):4-14.

[19] Blanchard P, Baujat B, Holostenco V, Bourredjem A, Baey C, Bourhis J, et al. Meta-analysis of chemotherapy in head and neck cancer (MACH-NC): a comprehensive analysis by tumour site. Radiother Oncol. 2011;100(1):33-40.

[20] Forastiere AA, Goepfert H, Maor M, Pajak TF, Weber R, Morrison W, et al. Concurrent chemotherapy and radiotherapy for organ preservation in advanced laryngeal cancer. N Engl J Med. 2003;349(22):2091-8.

[21] Forastiere AA, Maor M, Weber RS, Pajak T, Glisson B, Trotti A, et al. Long-term results of Intergroup RTOG 91-11: A phase III trial to preserve the larynx—Induction cisplatin/5-FU and radiation therapy versus concurrent cisplatin and radiation therapy versus radiation therapy. Journal of Clinical Oncology. 2006;24(18_suppl):5517-.

[22] Prades JM, Lallemant B, Garrel R, Reyt E, Righini C, Schmitt T, et al. Randomized phase III trial comparing induction chemotherapy followed by radiotherapy to concomitant chemoradiotherapy for laryngeal preservation in T3M0 pyriform sinus carcinoma. Acta Otolaryngol. 2010;130(1):150-5.

[23] Argiris A, Lefebvre JL. Laryngeal Preservation Strategies in Locally Advanced Laryngeal and Hypopharyngeal Cancers. Front Oncol. 2019;9:419.

[24] Cohen EEW, Karrison T, Kocherginsky M, Huang CH, Agulnik M, Mittal BB, et al. DeCIDE: A phase III randomized trial of docetaxel (D), cisplatin (P), 5-fluorouracil (F) (TPF) induction chemotherapy (IC) in patients with N2/N3 locally advanced squamous cell carcinoma of the head and neck (SCCHN). Journal of Clinical Oncology. 2012;30(15_suppl):5500-.

[25] Haddad R, O'Neill A, Rabinowits G, Tishler R, Khuri F, Adkins D, et al. Induction chemotherapy followed by concurrent chemoradiotherapy (sequential chemoradiotherapy) versus concurrent chemoradiotherapy alone in locally advanced head and neck cancer (PARADIGM): a randomized phase 3 trial. Lancet Oncol. 2013;14(3):257-64.

[26] Hitt R, Grau JJ, Lopez-Pousa A, Berrocal A, Garcia-Giron C, Irigoyen A, et al. A randomized phase III trial comparing induction chemotherapy followed by chemoradiotherapy versus chemoradiotherapy alone as treatment of unresectable head and neck cancer. Ann Oncol. 2014;25(1):216-25.

[27] Budach W, Bolke E, Kammers K, Gerber PA, Orth K, Gripp S, et al. Induction chemotherapy followed by

concurrent radio-chemotherapy versus concurrent radio-chemotherapy alone as treatment of locally advanced squamous cell carcinoma of the head and neck (HNSCC): A meta-analysis of randomized trials. Radiother Oncol. 2016;118(2):238-43.

[28] Bonner JA, Harari PM, Giralt J, Azarnia N, Shin DM, Cohen RB, et al. Radiotherapy plus cetuximab for squamous-cell carcinoma of the head and neck. N Engl J Med. 2006;354(6):567-78.

[29] Bonner JA, Harari PM, Giralt J, Cohen RB, Jones CU, Sur RK, et al. Radiotherapy plus cetuximab for locoregionally advanced head and neck cancer: 5-year survival data from a phase 3 randomized trial, and relation between cetuximab-induced rash and survival. Lancet Oncol. 2010;11(1):21-8.

[30] Ang KK, Zhang Q, Rosenthal DI, Nguyen-Tan PF, Sherman EJ, Weber RS, et al. Randomized phase III trial of concurrent accelerated radiation plus cisplatin with or without cetuximab for stage III to IV head and neck carcinoma: RTOG 0522. J Clin Oncol. 2014;32(27):2940-50.

[31] Patil VM, Noronha V, Joshi A, Agarwal J, Ghosh-Laskar S, Budrukkar A, et al. A randomized phase 3 trial comparing nimotuzumab plus cisplatin chemoradiotherapy versus cisplatin chemoradiotherapy alone in locally advanced head and neck cancer. Cancer. 2019;125(18):3184-97.

[32] Evensen JF, Sand Hansen H, Overgaard M, Johansen J, Andersen LJ, Overgaard J. DAHANCA 9 - a randomized multicenter study to compare accelerated normo-fractionated radiotherapy with accelerated hyperfractionated radiotherapy in patients with primary squamous cell carcinoma of the head and neck (HNSCC). Acta Oncol. 2019;58(10):1502-5.

[33] Tao Y, Auperin A, Sire C, Martin L, Khoury C, Maingon P, et al. Improved Outcome by Adding Concurrent Chemotherapy to Cetuximab and Radiotherapy for Locally Advanced Head and Neck Carcinomas: Results of the GORTEC 2007-01 Phase III Randomized Trial. J Clin Oncol. 2018:JCO2017762518.

[34] Gebre-Medhin M, Brun E, Engstrom P, Haugen Cange H, Hammarstedt-Nordenvall L, Reizenstein J, et al. ARTSCAN III: A Randomized Phase III Study Comparing Chemoradiotherapy With Cisplatin Versus Cetuximab in Patients With Locoregionally Advanced Head and Neck Squamous Cell Cancer. J Clin Oncol. 2021;39(1):38-47.

[35] Mehanna H, Robinson M, Hartley A, Kong A, Foran B, Fulton-Lieuw T, et al. Radiotherapy plus cisplatin or cetuximab in low-risk human papillomavirus-positive oropharyngeal cancer (De-ESCALaTE HPV): an open-label randomized controlled phase 3 trial. Lancet. 2019;393(10166):51-60.

[36] Gillison ML, Trotti AM, Harris J, Eisbruch A, Harari PM, Adelstein DJ, et al. Radiotherapy plus cetuximab or cisplatin in human papillomavirus-positive oropharyngeal cancer (NRG Oncology RTOG 1016): a randomized, multicentre, non-inferiority trial. Lancet. 2019;393(10166):40-50.

[37] Geoffrois L, Martin L, De Raucourt D, Sun XS, Tao Y, Maingon P, et al. Induction Chemotherapy Followed by Cetuximab Radiotherapy Is Not Superior to Concurrent Chemoradiotherapy for Head and Neck Carcinomas: Results of the GORTEC 2007-02 Phase III Randomized Trial. J Clin Oncol. 2018;36(31):3077-83.

[38] Yu Y, Lee NY. JAVELIN Head and Neck 100: a Phase III trial of avelumab and chemoradiation for locally

advanced head and neck cancer. Future Oncol. 2019;15(7):687-94.

[39] Lefebvre JL. Surgery for Laryngopharyngeal SCC in the Era of Organ Preservation. Clin Exp Otorhinolaryngol. 2009;2(4):159-63.

[40] Martin A, Jackel MC, Christiansen H, Mahmoodzada M, Kron M, Steiner W. Organ preserving transoral laser microsurgery for cancer of the hypopharynx. Laryngoscope. 2008;118(3):398-402.

[41] Durmus K, Kucur C, Uysal IO, Dziegielewski PT, Ozer E. Feasibility and clinical outcomes of transoral robotic surgery and transoral robot-assisted carbon dioxide laser for hypopharyngeal carcinoma. J Craniofac Surg. 2015;26(1):235-7.

[42] Park YM, Kim WS, Byeon HK, De Virgilio A, Jung JS, Kim SH. Feasiblity of transoral robotic hypopharyngectomy for early-stage hypopharyngeal carcinoma. Oral Oncol. 2010;46(8):597-602.

[43] Dziegielewski PT, Kang SY, Ozer E. Transoral robotic surgery (TORS) for laryngeal and hypopharyngeal cancers. J Surg Oncol. 2015;112(7):702-6.

[44] Stoeckli SJ, Pawlik AB, Lipp M, Huber A, Schmid S. Salvage surgery after failure of nonsurgical therapy for carcinoma of the larynx and hypopharynx. Arch Otolaryngol Head Neck Surg. 2000;126(12):1473-7.

[45] Research ICoM. Consensus Document for Management of Larynx and Hypopharynx Cancers: Prepared as an outcome of ICMR Subcommittee on Larynx & Hypopharynx Cancers: Indian Council of Medical Research; 2017 [Available from: https://main.icmr.nic.in/sites/default/files/guidelines/Larynx%20and%20Hypopharynx%20Cancers_0.pdf.

[46] Garneau JC, Bakst RL, Miles BA. Hypopharyngeal cancer: A state of the art review. Oral Oncol. 2018;86:244-50.

[47] Chow LQM, Haddad R, Gupta S, Mahipal A, Mehra R, Tahara M, et al. Antitumor Activity of Pembrolizumab in Biomarker-Unselected Patients With Recurrent and/or Metastatic Head and Neck Squamous Cell Carcinoma: Results From the Phase Ib KEYNOTE-012 Expansion Cohort. J Clin Oncol. 2016;34(32):3838-45.

[48] Ferris RL, Blumenschein G, Jr., Fayette J, Guigay J, Colevas AD, Licitra L, et al. Nivolumab for Recurrent Squamous-Cell Carcinoma of the Head and Neck. N Engl J Med. 2016;375(19):1856-67.

[49] Hasegawa Y, Goto M, Hanai N, Ozawa T, Hirakawa H. Predictive biomarkers for combined chemotherapy with 5-fluorouracil and cisplatin in oro- and hypopharyngeal cancers. Mol Clin Oncol. 2018;8(2):378-86.

Chapter 9

Premalignant Conditions of Larynx

Nitika Mehta and Saima Tabassum

Abstract

Premalignant conditions of larynx encompass a variety of lesions that have the potential to evolve into malignant changes. The dysplastic premalignant epithelial changes of larynx have significantly increased Risk of developing in cancer than the hyperplastic stage of epithelial changes and this transformation significantly depends on the grade of dysplasia. Therefore, early diagnosis & prompt treatment should thus prevent the development of invasive carcinoma requiring more debilitating surgical resection. The histopathological examination is diagnostic & the evolution of advanced laryngoscopic surgical procedures including CO2 laser and newer treatment methods such as photodynamic therapy has shown promising results in their management.

Keywords: Premalignant lesions, larynx, keratosis, erythroplakia, leukoplakia

1. Introduction

The location of larynx is quiet unique that is it lies at the crossroads of air and food passages often referred to as part of the upper aerodigestive tract. It is also known as the organ of phonation, owing to its anatomical evolution & ability to produce voice. Indeed, from a physiologic point of view, it is essentially a valve or sphincter with a triple function: that of an open valve in respiration; that of a partially closed valve whose orifice can be modulated in phonation; that of a closed valve, protecting the trachea and bronchial tree during deglutition [1].

The larynx commences at the laryngeal inlet, (consisting of epiglottis anteriorly, aryepiglottic folds on either sides and interarytenoid fold posteriorly) and extends to the inferior border of cricoid cartilage, lying opposite the 3rd to 6th cervical vertebrae in adults and is somewhat higher in children. Structurally, it can be divided into three subsites, namely, the supraglottis, glottis and the subglottis by true and false vocal folds.

There are certain areas of larynx which are difficult to visualize through routine outpatient procedures like indirect laryngoscopy and these areas are of great clinical importance since many a times tumors tend to involve these subsites and are missed due to their anatomical location. Hence these areas require a special mention when discussing the anatomy.

Anterior commissure (anterior convergence of vocal folds and its insertion into the laminae of thyroid cartilage) is difficult to visualize through indirect laryngoscopy, it is located at the anterior junction of the two vocal folds, many a times a residual tumor is left behind during the surgical management; and if not managed properly, causes notable post-op morbidity. Between the two arytenoid cartilages is present the posterior commissure. The vocal folds extend anteriorly to form a concentration of collagen fibres, known as anterior commissure tendon or Broyle's ligament which is attached to the deep layer of lamina propria and the inner perichondrium of the thyroid cartilage. Broyle's ligament, being devoid of glands, is resistant to the spread of tumors and hence acts as an effective safety barrier for further spread of malignancy. On the other hand, the mucosa of the glottis, lying superior and inferior to this ligament, is thrown back on the bare areas of thyroid cartilage, which can gave way to malignancies to invade the thyroid cartilage.

Histologically, two types of mucosal linings can be seen in larynx. Most of it is lined by pseudostratified ciliated columnar (respiratory) epithelium, except the vocal folds, the posterior glottis, a part of aryepiglottic folds and half of posterior surface of epiglottis, which are lined by non-keratinizing stratified squamous epithelium. The transition between the two epithelia, marked by the inferior arcuate line (present on the upper surface of vocal folds), is a common site for squamous cell carcinoma in larynx. The mucous glands, though freely dispersed throughout the mucosa of the larynx, are exceptionally numerous on the posterior surface of epiglottis and in the saccule. The mucus from the glands in the saccule are responsible for the lubrication of the vocal folds [2].

The malignancy was recognized long back in ancient times but the concept of premalignancy was not introduced till the end of 19th century. The term premalignant/precancer was introduced by Dubreuilh in 1896 for skin lesion and during the same era Durant described the first documented cases of laryngeal leukoplakia as "white cicatrices" adjacent to a malignant laryngeal lesion [3]. Later after almost 4 decades Jackson in 1923 conceptulized premalignancy of larynx as similar to a "large no. of citizens leaving their regular daily routine & mobilizing preparatory to invasion" [4].

Laryngeal cancer is the most common cause of head neck cancer in United States of America & is responsible for thousands of death each year [5]. The best chance of curing any cancer is via its early detection and eradication as morbidity and mortality are proportionately related to stage. Thus, appropriate management of precancerous laryngeal lesions in those patients fortunate enough to present at this stage is obviously vital.

The premalignant lesions of larynx are the identifiable local features that with time has a tendency to transform into invasive carcinoma. This change in the local sign occurs basically due to changes in the laryngeal cell that may lead to dysplastic or hyperplastic epithelial changes. WHO (World Health Organization) has defined premalignant lesions of larynx as morphological alterations of the mucosa caused by chronic local irritative factors as referable to local expression of generalized illness, presenting a higher probability of degeneration into the carcinoma with respect to surrounding mucosa. Moreover, WHO has classified these lesions on the basis of hyperplasia & various degree of dysplastic changes into simple squamous cell hyperplasia, mild dysplasia, moderate dysplasia, severe dysplasia & carcinoma in situ [6].

The epidemiology of premalignant lesions, reveals a scarce data. However, it is known that these lesions are more prevalent in males and are frequently seen in patients above 50 years of age.

A wide array of conditions have been implicated in the development & rapid transformation of premalignant lesions into an invasive cancer, including long-term tobacco exposure and alcohol abuse, various occupational professions related to the textile industry, chemical industries dealing with wood processing. A small proportion of carcinomas appears to be related to transcriptionally active human papillomavirus infection. So these factors basically changes the morphology of the glottis epithelial cells into hyperplastic & dysplastic changes. To understand this we must know the normal epithelial spread of larynx (**Table 1**) (**Figures 1** and 2).

Nonkeratinized stratified squamous epithelium	Pseudostratified ciliated columnar epithelium with globet cells	Seromucinous glands
Anterior epiglottic surface	Ventricular folds	Posterior epiglottic surface
Upper half of the posterior epiglottic surface	Ventricle	False vocal cords
Superior margin of A-E folds	Saccule	Ventricle
Vocal cords	Subglottic region	Saccule & subglottis

Table 1.
Normal histology of larynx.

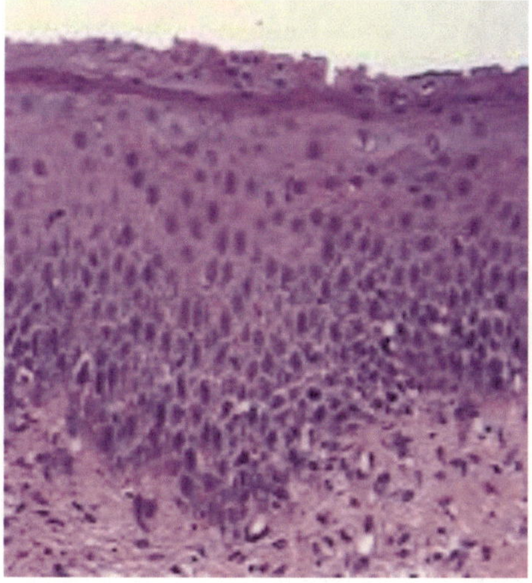

Figure 1.
Histological view of larynx (Nonkeratinized stratified squamous epithelium).

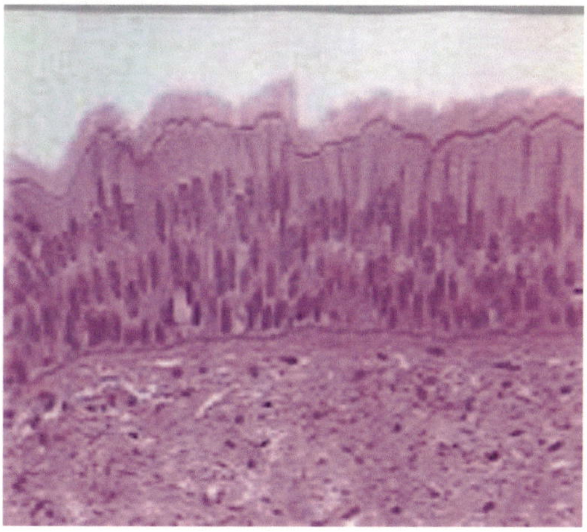

Figure 2.
Histological view of larynx (Pseudostratified ciliated columnar epithelium).

Although we are concerned about premalignant lesion only but this is important to understand the possible histological variety of malignant neoplasms that may arise in the larynx (**Table 2**) reflecting the different tissues from which they

Histological types	Squamous cell carcinoma	Muco epidermoid	Adenoid cystic	Sarcomas	Lymphoma	Neuroendocrine
Variants	1. Verrucous type 2. Spindle type 3. Basaloid type			1. Rhabdo myosarcoma 2. Chondro sarcoma		1. Carcinoid 2. Small cell

Table 2.
Histological Subtypes of Laryngeal Malignancies and their variants.

originate. The vast majority, however, are squamous carcinomas (up to 95%) and predominantly arise on the true vocal folds. All other histological subtypes will necessarily develop via a premalignant phase, but due to the paucity of such cases in the literature they have not been studied and characterized to the same extent as premalignant squamous carcinomatous lesions [7].

So it is the normal histological pattern which undergoes these various changes at the cellular & genetic level under the influence of various factors as already mentioned above, thus changes into a dysplastic or hyperplastic variation may occur, making it vulnerable to transform into a cancerous lesion.

The macroscopic changes of the lesions have no appearance & hence in clinical practice are commonly referred as: leukoplakia, erythroplakia, erythroleukoplakia, keratosis and chronic laryngitis although there is no consensus on this issue. The current laryngeal investigation systems for obtaining the high quality & resolution images so as to reveal the detailed morphology of glottis structures is one of the main task in laryngeal imaging & helps in diagnosis. These includes:

- Endoscopy–white light laryngoscopy
- Stroboscopy
- Contact endoscopy
- Autofluorescence
- Narrow band imaging (NBI)
- Ultrasound
- Computed axial tomography (CAT)/Magnetic resonance imaging (MRI)

So the appearance of lesion with these mentioned investigation system is no doubt of great help in diagnosis & prognosis of lesion but histopathological appearance is always diagnostic.

2. Etiology

The risk factors for pre malignant tumors of larynx are primarily similar to those of laryngeal carcinoma. These risk factors may cause conversion of a dysplastic lesion into metaplasia and eventually may lead to malignancy but the laryngeal neoplasia is a preventable disease in the vast majority of cases, which points out the role of various environmental and social factors. The most commonly and strongly implicated factor remains smoking. Burning cigarettes release tar that contains polycyclic aromatic hydrocarbons which have been proven to be carcinogenic and act by damaging the nucleic acids in the cells. Similarly, alcohol consumption may be an independent risk factor & in such people, supraglottic carcinoma is frequently seen. Though alcohol is directly implicated in carcinogenesis, it may be associated with other co morbidities and deficiencies as in malnutrition or vitamin deficiencies. When alcohol consumption is combined with smoking, the risk of neoplasia multiplies.

Other known etiological factor for oropharyngeal carcinoma includes the Human Papilloma Virus or the HPV; the serotypes strongly associated with oropharyngeal carcinoma are 16 and 18 (as seen in carcinoma cervix) [8].

In most HPV positive laryngeal carcinomas, serotype 16 is frequently isolated, while in recurrent respiratory papillomatosis, serotypes 6 and 11 are commonly isolated.

Recurrent respiratory papillomatosis does not usually turn into squamous carcinoma, owing to different pathogenesis, however this transformation may be seen in patients who have a history of exposure to radiation.

The epidemiological studies have shown that the prevalence of HPV in patients of laryngeal carcinoma varies greatly i.e., between 0% to 58% (grossly around 25%), depending upon the investigations and the population [9]. Lately, studies have shown that HPV and carcinoma larynx are not strongly co related. On the other hand, it has been seen that HPV can be present in people with otherwise histologically normal epithelium of larynx and with no signs or symptoms [10].

The association of GERD (Gastro Esophageal Reflux Disorder) with laryngeal malignancy has been explored by many researchers. Olson in 1983 was the pioneer to study the role of chronic laryngopharyngeal reflux (LPR) in laryngeal carcinoma [11]. He found a significant relationship between these two pathologies, where the incidence of laryngeal carcinoma was higher in patients suffering from LPR [7]. On the contrary Chen et al. found no association between GERD and laryngeal neoplasia [12].

Many other environmental factors have been known to increase the risk of laryngeal malignancy such as industrial pollutants like asbestos, malnutrition, lower socioeconomic status etc. [13]. Exposure to radiation for managing other neck tumors like thyroid cancer can also predispose to laryngeal malignancies [14].

Even the role of genetic factors have been implicated to increase the susceptibility of an individual to develop laryngeal neoplasia such as enzymatic polymorphisms in elimination and detoxification of alcohol and smoke produced carcinogens [15].

3. Molecular genetics

The concept of field cancerization was introduced by Slaughter et al in a study of oral cancer [16]. He found that there occurred histopathological abnormalities in the epithelium surrounding the invasive cancer and the abnormalities ranged from keratosis, dysplasia and hyperkeratosis, epithelial hyperplasia etc. With this concept many researchers tried to study the genetics around the tumor site and premalignant conditions to predict their clinical outcome. In many tumor types, including HNSCC (Head and Neck squamous cell carcinoma), p53 inactivation apparently occurs in the transition from the preinvasive to the invasive state [17]. A second

17p13 locus may be altered earlier in progression. Existence of an alternate gene in this region has been implied in the genetic progression of brain and breast cancer [18, 19]. In a study by Califano et al the analysis of premalignant lesions was carried out a genetic level, they concluded that early genetic study of a premalignant lesion could aid and influence our treatment strategies from a conservative to a more aggressive one according to the genetic events detected [20].

4. Classification

Various classification of premalignant laryngeal lesions have been given by various authors, still it continues to be a controversial topic of laryngeal pathology for decades now, considering the classification, histological diagnosis and the treatment aspect as well. For clinical management of these lesions system based on the evaluation of the grade of hyperplasia and/or dysplasia of epithelium have been established (**Table 2**).

According to Hellquist et al [21] a distinction can be made between various lesions:

- Grade I lesions, presenting hyperplasia and/or keratosis with or without mild dysplasia where stratification is preserved and superficial cellular layers show cytoplasmic differentiation.

  The cellular and architectural atypia occur in the lower third part with nuclear crowding, cellular and nuclear pleomorphism with increased nuclear/cytoplasmic ratio.

- Grade II lesions characterized by moderate dysplasia. Histologic changes are similar to grade I but abnormalities extend up to two-third of the thickness of the epithelium, hence the differentiation & stratification is seen in superficial layers with numerous mitotic features.

- Grade III lesions, in which dysplasia is severe or of such type as to configure carcinoma in situ. Here, non-stratified & undifferentiated cells occupy from more than two-third up to the full thickness of the epithelium in majority of the cases there is no keratinization. Nuclear pleomorphism is seen with-bizarre large nuclei & the lesion is always contained by the basal lamina.

This grading is based on the classification proposed by the Kleinsasser in 19631 and later, by Delemarre, distinguishing a first class characterized by simple squamous cell hyperplasia, a second class represented by squamous cell hyperplasia with atypia and third class represented by carcinoma in situ.

The modified Ljubljana [22, 23] classification, the modification done by a working group of European society of pathology in November 1997 in London, United Kingdom (UK) devised the classification to cater to specific clinical and histological laryngeal problems, as it does not follow the three grade criteria, so was divided it into four grades as follows:

1. Simple hyperplasia (SH) is benign group.

2. Abnormal hyperplasia (AbH) is benign group.

3. Atypical hyperplasia (AtH) is potentially malignant.

4. Carcinoma in situ is malignant.

The term dysplasia was accepted in laryngeal pathology first after the Toronto Centennial Conference on Laryngeal Cancer in 1974, almost after 11 years of proposed Kleinsasser classification. Several terms such as squamous intraepithelial neoplasia (SIN) and laryngeal intraepithelial neoplasia (LIN) were introduced. The term squamous intraepithelial neoplasia (SIN) was used for laryngeal precursor lesions by Friedmann and Osborn in 1976, and 10 years later Crissman and Fu opted for intraepithelial neoplasia of the larynx [24]. In addition, Friedmann and Ferlito used laryngeal intraepithelial neoplasia (LIN) [25]. An attempt to reconcile different schemes showed:

1. LIN I is regarded the equivalent of mild dysplasia

2. LIN II of moderate dysplasia and

3. LIN III of severe dysplasia and carcinoma in situ.

After that many editions of the World Health Organization (WHO) classification have been proposed & all such terms like as squamous intraepithelial neoplasia (SIN) and laryngeal intraepithelial neoplasia (LIN) were used but are now being abandoned and replaced by squamous intraepithelial lesions (SIL) [26, 27]. The essential update in the four editions of WHO was the attempt to induce a simplification from a four- to a two-tier system. The current WHO classification (2017) thus recommends the use of a two-tier system with reasonably clear histopathological criteria for the two groups:

1. Low-grade and

2. High-grade dysplasia.

Although the disadvantages like inter observer variability apart, subjectivities and uncertainties still remains but to a lesser degree.

Hence, it is very difficult to predict accurately which lesions will progress into invasive malignancy based only on clinical appearance. The diagnosis, treatment and prognosis of these lesions depend almost entirely on their histological abnormalities. In **Table 3** we have compared the different classifications given by different authors.

4.1 Clinical features

The most common presentation of patients harboring premalignant lesions is dysphonia which can be progressive or fluctuating. Rarely patients may even present with breathing difficulty or foreign body sensation throat.

The diagnosis is made by doing a flexible endoscopy. These lesions either appear as white keratotic patches, single, multiple or confluent (**Figures 3-5**). They are also seen as erythroplakia (red), mixed leucoerythroplakic (speckled) patches.

In general clinical appearance has shown to have poor correlation with the state of underlying epithelium [28, 29]. Still a few authors have found higher chances of malignancy and dysplasia with certain types of lesions. Following features in decreasing order of importance, ulceration, erythroplasia, surface granularity, increased keratin thickness (verrucous appearance), increased size, recurrence after excisional biopsies and long duration have all been associated with carcinoma [30].

Kleinsasser classification	WHO classification	Ljubljana classification	Modified Ljubljana classification	Freidmann and Ferlito (Laryngeal intraepithelial neoplasia)
Grade-I	Simple squamous cell hyperplasia	Simple hyperplasia	Simple hyperplasia	
Grade-II	Mild dysplasia	Abnormal hyperplasia (AbH)	Abnormal hyperplasia (AbH)	Laryngeal intraepithelial neoplasia- Grade-I
Grade III	Moderate dysplasia	Atypical hyperplasia (AtH)	Atypical hyperplasia (AtH)	Laryngeal intraepithelial neoplasia- Grade-II
	Severe dysplasia	Atypical hyperplasia (AtH)	Carcinoma in situ	Laryngeal intraepithelial neoplasia- Grade-III
	Carcinoma in situ	Carcinoma in situ		

Table 3.
Various classifications of laryngeal precancerous conditions.

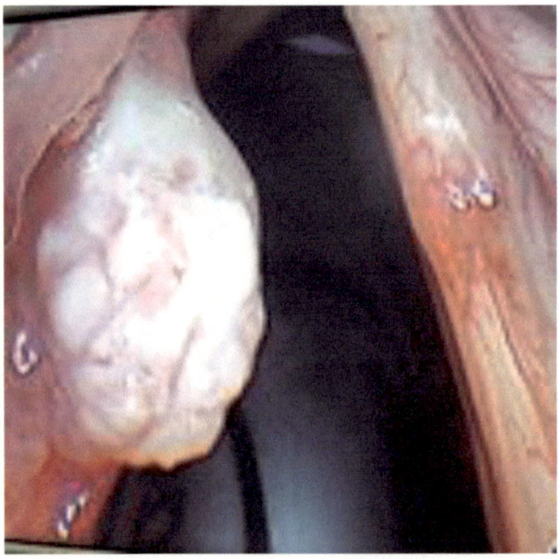

Figure 3.
Single keratotic lesion seen involving the left true vocal fold.

4.2 Management

The management of premalignant lesions is challenging for a clinician as it poses a diagnostic challenge and also because it requires close monitoring and follow up due to underlying risk of malignancy.

The laryngeal cancer represents about 1–2% of all malignant tumors. In 90% of cases carcinomas develop from precancerous epithelial lesions [31]. Prompt treatment after an early diagnosis is capable to prevent the development of an invasive neoplasm and the consequent recourse to more invasive laryngeal surgery [32, 33]. Lack of valid protocol or guidelines to manage such precancerous conditions makes it tough for an ENT surgeon to make a decision plan for their management.

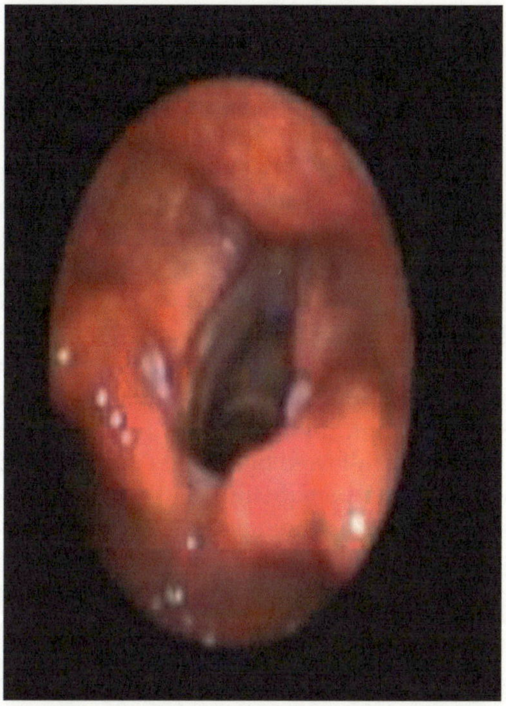

Figure 4.
Multiple Keratotic Lesion involving the bilateral arytenoids.

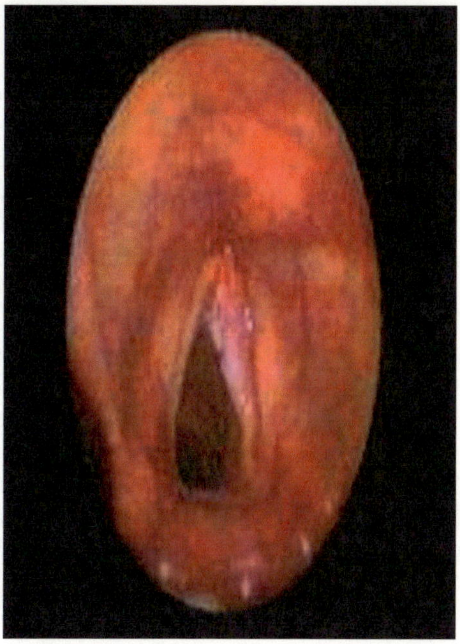

Figure 5.
Endoscopic image depicting a single confluent lesion involving the right Vocal Fold.

The dilemma in managing premalignant conditions lies in whether to manage it conservatively with close follow up or to do a biopsy. The invasiveness of the lesion and the prediction whether a lesion has a malignant potential cannot be assessed by clinical examination. Even various investigation modalities like endoscopy, stroboscopy fail to analyse the invasiveness of lesion. Newer techniques such as contact endoscopy using highly magnified images (up to 150 X) using a rigid endoscope which is placed in direct contact with vocal fold epithelium and staining is done using 1% methylene blue dye. Though it has been found to have a high sensitivity and specificity still its limitation to unable to detect the dysplasia in deeper layers and the learning curve associated with it and requiring an expertise of a pathologist has made its application limited in the field of otorhinolaryngology [28, 32, 34].

In an attempt to formulate a plan a meeting of UK otolaryngologists and pathologists involved in the care of Head and Neck cancer was held and guidance in relation to premalignant conditions was issued [35]. In case of single (**Figure 3**) and multiple foci (**Figure 4**) they should be completely excised to all visible margins, if possible and in the presence of widespread, confluent leukoplakia (**Figure 5**), histopathological mapping of the lesion with multiple biopsies should be initially performed, followed by staged resection, if feasible. Once sending the biopsy specimen proper labelling and anatomical orientation should be presented on a template to the pathologist with photo documentation prior to histological analysis.

The patient's general condition and fitness for surgery, physiological age, comorbidity and the presence of other risk factors also play a vital role in planning a surgical procedure. The most essential step to be taken before planning the surgical procedure is a detailed and vivid discussion with the patient to inform him/her about the potential risks of hoarseness and change in voice quality postoperatively and about the possibility of recurrence.

4.3 Surgical treatment

The surgical procedure options are in the form of cold steel or carbon dioxide (CO_2) laser resection. Both are taken up via an endoscopic approach. If laser excision is planned, CO_2 laser is a preferred laser type. The use of the laser for ablation is to be discouraged, because no specimen is provided for diagnosis and it may be Associated with a possible higher risk of damage and impact on voice production. Hence, stripping of the cord is also not recommended due to the poor quality voice issues.

There are a few vital points which should be borne in mind while dissecting these lesions and they are as following: A proper plane of dissection should be achieved and the vocal ligament should be preserved so as to attain a good postoperative voice quality. An overzealous dissection can lead to postoperative scarring and poor voice outcomes. In such cases excision biopsy is performed with special care so as to preserve the deeper layers of vocal cords and the surrounding normal mucosa.

In case of anterior commissure lesions there is a risk of recurrence and their progression to cancer is reported in literature so adequate clearance and regular follow up is required in case the disease is progressing to anterior commissure.

4.4 Radiotherapy

Role of radiotherapy in premalignant conditions is only reserved for those patients, in whom the surgical intervention is contraindicated due to morbidity. Many studies have shown that radiation therapy to be ineffective in preventing the progression of dysplastic lesions to carcinoma; in fact, it may even precipitate malignant degeneration [30]. Therefore, the application of radiation therapy should be reserved for invasive carcinoma only.

4.5 Follow up

The follow up of such patients is the most vital part of their management since there is always a risk of recurrence and malignant transformation. In the literature no fixed protocol has been designed for the follow up plan of premalignant lesions but it has been noted that malignant transformation rate is higher with moderate to severe dysplasia as compared to mild dysplasia [15]. To simplify things we follow a self-designed protocol according to which we divide the patients into two groups that is the high risk and low risk group. Now patients in high risk group are those who have moderate, severe dysplasia and carcinoma in situ (according to WHO classification) and patients even with mild dysplasia but who are cigarette smokers, heavy alcohol consumers are included in this group. In high risk we follow the same protocol as T1 carcinoma that is for initial 2 years every month follow up, 2 monthly in the second year, 3 monthly in the third year and 6 monthly in fourth and fifth year.

In cases of low risk group the follow up plan was to do a regular monthly check up for at least 6 months. Following that clear instructions to the patient to revert back, if there is change in voice and on appearance of any suspicious symptoms.

4.6 Other treatment options

Photodynamic Therapy (PDT) is a minimally invasive treatment that involves the activation by light of a drug (photosensitizer) that generates cytotoxic reactive oxygen species. This therapy has been specially studied in cases of premalignant laryngeal lesions. A clinical trial was conducted in 2014 using a compound named 3-(1'-hexyloxyethyl) pyropheophorbide (HPPH) mediated photodynamic therapy [36]. The results of this phase I b trials were very promising with a fewer complications rate. Though this clinical trial is still underway and hence awaiting its approval. Its use in oral cancer lesions, especially for the recurrent ones has been established by many authors [37].

5. Conclusion

Early diagnosis, timely management and a regular follow of patients harboring premalignant lesions can prevent its progression to full blown laryngeal carcinoma. The newer treatment modalities in the form of photodynamic therapy though are in their initial phase of testing but they do show a potential in future management of such lesions.

Conflict of interest

The authors declare no conflict of interest.

Abbreviations

HPV	Human papilloma virus
LPR	Laryngopharyngeal Reflux
SH	Simple Hyperplasia
AbH	Abnormal Hyperplasia
AtH	Atypical Hyperplasia

SIN	Squamous intraepithelial neoplasia
LIN	Laryngeal intraepithelial neoplasia
WHO	World Health Organization
PDT	Photodynamic therapy
HNSCC	Head and Neck Squamous cell carcinoma
HPPH	3- (1'-hexyloxyethyl) pyropheophorbide

Author details

Nitika Mehta* and Saima Tabassum
ASCOMS, Jammu, India

*Address all correspondence to: nitikamehta22@gmail.com

References

[1] Armstrong WB, Netterville JL Anatomy of the larynx, trachea, and bronchi. Otolaryngol Clin N Am (1995).28:685-99.

[2] Thiagarajan, Balasubramanian. Anatomy of Larynx A Review; Otolaryngology Online Journal. 2015;5:5-12.

[3] Horhat R, Horhat D, Poenaru M, et al. Histopathological aspects in laryngeal precancerous lesions. *Studia Universitatis Vasile Goldis (Seria Ştiințele Vieții)* 2009; 19:241-245.

[4] Sadri, Maziar, Jeremy McMahon, and Andrew Parker. "Management of laryngeal dysplasia: a review." European Archives of Oto-Rhino-Laryngology 263.9 (2006): 843-852.

[5] Meganne H, Paleri V, West C M L, Nutting C. Head and neck cancer- Part 1: Epidemiology, presentation, and prevention. BMJ 2010; 341: c4684.

[6] Kramer IR, Lucas RB, Pindborg JJ, Sobin LH. Definition of leukoplakia and related lesions: an aid to studies on oral precancer. Oral Surg Oral Med Oral Pathol. 1978 Oct;46(4):518-39. PMID: 280847.

[7] Jahangir.A, Khalid.G, Premalignant Lesions of the Larynx, Laryngology, Otorhinolaryngology-Head and Neck Surgery Series. India, 2014, 223-233.

[8] Hobbs CG, Sterne JA, Bailey M, Heyderman RS, Birchall MA, Thomas SJ. Human papillomavirus and head and neck cancer: a systematic review and meta-analysis. Clin Otolaryngol 2006;31(4):259-266.

[9] Gale N, Michaels L, Luzar B, et al. Current review on squamous intraepithelial lesions of the larynx. Histopathology 2009;54(6):639-656.

[10] Nunez DA, Astley SM, Lewis FA, Wells M. Human papilloma viruses: a study of their prevalence in the normal larynx. J Laryngol Otol 1994;108(4):319-320.

[11] Olson NR. Effects of stomach acid on the larynx. Proc Am Laryngol Assoc 1983;104:108-112.

[12] Chen MY, Ott DJ, Casolo BJ, Moghazy KM, Koufman JA. Correlation of laryngeal and pharyngeal carcinomas and 24-hour pH monitoring of the esophagus and pharynx. Otolaryngol Head Neck Surg. 1998;119: 460-462) (retraction in Chen MY, Ott DJ, Koufman JA. Otolaryngol Head Neck Surg. 1999;121:168).

[13] Sheahan P, Ganly I, Rhy Evans PH, Patel SG. Tumours of the larynx. In Montgomery PQ, Rhys Evans PH, Gullane PJ (eds). Principles and Practice of Head and Neck Surgery and Oncology. 2nd ed. London, UK: Informa Health Care; 2009:257-290.

[14] Baker DC Jr, Weissman B. Postirradiation carcinoma of the larynx. Ann Otol Rhinol Laryngol 1971;80(5):634-637.

[15] Geisler SA, Olshan AF, Cai J, Weissler M, Smith J, Bell D. Glutathione S-transferase polymorphisms and survival from head and neck cancer. Head Neck 2005;27(3):232-242

[16] Slaughter DP, Southwick HW, Smejkal W. Field cancerization in oral stratified squamous epithelium; clinical implications of multicentric origin. Cancer. 1953 Sep;6(5):963-8. doi: 10.1002/1097-0142(195309)6:5<963:: aid-cncr2820060515>3.0.co;2-q. PMID: 13094644.

[17] Boyle Jo, Hakim J, Koch W, van der Riet P,Hruban RH, Roa RA, Correo R, Eby YJ, Ruppert JM, Sidransky D. The

incidence of p53 mutations increases with progression of head and neck cancer. Cancer Res. 1993 Oct 1; 53 (19):4477-80.PMID:8402617.

[18] Saxena, A., Clark, W. C., Robertson, J. T., Ikejiri, B., Oldfield, E. H., and All, I. U. Evidence for the involvement of a potential second tumor suppressor gene on chromosome 17 distinct from p53 in malignant astrocytomas. Cancer Res., 52: 6716â€”6721, 1992.

[19] Merlo, G. R., Venesio, T., Bernardi, A., Cropp, C. S., Diella, F., Cappa, A. P., Callahan, R., and Uscia, D. S. Evidence for a second tumor suppressor gene on l'lp linked to high S-phase index in primary human breast carcinomas. Cancer Genet. Cytogenet., 76: 106â€”11, 1994.

[20] Califano J, van der Riet P, Westra W, Nawroz H, Clayman G, Piantadosi S, Corio R, Lee D, Greenberg B, Koch, Sidransky D. Genetic progression model for head and neck cancer: implications for field cancerization. Cancer Res. 1996 Jun 1;56 (11):2488-92. PMID: 8653682.

[21] Hellquist H, Lundgren J, Oloffson J. Hyperplasia, keratosis, dysplasia and carcinoma in situ of the vocal cords- a follow up study. Clin Otolaryngol allied Sci. 1982;7(1): 11-27.PMID: 7037233.

[22] Poljak M, Gale N Kambic V. Human papillomaviruses: a study of their prevalence in the epithelial hyperplastic lesions of the larynx. Acta Otolaryngol Suppl. 1997; 527:66-9. doi:10.3109/00016489709124038. PMID:9197485.

[23] Kambic V, Lenart I. Our classification of hyperplasia of the laryngeal epithelium from the prognostic point of view. Journal Francais D'oto-rhino-laryngologie, Audio-phonologie et Chirurgie Maxillo-faciale. 1971 Dec;20(10):1145-1150.

[24] Friedmann I, Osborn DA. The larynx. In: Symmers WSTC, editor. Systemic pathology. 3rd ed. Edinburgh:Churchill Livingstone; 1976.

[25] Crissman JD, Fu YS. Intraepithelial neoplasia of the larynx. A clinicopathologic study of six cases with DNA analysis. Arch Otolaryngol Head Neck Surg. 1986;112:522-8. doi:10.1001/archotol.1986.03780050046008

[26] Gale N, Pilch BZ, Sidransky D, Westra WH, Califano J. Epithelial precursor lesions. In: Barnes L, Eveson JW, Reichart P, Sidransky D, editors. Pathology and genetics head and neck tumours WHO classification of tumours. Lyon: IARC Press; 2005. p. 177-179.

[27] El-Naggar AK, Chan JKC, Grandis JR, Takata T, Slootweg PJ, editors. WHO classification of head and neck tumours. Lyon: IARC; 2017.

[28] Gale, N., Michaels, L., Luzar, B., Poljak, M., Zidar, N., Fischinger, J. and Cardesa, A. (2009), Current review on squamous intraepithelial lesions of the larynx. Histopathology, 54: 639-656. doi:10.1111/j.1365-2559.2008.03111.x.

[29] Hrvoje Čupic, Božo Krušlin & Mladen Belicza (1997) Epithelial Hyperplastic Lesions of the Larynx in Biopsy Specimens, Acta Oto Laryngologica, 117:sup527, 103,104, doi: 10.3109/00016489709124047.

[30] Hakeem AH, Hakeem IH, Pradhan SA. Premalignant lesions of the larynx and their management. Otorhinolaryngol Clin Int J.2010;2:161-5.

[31] Minni A, Barbaro M, Rispoli G, Diaferia F, Bernardeschi D, Filipo R. Treatment with laser CO2 cordectomy and clinical implications in management of mild and moderate laryngeal precancerosis. Eur Arch Otolaryngol 2008;265: 189-93.

[32] Kleinsasser O. [The classification and differential diagnosis of epithelial hyperplasia of the laryngeal mucosa on the basis of histomorphological features. II] Z Laryngol Rhinol Otol.1963;42:339-62.

[33] Malzahn K, Dreyer T, Glanz H, Arens C. Autofluorescence endoscopy in the diagnosis of early laryngeal cancer and its precursor lesions. Laryngoscope 2002;112:488-93.

[34] Ferlay J, Shin HR, Bray F, Forman D, Mathers C, Parkin DM. Estimates of worldwide burden of cancer in 2008: GLOBACON 2008. Int J Cancer 2010; 127 (12);2893-2917.

[35] Mehanna H, Paleri V, Robson A, Wight R, Helliwell T. Consensus statement by otorhinolaryngologists and pathologists on the diagnosis and management of laryngeal dysplasia. *Clin Otolaryngol*. 2010;35(3):170-176. doi:10.1111/j.1749-4486.2010.02119.x.

[36] Rigual N, Shafirstein G, Cooper MT, et al. Photodynamic therapy with 3-(1'-hexyloxyethyl) pyropheophorbide a for cancer of the oral cavity. *Clin Cancer Res*. 2013;19(23):6605-6613. doi:10.1158/1078-0432.CCR-13-1735.

[37] Mimikos C, Shafirstein G, Arshad H. Current state and future of photodynamic therapy for the treatment of head and neck squamous cell carcinoma. *World J Otorhinolaryngol Head Neck Surg*. 2016;2(2):126-129. doi:10.1016/j.wjorl.2016.05.011.

Chapter 10

Transoral Videolaryngoscopic Surgery (TOVS)

Koji Araki and Akihiro Shiotani

Abstract

Transoral videolaryngoscopic surgery (TOVS) for laryngopharyngeal cancer developed by Shiotani et al., uses the laparoscopic surgical system and distending laryngoscope. This method enables precise procedures and en bloc resection under a good view with videoendoscope in the structurally complex laryngopharynx. The major indications are Tis-2, and selected T3 lesions of hypopharyngeal, oropharyngeal, and supraglottic laryngeal cancer. TOVS is also considered for resectable rT1 and rT2 radiation failure cases and selected T3–4 advanced cases following neoadjuvant chemotherapy. Patients with resectable lymph node metastases are treated by neck dissection. Major contraindications are crico-arytenoid joint fixation, circumferential invasion of more than half, bilateral arytenoid invasion, and invasion to the thyroid cartilage, cricoid cartilage, hyoid bone, deep pharyngeal constrictor muscle. Oncological outcomes are good in long-term survival and larynx preservation rates with sparing radiation in half of the patients. However, advanced T stage and N3 cases showed a worse prognosis. Regarding functional outcome, swallowing function can maintain in most patients. Postoperative voice impairment can occur after wound healing. TOVS has some advantages particularly for hypopharyngeal cancer, in maneuver with smaller diameter instruments and tactile sense, and in less invasiveness without a tracheostomy, compared to other transoral surgeries.

Keywords: Transoral videolaryngoscopic surgery (TOVS), transoral surgery, hypopharyngeal cancer, swallowing function, voice impairment, sentinel node navigation surgery, conversion surgery, neoadjuvant chemotherapy

1. Introduction

Transoral videolaryngoscopic surgery (TOVS) for laryngopharyngeal cancer was developed by Shiotani and his colleagues in Japan since 2004 and the first report was published in 2010 [1–4]. This novel endoscopic transoral surgical system uses the laparoscopic surgical system and distending laryngoscope which enables en bloc resection under a good view with videoendoscope. Recently, surgical instruments used in TOVS have been modified to some extent. Good long-term survival, larynx preservation, and functional outcomes were reported [5]. In this chapter, the tips and the pearls of TOVS including detail of the surgical procedures, managements, and outcomes are described.

2. The feature of TOVS

The break out of transoral surgery for laryngopharyngeal cancer was started from transoral laser microsurgery (TLM), developed by Steiner et al. [6]. TLM is suitable for glottic lesions which are required fine and precise maneuver in a limited narrow space. Although TLM yields good oncological outcomes, the microscopic view through a rigid laryngoscope is linear and is not wide enough to observe the entire laryngopharynx. Particularly when observing the postcricoid area and inner surface of the epiglottis, it is often hidden by the blade of the laryngoscope. Multiple repositioning of the laryngoscope is also needed when the lesion is relatively large. In addition, pathological workup is difficult when piece-by-piece resection is performed.

To overcome these drawbacks, TOVS was developed. The endoscopic view under a flexible videoscope is wider than that under a microscope, and a wide working space can be achieved by using the FKWO retractor. This method enables detailed observation, precise procedures, and en bloc resection in the structurally complex laryngopharynx.

Although transoral robotic surgery (TORS) is actively performed for hypopharyngeal cancer in South Korea, tracheostomy is required because the intubation tube interferes with the arms of the robot [7]. In TOVS, a videoscope and forceps with a smaller diameter than the arms of the robot are used; hence, surgical procedure without tracheostomy is possible even in the narrow and distal spaces such as the hypopharynx. In addition, the surgeon has tactile sense through instruments. Therefore, TOVS has some advantages in maneuver and is less invasive compared to TLM and TORS, particularly for hypopharyngeal cancer.

3. Indications

The major indications for TOVS are Tis, T1, and T2 lesions of hypopharyngeal, oropharyngeal, and supraglottic laryngeal cancer. TOVS is also indicated for selected T3 lesions without deep invasion. Furthermore, TOVS is considered for small radiation failure cases (rT1 and rT2) if the lesions are resected with enough margins [8]. TOVS is also considered in advanced T3 or T4 cases after the tumor shrinks to a limited area following neoadjuvant chemotherapy (NAC). However, it is not a standard indication due to issues in the resection area, possibly leading to oncologically inadequate resection, as described in Section 11.3 (**Table 1**).

Anatomical contraindications for TOVS are cricoarytenoid joint fixation due to cancer invasion, circumferential invasion of more than half of the esophageal inlet, bilateral arytenoid invasion, and invasion to the thyroid cartilage, cricoid cartilage, hyoid bone, deep pharyngeal constrictor muscle, hard palate, and pterygoid hamulus. Oncologically sufficient resection is technically difficult, and functional preservation may not be excellent because of dysphagia and respiratory disorders due to postoperative stenosis and vocal cord movement restriction.

Patients with resectable lymph node metastases are treated by neck dissection (ND) along with TOVS on the same day or 1–2 weeks later. TOVS is generally performed in N1–N2 cases; however, although they are technically resectable, TOVS is not generally indicated in N3 cases due to poor prognosis [5]. Considering that postoperative chemoradiotherapy is needed in most N3 cases, transoral surgery has little significance due to increased invasiveness without improvement in oncological outcomes.

Although the extent of lesions is the basis of decision making for surgical indications, the final decision is made by considering the systemic condition. Preoperative swallowing function should be evaluated in cases predisposed to dysphagia, and surgical indication should be conservatively decided. Age; performance status;

Primary site	Hypopharynx, oropharynx, supraglottic cancer Tis-T2, selected T3 cases Resectable rT1–2 cases Seleted advanced T cases following NAC Contraindications Cricoarytenoid joint fixation Circumferential invasion of more than half Bilateral arytenoid invasion Invasion to the thyroid cartilage, cricoid cartilage, hyoid bone, deep pharyngeal constrictor muscle etc.
Cervical lymph node metastases	N1–2 cases Neck dissection along with TOVS
Other factors	Preoperative swallowing function Radiation history, Comorbidity (cardiorespiratory diseases, diabetes etc.) Age, Performance status, Family environments

Table 1.
Indications for TOVS.

medical history including radiation history; comorbidities such as respiratory diseases, cardiovascular diseases, and diabetes; and family environments should also be considered.

4. Devices

The FKWO retractor (**Figure 1a**, Olympus medical systems, Tokyo, Japan) with various blades is used to expose the laryngo-hypopharynx and widen the operative field of view in most cases. Weerda distending video laryngoscope (8588BV; Karl Storz, Tuttlingen, Germany) is also useful.

Endoeye flex (LTE-S190–5, Olympus Medical Systems, Tokyo, Japan; **Figure 1b**), an HD videoendoscope with a thin 5-mm diameter and an articulating tip that can bend in all directions up to 100°, is used to observe the surgical field in most cases. This endoscope is suitable to observe the structurally complex laryngopharynx with minimal device conflict during transoral surgery. In addition, it has the function of image-enhanced endoscopy (narrow-band imaging: NBI), which is useful for evaluating the extent of mucosal lesions. A rigid laryngeal endoscope (8575AV; Karl Storz), connected to a high-definition camera set (22220150–3; Karl Storz), also provides a wide and clear view.

For forceps, scissors, electrocautery electrodes, suction coagulators, and clip applicators, reusable straight devices are used. Incision and separation are performed using laparoscopic surgical instruments measuring 3 mm in diameter connected to an ordinary electrocautery unit, including separating (30721MD; Karl Storz) or scissor-type (30721 MW; Karl Storz) tip forceps and hook-type (26870UF; Karl Storz) or needle-type (26167NX; Karl Storz) scalpels. For hemostasis, a suction coagulator (8606E; Karl Storz) or hemostatic clips (8665 L and 8665R; Karl Storz) are used (**Figure 1c**).

New malleable or curved devices, including LaryngoFIT forceps and scissors (8791GHZ, 8793AZ, 8791AZ, and 8794AZ, Karl Storz, Tuttlingen, Germany), a malleable needle electrocautery electrode (KD600, Olympus medical systems, Tokyo, Japan), a fiber guide CO2 laser (AcuPulse DUO, Lumenis, Yokneam Illit, Israel), and a malleable suction coagulator (7030010, Amco, Tokyo, Japan), have been recently shown to be very helpful (**Figure 1d**). Most of these devices have a

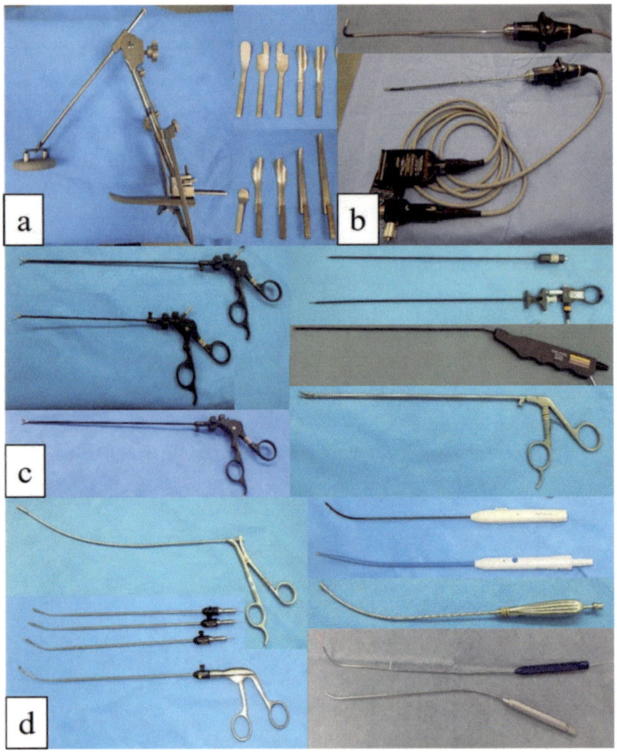

Figure 1.
Devices for TOVS. a. FKWO retractor, b. Endoeye flex, c. straight devices - forceps, scissors, electrocautery electrodes, suction coagulators, and clip applicators, d. malleable and curved devices - curved forceps, malleable forceps and scissors, malleable needle electrocautery electrode, malleable suction coagulator, curved suction, malleable and curved handpieces of fiber guide CO2 laser.

thin shaft of approximately 3 mm in diameter, except for the malleable suction coagulator, which has a thin shaft measuring 5 mm in diameter. These devices are effective for approaching from any direction in the view of the endoscope, allowing the surgeon to make parallel or perpendicular cuts along the line of sight [5].

5. Surgical procedures

5.1 Setting

TOVS is performed under general anesthesia by orotracheal intubation using a small diameter (6–7 mm) reinforced endotracheal tube. When the resection area includes the epiglottis and tongue base, nasotracheal intubation is recommended.

To expose the surgical fields, a FKWO retractor with various blades, including large blade, laryngeal blade, and tongue base blades, is the most useful for laryngo-pharyngeal lesions. Attaching pre-made mouthpieces to prevent tooth injury is also recommended. Although surgical field exposure is the most principal and important step to complete transoral surgery successfully, it is one of the most difficult steps that requires extensive experience and many learning curves.

Basic techniques for obtaining good surgical field exposure are as follows. For piriform sinus lesions, the laryngeal blade or tongue base blade is inserted into the glottis, vallecula of the epiglottis, or anterior end of the piriform sinus lateral of the pharyngoepiglottic fold and the aryepiglottic fold (**Figure 2a, b**). For posterior wall

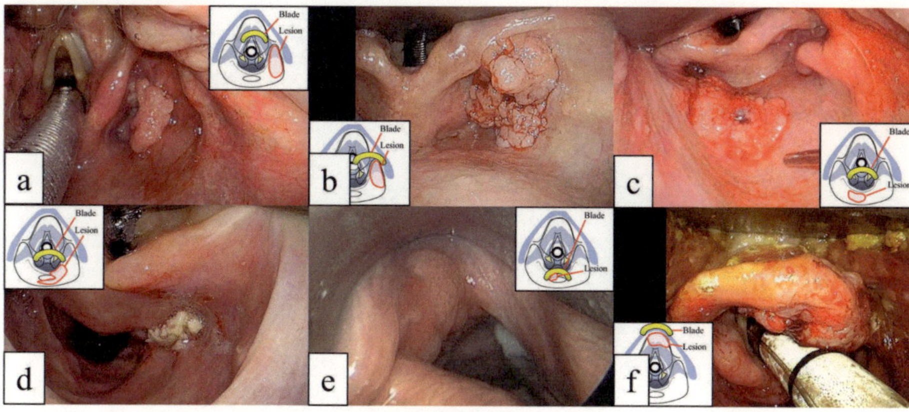

Figure 2.
Technique of surgical field exposure. a. Right piriform sinus lesion, b. right piriform sinus lesion, c. posterior wall lesion, d. Postcricoid lesion, e. esophageal inlet lesion, f. Epiglottic lesion.

lesions, the laryngeal blade is inserted into the glottis or postcricoid area (**Figure 2c**). In some of these cases, it is effective and helpful to obtain good surgical fields that the blade is inserted behind the endotracheal tube, and the tube is pushed forward (**Figure 2b, c**). For postcricoid and esophageal inlet lesions, the laryngeal blade is inserted into the glottis or postcricoid area behind the endotracheal tube, and the tube is pushed forward (**Figure 2d, e**). For epiglottic and tongue-based lesions, the tongue base blade is inserted into the tongue base (**Figure 2f**). Poor ventilation by kinking of the tracheal tube can occur due to compression by the blade, and a careful procedure is needed.

These instruments can expose most lesions; however, some patients have poor laryngopharyngeal exposure. For patents who have poor laryngopharyngeal exposure by conventional blades, novel prototypes of curved blades are currently under development (**Figure 3**). These new blades are effective to expose the distal hypopharynx to the esophageal inlet [5].

5.2 Evaluation

TOVS is performed by two head and neck surgeons. The operator manipulates instruments bimanually, and the assistant holds the videoscope to maintain an appropriate view of the surgical fields (**Figure 4a**). Occasionally, the assistant holds another pair of forceps or a suction device to support operator (**Figure 4**).

To evaluate the extent of the lesions and mark the resection area of the laryngopharynx, Endoeye flex with the function of image-enhanced endoscopy (NBI) is an ideal tool for this surgery. After meticulous washing of the laryngopharynx to remove blood and saliva with physiological saline, the lesion extent is evaluated by endoscopic vision with normal light and NBI (**Figure 4b, c**). Subsequently, iodine staining is performed to show the mucosal extent of the lesions. After 1% iodine solution is sprayed around the lesions and rinsed with physiological saline, superficial lesions can be clearly demarcated as iodine-unstained areas (**Figure 4d**). This procedure is particularly effective in identifying the boundary of lesions in hypopharyngeal cancer and oropharyngeal cancer, except that of tongue base lesions.

Palpation using forceps is also an important procedure to evaluate tumor size and deep infiltration and determine whether the lesions can be resected. In the case of lesion immovability and/or finding anatomical contraindications during the evaluation process, discontinuation of TOVS should be considered.

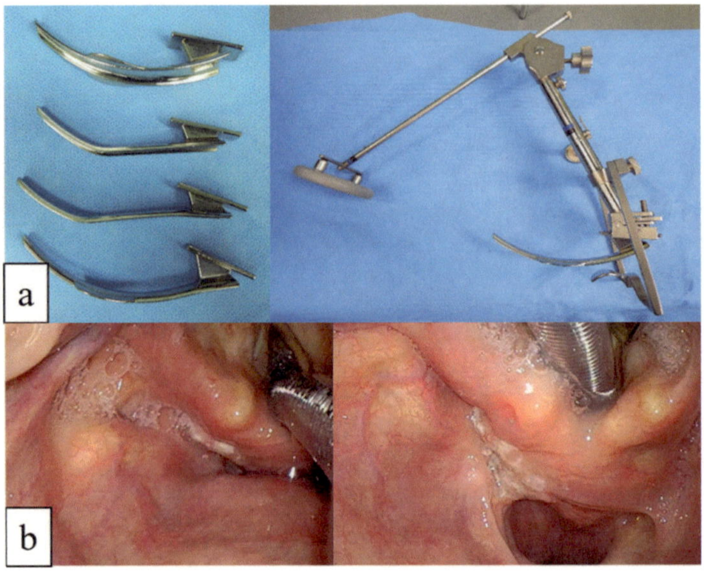

Figure 3.
Novel blades for FKWO retractor. A: Prototype of curved blades, b: Representative case (Postcricoid lesion), conventional blade (left), curved blade (right).

Thereafter, the incision line of the mucosa around the lesions is marked with a safety margin of 5–10 mm using needle-type electrocautery (**Figure 4e**). Due to cases of multiple sporadic mucosal lesions, evaluation of the entire laryngopharynx is recommended.

5.3 Resection

A soft suction tube is placed transnasally to prevent blurry vision by smoke and blood. After circumferential mucosal incision, the operator manipulates the grasping forceps to grasp and retract the edge of the lesion. Appropriate counter traction is applied to determine the appropriate incision layer and enables resection of appropriate tissue by electrocautery. In many cases, resection from the periphery to the inside enables en block resection (**Figure 4f–j**). It is important to confirm deep infiltration by palpation during the procedure. Representative cases are presented in Section 9.

Although hemostasis can be performed with a suction coagulator in most cases, multiple vessel clips should be used when thick blood vessels can be confirmed (**Figure 4k**). Bleeding from the posterior wall, the branch of the superior laryngeal artery running from the upper outside of the thyroid cartilage, or the branch of the lingual artery, is occasionally difficult to control.

Frozen section pathological analysis with the stumps of surgical margins in at least four horizontal directions and a deep margin is performed. In addition, the extracted specimen is stained with iodine to confirm the sufficiency of safety margin. Additional resection is performed based on these results when necessary.

5.4 End of surgery

In some cases, fibrin glue is sprayed to the wound to prevent bleeding (**Figure 4l**). However, it is not necessary due to the possibility of it becoming a foreign body in the airways. A nasogastric tube is inserted in cases with a high possibility of postoperative dysphagia (**Figure 4**).

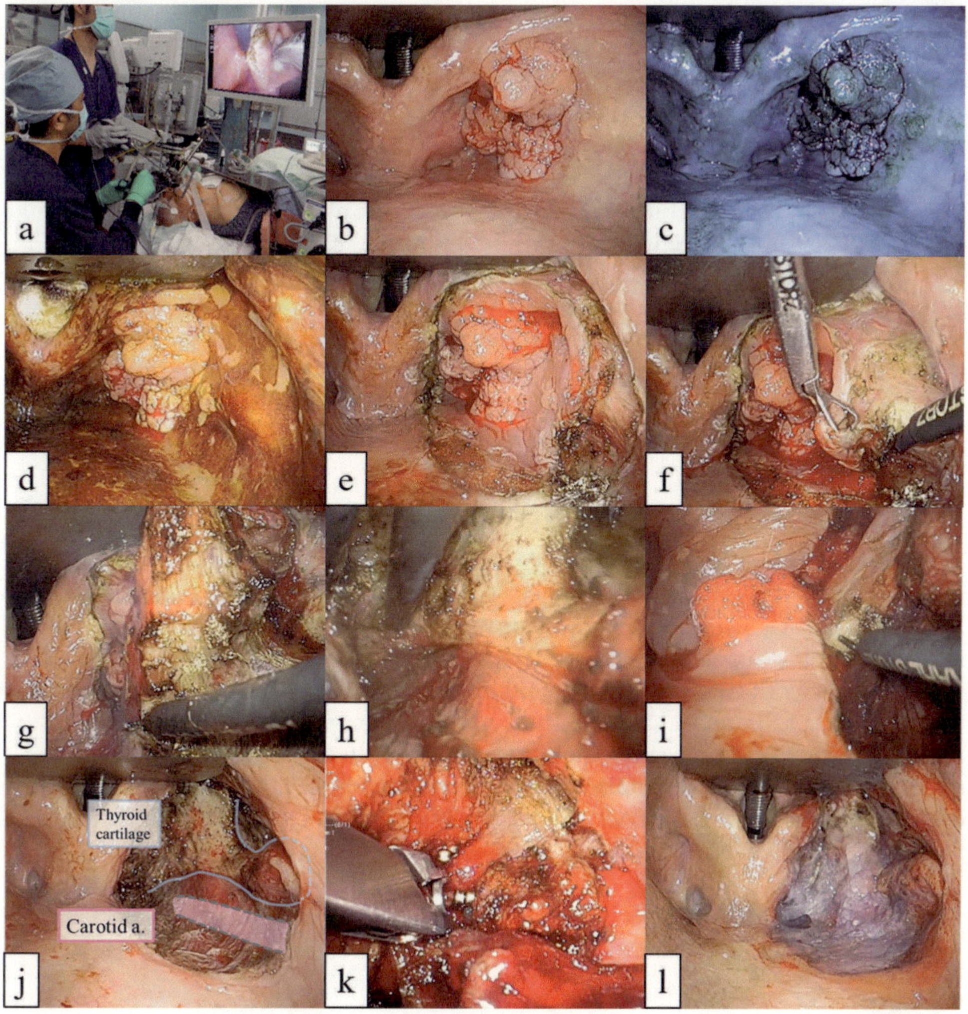

Figure 4.
Step-by-step procedure (Hypopharyngeal cancer, Rt. piriform sinus lesion). a. outside view of TOVS, b. observation with normal light, c. observation with NBI, d. observation after iodine staining, e. marking of the mucosal incision line, f. resection from the oral side, g. resection of the muscular layer, h. resection of the inner border of the thyroid cartilage, i. resection of the caudal end, j. view after resection, k. hemostasis using vessel clip, l. view after spraying of fibrin glue.

Local steroid injection (triamcinolone acetonide) is also performed to reduce the degree of postoperative scar contracture in selected non-irradiated cases. In deeply invasive tumors and previously irradiated patients, this procedure may cause wound healing complications; hence, local steroid injection should be considered in only new cases with extensive excision of the pyriform sinus, postcricoid, and/or esophageal inlet lesions [9].

TOVS can be completed without tracheostomy if no bleeding and no severe airway stenosis due to laryngopharyngeal edema is confirmed. The endotracheal tube is basically extubated immediately after surgery. In cases with suspected airway stenosis risk, extubation should be performed under preparation for immediate reintubation using a tube exchanger. Patients who have a high risk of bleeding after surgery or severe laryngopharyngeal swelling due to long surgery or neck dissection should be kept intubated or should undergo tracheostomy without hesitation.

6. Management of lymph node metastasis

For patients with node-positive disease, ND is performed after TOVS on the same day. Some patients may undergo ND separately within 1–2 weeks of TOVS.

The veins around the laryngopharynx should be preserved whenever possible to reduce postoperative laryngeal edema due to temporal insufficiency of blood flow. In N2c cases treated with bilateral NDs, severe edema of the entire laryngopharynx can occur. Therefore, careful attention should be paid to postoperative airway management and prophylactic tracheostomy should be considered.

Perforation between the wound of the TOVS and the neck can occur during ND. In such cases, postoperative infections, particularly around the carotid artery or retropharyngeal space, might be a fatal complication. Therefore, closure using a muscular flap should be performed and careful and intensive postoperative management to prevent subcutaneous emphysema and infections are necessary.

7. Anatomical tips for TOVS in hypopharyngeal cancer

The tips of the inside-out anatomy of the larynx and hypopharynx are shown in **Figure 5a**. The superior laryngeal artery and superior laryngeal nerve enter the laryngopharynx through the thyrohyoid membrane. The superior laryngeal nerve runs along the submucosal layer of the anterior wall of the pyriform sinus. The recurrent laryngeal nerve runs in a deep layer between the inferior cornu of the thyroid cartilage and the posterior cricoarytenoid muscle. The superficial branch of the recurrent laryngeal nerve usually causes anastomosis with the superficial laryngeal nerve (Galen's anastomosis).

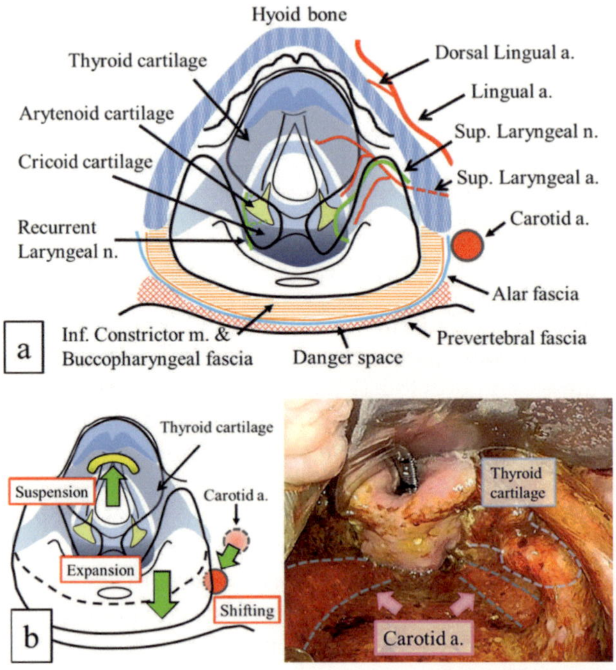

Figure 5.
Inside-out anatomy of the larynx and hypopharynx. a. Landmarks of the larynx and hypopharynx. b. Location of the carotid artery after surgical field exposure. a. Artery, n. nerve.

The carotid artery is close to the surgical field in some cases of angiectopia. The carotid artery is also close to the surgical field in cases of excessive laryngopharyngeal suspension to better expose the surgical field. The retractor opens the space between the alar of the thyroid cartilage and the prevertebral space, which causes the shift of the carotid artery from lateral to medial. As a result, the carotid artery becomes adjacent to the area between the posterior wall and the outer wall of the piriform sinus behind the alar of the thyroid cartilage (**Figure 5b**). Therefore, especially in the case that includes the pharyngeal constrictor muscle layer resection, the procedure should be performed with careful caution. Since this cannot be predicted by preoperative imaging, it is necessary to estimate the position of the carotid artery by careful observation of the arterial pulsation in the endoscopic view and the shift of the pulsating site by manual compression from the outside of the neck.

In the case of deeper infiltration in the posterior wall, the resection should also be performed with careful caution. When an excision of all layers of the pharyngeal constrictor muscle is performed, deeper damage from the buccopharyngeal fascia to the alar fascia causes perforation of the danger space in the retropharyngeal space (**Figure 5a**). This damage may cause severe postoperative complications such as cervical spondylitis and/or mediastinitis. In particular, post-irradiated cases have a high risk of developing complications due to poor wound healing and increased susceptibility to infection. Therefore, it is important to preserve the buccopharyngeal fascia and alar fascia whenever possible.

To perform better and safer transoral surgery, the surgeon should understand and familiarize themselves with the anatomical landmarks inside the laryngopharynx, check the preoperative endoscopic and imaging findings, observe surgical fields in detail under videoscopic view, and manipulate a careful procedure for each case.

8. Postoperative management

8.1 Perioperative management

Since tracheostomies are not performed in most cases, careful attention should be focused on airway management and postoperative bleeding. Laryngopharyngeal edema may worsen for a few days after surgery, although problems may not arise at the time of extubation. Routine endoscopic observation over time should be performed, and steroid administration should be considered if needed. Postoperative bleeding can occur not only immediately but also for more than 2 weeks after surgery due to crust removal during the wound healing process. Therefore, careful follow-up with a ready for emergency airway management, including tracheostomy, is necessary for more than 2 weeks after surgery.

For nutritional management, resurgence of oral intake is considered according to the extent of resection and the risk factors of dysphagia (such as age, performance status, preoperative swallowing function, and irradiation history). However, in cases with small lesions and low risk of dysphagia, oral intake can be resumed from the next day. In many cases with extensive, muscular layer resection and/or arytenoid resection, nasogastric tubal feeding is needed. Swallowing examinations such as videofluorography and/or videoendoscopy are usually performed within 1 week of surgery. Assessment for oral intake should be judged based on these results, and swallowing rehabilitation (direct or indirect training) by a speech therapist should be performed, if necessary, with being appropriate re-evaluation. In most cases, a normal diet can be resumed within 1 week to 1 month of TOVS.

In cases without any postoperative complications such as airway, bleeding, infection, and dysphagia, the patient can be discharged from the hospital. Patients with small lesions are usually discharged within 1–2 weeks after TOVS.

8.2 Long-term management

It is important to consider the possibility of pneumonia due to silent aspiration. Only a few percent of patients have long-term dysphagia [5, 10]. If long-term oral intake is difficult, gastrostomy is considered.

Epithelization of the wound healing occurs 1–2 months after TOVS in most cases. However, wound healing is very slow and takes more than 6 months in some previously irradiated cases [8]. In such cases, the risk of infection is high. Serious complications such as cervical spondylitis and mediastinitis can occur after more than 6 months after surgery. Long-term antibiotic administration is required in some cases. In addition, it is difficult to discriminate infection/inflammation from recurrence; therefore, long-term follow-up with careful observation is necessary.

Wound adhesion and scar formation due to wound healing causes fixation of the cricoarytenoid joint in some cases of extensive pyriform sinus resection. In such cases, restriction of vocal fold movement and insufficient glottic closure may occur several months after TOVS. Although there is no problem with laryngeal function immediately after surgery, dysphagia and voice disorder might worsen over a few months after TOVS. Intraoperative local steroid injection (triamcinolone acetonide) is effective; however, its indications should be limited only to new cases with extensive excision of the pyriform sinus, postcricoid, and/or esophageal inlet lesions, as described in Section 5.4 [9].

8.3 Oncological management and additional treatments

The pathological assessment of surgical margins in the resected permanent specimen is often difficult due to cauterization. Therefore, the margins are uncertain in some cases. In cases with horizontal margins, careful follow-up enables early detection, even in the case of recurrence. However, in cases with deep margins, early detection of recurrent lesions may be difficult after wound healing. In such cases, a second-look operation after 2–3 months of TOVS or postoperative irradiation should be considered.

According to pathological findings, patients might undergo postoperative radiation therapy (RT) or chemoradiation therapy (CRT). Definite positive margins, multiple lymph node metastases, extranodal extension, and perineural invasion are indications for RT or CRT.

9. Representative cases

9.1 Case 1: 64-year-old male, hypopharynx cancer, pT3N0M0

The lesion was extended from the left pyriform sinus to the posterior wall and anterior surface of the epiglottis (**Figure 6**).

9.2 Case2: 58 years-old male, hypopharyngeal cancer, rT2N0M0

Chemoradiotherapy for hypopharyngeal cancer (T3N0M0), was performed 2 years before TOVS. The recurrent lesion was located more than half of the posterior wall to the esophageal inlet (**Figure** 7).

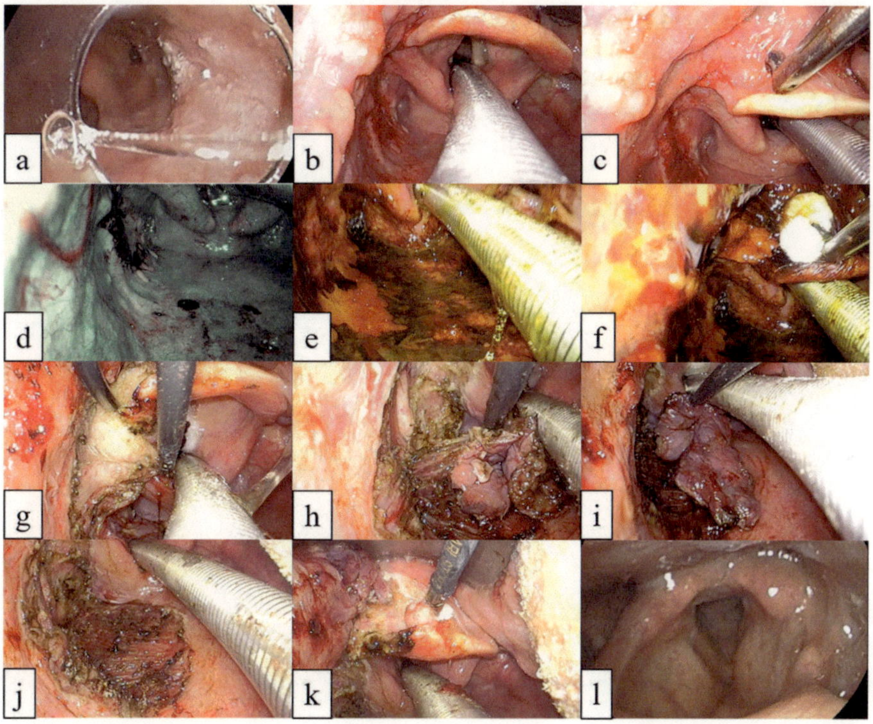

Figure 6.
Case 1. a. Pre-operative endoscopic view, b. observation with Normal light: Lesion was extended from left piriform sinus to posterior wall. c. Observation with Normal light: Lesion was extended to the left side of the anterior surface of the epiglottis. d. Observation with NBI, e. observation after iodine staining: Left piriform sinus to the posterior wall, f. observation after iodine staining: Anterior surface of epiglottis, g. resection from the left side of the anterior surface of the epiglottis to the upper side of the piriform sinus. h. Resection of the left piriform sinus to the lateral wall, i. removal of resected en block specimen, j. view after resection: Left piriform sinus to posterior wall, k. view after resection: Resected anterior surface and left edge of epiglottis, l. postoperative endoscopic view (2 months after TOVS).

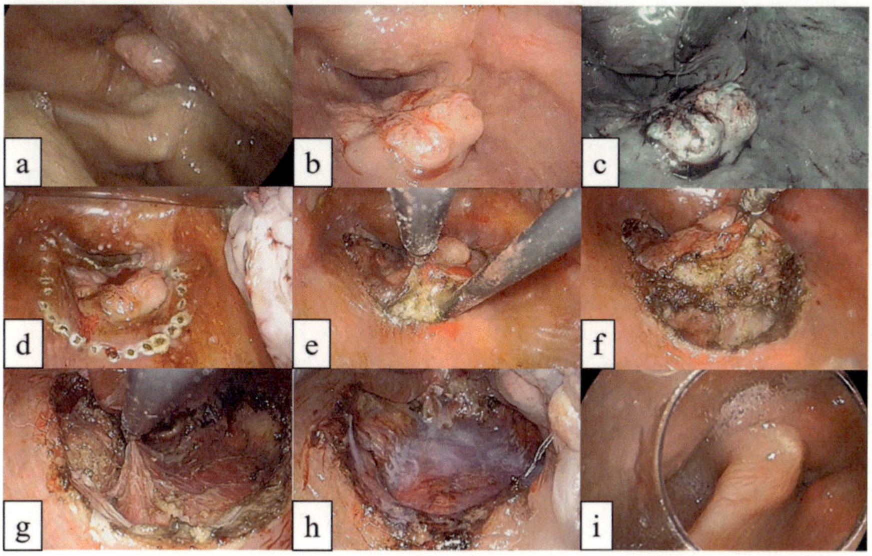

Figure 7.
Case 2. a. Pre-operative endoscopic view, b. observation with Normal light, c. observation with NBI, d. marking of the mucosal incision line, e. resection from Musclar layer of oral side, f. resection of the whole layer of pharyngeal constrictor muscle, g. view after resection: Ara fascia was preserved. h. View after spraying fibrin grue, i. postoperative endoscopic view (9 months after TOVS).

9.3 Case3: 72-year-old male, hypopharynx cancer, rT3N0M0

Chemoradiotherapy for hypopharyngeal cancer (T2NM0) was performed 10 years before TOVS. The recurrent lesion was located from the right side of postcricoid to left side posterior wall, esophageal inlet (**Figure 8**).

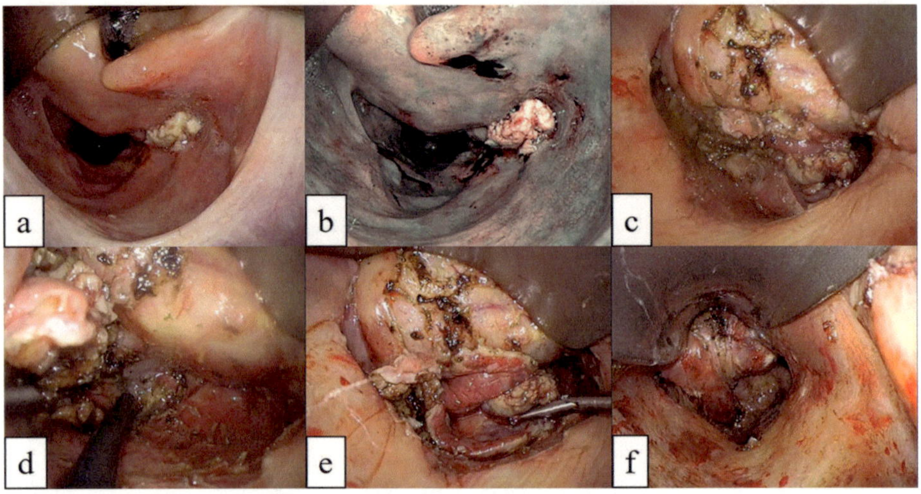

Figure 8.
Case 3. a. Observation with normal light, b. observation with NBI, c. marking of the mucosal incision line, d. resection right side of postcricoid to esophageal inlet, e. removal of resected en block specimen, f. view after resection: More than half of the posterior wall and the esophageal inlet were resected.

10. Outcomes

10.1 Oncological outcome

A recent report by Tomifuji et al. demonstrated excellent outcomes of TOVS for both new and salvage cases [5]. In 83 new hypopharyngeal cancer cases, the 2-year overall survival (OS), disease-specific survival (DSS), local control rate (LCR), laryngeal preservation rate (LPR), and disease-free survival (DFS) were 90.6%, 97.4%, 96.3%, 96.9%, and 80.40%, respectively, and the 5-year OS, DSS, LCR, LPR, and DFS were 83.2%, 94.3%, 94.7%, 94.6%, and 73.0%, respectively. In 12 salvage cases of hypopharyngeal and supraglottic cancer after RT or CRT, the 2-year OS, DSS, LCR, LPR, and DFS were 100%, 100%, 75%, 91.7%, and 75%, respectively, and the 5-year OS, DSS, LCR, LPR, and DFS were 87.5%, 87.5%, 75%, 82.5%, and 75%, respectively. Regarding T classification, advanced T stage showed worse OS and DSS outcomes than early stage. Regarding N classification, patients with N3 neck disease showed a significantly worse prognosis in terms of OS and DSS.

Among 115 cases of hypopharyngeal and supraglottic cancer, 20.8% of patients had a previous history of RT or CRT in the neck, 28.7% of patients were performed postoperative RT or CRT. As the result, 50.4% of patients could be spared RT or CRT [5].

10.2 Functional outcome

Regarding swallowing functional outcomes, most patients maintain good oral food intake. Among 115 patients more than 6 months after TOVS, the functional outcome swallowing scale (FOSS) score, which divides the swallowing function into six stages, was 0 in 65% patients, 1 in 20% patients, 2 in 4.3% patients, 3 in 7.0% patients, and 4 in 3.5% patients (0–2, stable status; 3, unstable status requiring occasional follow-up of swallowing function; and 4–5, life-threatening status requiring tube feeding or surgical intervention). In 3.4% of patients, oral food intake could not be achieved within 6 months of surgery and required tube feeding, total pharyngolaryngectomy due to severe pharyngeal stenosis, or laryngotracheal separation surgery. Another 1.7% of patients had deteriorated swallowing function after 4.5 years and 7 years of TOVS and underwent laryngotracheal separation surgery to prevent aspiration pneumonia. Therefore, 5.2% of patients could not maintain oral intake during the long-term follow-up [5]. The risk factors associated with postoperative severe dysphagia include patient age (particularly >80 years), large resection area, arytenoid and/or pyriform sinus resection, pulmonary dysfunction, and tracheostomy [10].

Postoperative voice impairment was found in 29.1% of hypopharyngeal and supraglottic cancer cases 6–12 months after TOVS. Scar contracture after wound healing was the mechanism described in Section 8.2. Large resection area including the medial and lateral pyriform sinuses was the risk factor [11]. Surgeons should inform the patients regarding the risk of postoperative voice impairment during pre-operative counseling.

10.3 Complications

In 115 cases of hypopharyngeal and supraglottic cancer, the major complications related to TOVS were neck emphysema (7.8%, conservative observation: 100%), airway edema (6.9%, steroid treatment: 88%, tracheostomy: 12%), bleeding (2.6%, tracheostomy: 67%, reoperation: 33%), partial laryngopharyngeal necrosis due to postoperative RT and CRT (1.7%), perforation of the neck (0.86%), and laryngeal chondritis (0.86%) [5].

The proportion of patients avoiding endotracheal tube extubation immediately after surgery and maintain intubation for 1 day due to long operation time or poor oxygenation was 1.7%. Tracheostomy was performed in 9.5% of patients—in 4.3% of patients, prophylactic tracheostomy was performed; in 3.4% of patients, emergency tracheostomy was performed; and in 1.7% of patients, preoperative tracheostomy was performed due to dyspnea or difficulty of intubation. Tracheostomy could not be closed due to persistent laryngeal stenosis and persistent dysphagia in 3.4% of all patients undergoing TOVS [5].

11. Future directions

11.1 Development of devices

In the early phase of TOVS establishment, a major problem in the surgical procedure was the conflict of instruments in the narrow laryngopharyngeal cavity due to the straight shape of the endoscope and forceps. In recent years, endoscopes, forceps, CO2 lasers, and electrocautery with flexibility have been commercially available (**Figure 1d**).

The currently available endoscopes are designed for two-dimensional imaging. Therefore, TORS, which uses three-dimensional (3D) imaging, is considered superior to TOVS. However, the newly developed 3D endoscopes that can be used for TOVS will be commercially available soon. TOVS has the advantage of having tactile sense; hence, it can be a more suitable surgery for hypopharyngeal lesions using a 3D endoscope than TORS.

In addition, new curved blades for the FK-WO retractor have been developed (**Figure 3**). In a trial conducted in our department, new curved blades enabled appropriate exposure of surgical fields in the pyriform sinus apex and esophageal inlet in five cases with poor surgical field exposure using conventional blades, and surgical procedures could be accomplished in all cases. While using curved blades, the surgical maneuver is occasionally difficult with straight devices; however, malleable devices fit well [5].

With the continuous development of devices and by combining devices such as 3D endoscopes, malleable devices, and new curved blades, TOVS will be an easier procedure with a broad indication of the entire laryngopharynx and will be a more accomplished surgery with better oncological outcomes and safety.

11.2 Management of lymph node metastasis

Cervical lymph node metastasis is one of the most important prognostic factors in head and neck squamous cell carcinoma. Although many cases of transoral surgery are in the early stage with a clinically node-negative (cN0) status, the rate of positive lymph node metastasis in patients with cN0 laryngopharyngeal cancer is approximate 20–30%. Therefore, it is debatable whether neck dissection should be performed immediately in cN0 cases.

Tomifuji et al. reported the relationship between the histological parameters of resected primary lesions of TOVS and lymph node metastasis in supraglottic and hypopharyngeal cancers. Tumor depth and venous invasion were the most useful parameters for predicting lymph node metastases. They recommended that elective ND should be considered when the tumor depth is >1 mm and/or there is a presence of venous invasion. Moreover, careful observation when the tumor depth is between 0.5 and 1 mm, and, regular clinical follow-up when <0.5 mm, are recommended, respectively [12].

Another promising strategy for the management of lymph node metastasis is sentinel node navigation surgery (SNNS). It enables a personalized evaluation for neck dissection in cN0 cases individually, thereby eliminating unnecessary ND. Araki et al. reported a multicenter feasibility study of the combination of transoral surgery with SNNS for laryngopharyngeal cancer using an intraoperative injection of indocyanine green. In 22 patients with cN0 hypopharynx, oropharynx, or supraglottic cancer, the accuracy, sensitivity, and specificity of the combination strategy were 95.5%, 75%, and 100%, respectively. The 5-year DSS rate was 100%, and OS was 72.3% [13]. This combination strategy holds promise as a feasible tool for personalized and minimally invasive treatment options for both primary lesions and lymph node metastasis with favorable oncological outcomes.

11.3 Conversion surgery with neoadjuvant chemotherapy (NAC)

While the major indications for TOVS are early-stage up to T2, TOVS can be performed in selected cases with advanced lesions when NAC is effective for shrinking the lesions. Tomifuji et al. reported good results of conversion surgery with NAC. In the cases of T3 and T4 hypopharyngeal cancer treated by NAC (cisplatin +5FU or docetaxel + cisplatin +5FU) followed by TOVS, the 5-year OS, DSS, LCR, LPR, and DFS were 75.0%, 82.5%, 91.7%, 100%, and 66.7%, respectively [5].

Although this strategy of conversion surgery seems to be effective, it also has an issue. When lesions shrink by NAC, the remaining lesion may be a single mass in some cases or multiple scattered lesions in other cases. When the resection area is limited to shrunk lesions, some of the scattered lesions outside the resection area might be missed despite the negative resection margin. The resection areas after NAC should be determined according to the initial lesions, and it is technically difficult to completely resect the entire area of the original advanced lesions. Hence, the indication of TOVS as a conversion surgery for advanced lesions should be limited to highly selected cases, and research on an appropriate and effective strategy for conversion surgery with NAC is necessary for the future.

11.4 Other than laryngopharyngeal cancer surgery

TOVS can be applied to any other surgery in addition to that for primary laryngopharyngeal cancer. Parapharyngeal and retropharyngeal metastatic lesions can be treated by TOVS in combination with a navigation system [14]. Less invasiveness surgery is needed for benign diseases in the laryngopharyngeal region compared to that for malignant diseases. The technique of TOVS has great benefits as a minimally invasive surgery for benign diseases including cysts, papilloma, benign

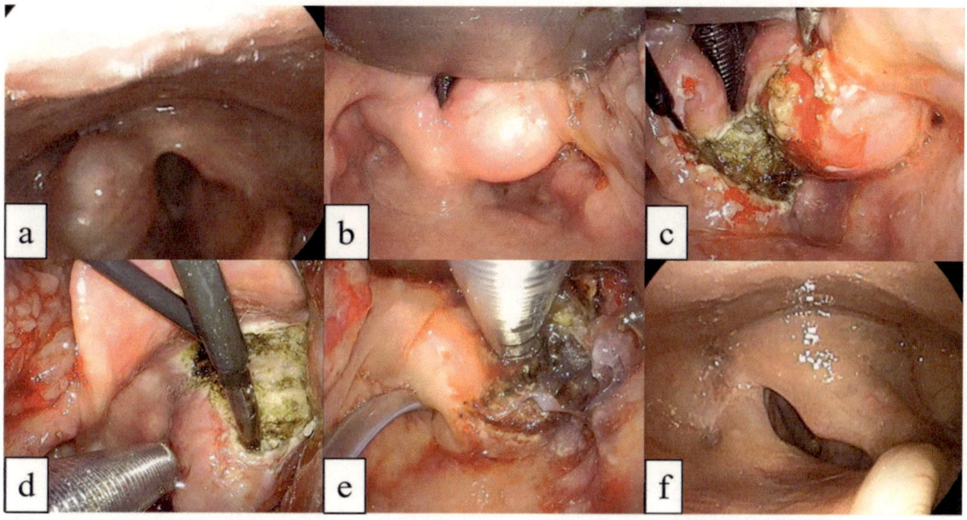

Figure 9.
56-year-old male, recurrent laryngeal pleomorphic adenoma. The orginal lesion was resected 1 year ago at another hospital. The recurrent lesion was located right arytenoid to aryepiglottic fold. a. Pre-operative endoscopic view, b. pre-operative view of surgical field, c. resection from inter arytenoid to right arytenoid, d. resection of right aryepiglottic fold, e. view after resection: Whole right arytenoid to aryepiglottic fold was resected and fibring grue is sprayed. f. Post-operative endoscopic view (9 months after TOVS).

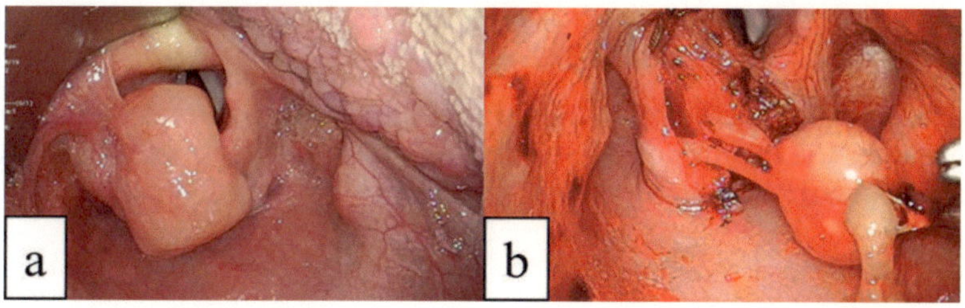

Figure 10.
19-year-old female, Neurofibromatosis type2. The lesion was located left arytenoid. a. Preoperative view of surgical field, b. resection of the lesion.

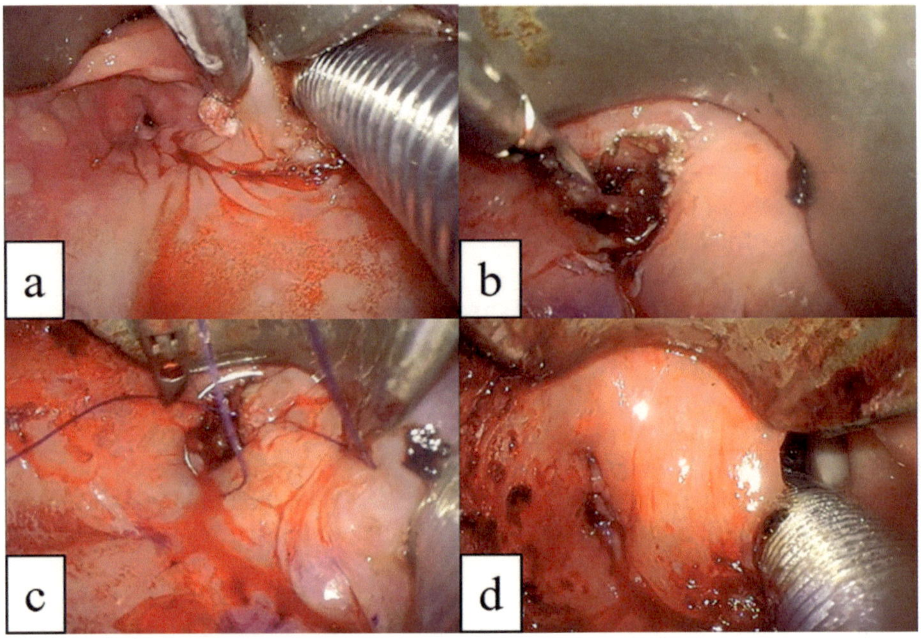

Figure 11.
30-year-old female, pyriform sinus fistula. a. Pre-operative view of surgical field, b. resection of the duct as far as possible, c. suture closure of mucosa, e. view after mucosal closure.

tumors (**Figures 9, 10**), pyriform sinus fistula [15] (**Figure 11**), foreign bodies, injection laryngoplasty for unilateral vocal cord palsy, cricopharyngeal myotomy for dysphagia, laryngopharyngeal dilatation surgery for stenosis and so on.

12. Conclusions

TOVS is a minimally invasive organ preservation surgery for laryngopharyngeal cancer with good oncological and functional outcomes. The procedure of this surgery has some advantage in maneuver and less invasiveness when compared to TLM and TORS, especially for hypopharyngeal cancer. It is expected that transoral surgery including TOVS will become increasingly popular as one of the standard treatments with the development of devices and establishing the evidence by accumulating cases.

Acknowledgements

This work was supported by a Grant-in-Aid for Scientific Research from the Japan Society for the Promotion of Science (JSPS KAKENHI grant no. 18 K09390), and a Special Research Grant on Defense Medicine from the Ministry of Defense of Japan.

Conflict of interest

The authors declare no conflict of interest.

Author details

Koji Araki* and Akihiro Shiotani
Department of Otorhinolaryngology-Head and Neck Surgery, National Defense Medical College, Tokorozawa, Saitama, Japan

*Address all correspondence to: kojaraki@ndmc.ac.jp

References

[1] Shiotani A, Tomifuji M, Araki K, Yamashita T, Saito K: Videolaryngoscopic transoral en bloc resection of supraglottic and hypopharyngeal cancers using laparoscopic surgical instruments. Ann Otol Rhinol Laryngol. 2010;119:225-232. doi: 10.1177/000348941011900403.

[2] Shiotani A, Tomifuji M, Araki K, Yamashita T: Transoral videolaryngoscopic surgery for en bloc resection of supraglottic and hypopharyngeal cancers. Otolaryngol Head Neck Surg. 2011;144:288-289. doi: 10.1177/0194599810392148.

[3] Yamashita T, Tomifuji M, Araki K, Kurioka T, Shiotani A: Endoscopic transoral oropharyngectomy using laparoscopic surgical instruments. Head Neck. 2011;33:1315-1321. doi: 10.1002/hed.21604.

[4] Tomifuji M, Araki K, Yamashita T, et al : Transoral Videolaryngoscopic surgery for oropharyngeal, hypopharyngeal, and supraglottic cancer. Eur Arch Otorhinolaryngol. 2014 ; 271 : 589-597. doi: 10.1007/s00405-013-2575-0.

[5] Tomifuji M, Araki K, Uno K, Kamide D, Tanaka S, Suzuki H, Tanaka Y, Kimura E, Hirokawa S, Taniai S, Shiotani A: Transoral videolaryngoscopic surgery for laryngeal and hypopharyngeal cancer - Technical updates and long-term results. Auris Nasus Larynx. 2020;47: 282-290. doi: 10.1016/j.anl.2019.09.003.

[6] Steiner W, Ambrosch P. Endoscopic laser surgery of the upper aerodigestive tract: With Special Emphasis on Cancer Surgery. 1st Edition. Stuttgart: Thieme; 2000. doi:10.1055/b-006-161074

[7] Park YM, Kim WS, De Virgilio A, et al : Transoral robotic surgery for hypopharyngeal squamous cell carcinoma: 3-year oncologic and functional analysis. Oral Oncol. 2012;48:560-566. doi: 10.1016/j.oraloncology.2011.12.011.

[8] Tomifuji M, Araki K, Yamashita T, Shiotani A. Salvage Transoral Videolaryngoscopic Surgery for radiorecurrent hypopharyngeal and supraglottic cancer. Auris Nasus Larynx. 2017;44:464-471. doi: 10.1016/j.anl.2016.10.006.

[9] Uno K, Tomifuji M, Araki K, Tanaka S, Taniai S, Tanaka Y, Kimura E, Ogawa K, Shiotani A: Scar contracture prevention with local steroid injections in transoral videolaryngoscopic surgery. Auris Nasus Larynx. 2020;47:856-863. doi: 10.1016/j.anl.2020.02.007.

[10] Tomifuji M, Araki K, Yamashita T, et al : Risk factors for dysphagia after transoral videolaryngoscopic surgery for laryngeal and pharyngeal cancer. Head Neck. 2016;38:196-201. doi: 10.1002/hed.23866.

[11] Tanaka S, Tomifuji M, Araki K, Uno K, Tanaka Y, Mizokami D, Suzuki H, Miyagawa Y, Taniai S, Shiotani A: Vocal function after transoral videolaryngoscopic surgery (TOVS) for hypopharyngeal and supraglottic cancer. Acta Otolaryngol. 2017;137:403-410. doi: 10.1080/00016489.2016.1266509.

[12] Tomifuji M, Imanishi Y, Araki K, Yamashita T, Yamamoto S, Kameyama K, Shiotani A: Tumor Depth as a Predictor of Lymph Node Metastasis of Supraglottic and Hypopharyngeal Cancers. Ann Surg Oncol. 2011;18:490-496. doi: 10.1245/s10434-010-1219-5.

[13] Araki K, Tomifuji M, Shiotani A, Hirano S, Yokoyama J, Tsukahara K, Homma A, Yoshimoto S, Hasegawa Y: Minimally invasive surgery for laryngopharyngeal cancer: a multicenter feasibility study of a combination strategy involving transoral surgery and real-time indocyanine green fluorescence-navigated sentinel node navigation surgery. Head Neck. 2020;42:254-261. doi: 10.1002/hed.25993.

[14] Kamide D, Tomifuji M, Maeda M, Utsunomiya K, Yamashita T, Araki K, Shiotani A: Minimally invasive surgery for pyriform sinus fistula by transoral videolaryngoscopic surgery. Am J Otolaryngol. 2015;36:601-605. doi: 10.1016/j.amjoto.2015.02.009.

[15] Tanaka Y, Tomifuji M, Suzuki H, Yamashita T, Araki K, Shiotani A: Transoral videolaryngoscopic surgery with a navigation system for excision of a metastatic retropharyngeal lymph node. ORL J Otorhinolaryngol Relat Spec. 2014;76:357-363. doi: 10.1159/000369626.

Section 2

Other Pharyngeal Diseases

Chapter 11

Factors of Nasopharynx that Favor the Colonization and Persistence of *Staphylococcus aureus*

Samuel González-García, Aída Hamdan-Partida, Anaíd Bustos-Hamdan and Jaime Bustos-Martínez

Abstract

Between 30 and 50% of the world population is permanently colonized in some anatomical site by *Staphylococcus aureus*, although the vast majority are asymptomatic carriers. The nose is its main niche and currently the colonization of *S. aureus* in the pharynx has become relevant due to the variety of reported carrier rates and the epidemiological importance of the dissemination of Methicillin-resistant *S. aureus* strains (MRSA) by pharyngeal carriers. For this bacterium to colonize a tissue successfully, it is necessary to establish many interactions with bacterial and host cell components such as bacterial wall teichoic acids (WTA) with the Scavenger SREC-1 host receptor and at the same time evade the defense mechanisms. On the other hand, there are host factors that will facilitate or complicate the colonization or persistence of *S. aureus* at these sites, such as physiological, genetic, immunological and microbiological factors.

Keywords: *Staphylococcus aureus*, colonization, nasopharynx, microbiota, SREC-1

1. Introduction

Staphylococcus aureus is a Gram-positive bacterium that lives in symbiosis with humans, it is an opportunistic and potentially lethal pathogen [1, 2] of great clinical importance due to the different virulence, invasiveness and resistance factors that it may possess [3]. In humans, it colonizes various tissues, forming part of the normal microbiota [3, 4], although it is also one of the principal cause of community-associated and nosocomial-associated infections; is one of the main causes of bacteremia and infective endocarditis, as well as skin, soft tissue and pleuropulmonary infections and contamination of medical devices [4]. Invasive disease is associated with a mortality rate of ≥20% [2]. Uncontrolled use of antibiotics, particularly their inappropriate and excessive use, has favored the emergence and maintenance of strains of *S. aureus* resistant to multiple antibiotics such as penicillin (penicillin-resistant *S. aureus*, PRSA), methicillin (methicillin-resistant *S. aureus*, MRSA) [5, 6] or vancomycin, strains with high rates of morbidity and mortality in many countries of the world [5]. The most studied primary reservoir site for *S. aureus* in humans is the nose, predominantly found in the anterior nasal vestibule [7]. Approximately 30% or more of the world population is colonized with *S. aureus* on the skin, mucous membranes, or in the nose [4, 5] (**Figure 1**).

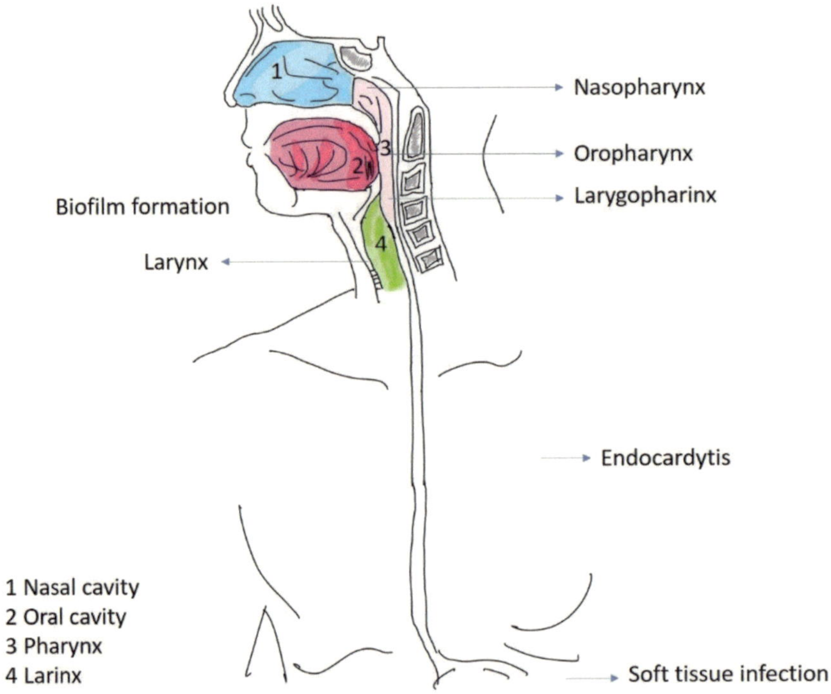

Figure 1.
S. aureus *can cause a wide range of diseases by spreading to various tissues, among the survival mechanisms being the formation of biofilms regulated by several genes such as the accessory regulatory gene* agr *and by intracellular infection mechanisms (Modified from Sasegbon and Hamdy. [49]).*

The mechanisms of colonization and persistence of *S. aureus* in the human nose have been extensively studied, however, it must be recognized that the clinical relevance of *S. aureus* carriers in the pharynx has not been sufficiently investigated [8]. This omission seems to be justified, if the nose is considered as the primary site of colonization of *S. aureus*, from there, other regions of the body are colonized by manual propagation [9]. However, in the adult population *S. aureus* can be commonly found in other parts of the body such as the armpits (8%), chest / abdomen (15%), perineum (22%), intestine (17–31%), vagina (5%) [10].

S. aureus carriers have been found in the pharynx and have been reported with high variability in different populations from 4 to 64% [11], some studies mention a higher rate of carriers in the pharynx than in the nose when samples are taken in parallel [10, 12, 13].

Colonization of *S. aureus* in the nose and pharynx is a multifactorial process that involves genetic aspects of the host, virulence factors of the pathogen, and possible interactions between the microbiota of the host [14], although in principle it is thinks that colonization of the pharynx is secondary to colonization of the nose, it is likely that both processes are independent [15].

2. Human determinants

The human determinants that allow bacterial colonization can be changes at the molecular level that alter the adhesiveness, recognition and eradication properties. Epidemiological studies present little information related to molecular studies [10].

The anterior nostrils are one of the main reservoir niches of *S. aureus*, however, the colonization of the nose begins from a cutaneous site, where the bacterium plays a role of commensal microbiota and, through contact with contaminated hands, spreads to the nose and other parts of the body [16].

Colonization of the nose begins a few days after birth [17]. Between 40 and 50% of newborns become carriers during the first eight weeks of life but decreases to 21% in the sixth month [18]. In another research, 80% of identical strains were found among mother–child pairs, and in 90% of newborns, *S. aureus* came from the maternal nose [16].

Days after birth, the hands are the main source of transmission of *S. aureus* from contaminated surfaces to the nose. Reagan et al. [19] demonstrated by means of a randomized, double-blind and placebo-controlled trial, the link between the passage from the hand to the nose of *S. aureus*, in addition they demonstrated that nasal decolonization with mupirocin decreased the carriage in the hands and nose [16].

Research in people living in the same household has found that they tend to carry genetically similar nasal strains, suggesting their horizontal transmission. Furthermore, it has been shown that the carriage of MRSA strains in various parts of the body increases the risk of nasal colonization by MRSA [16].

2.1 Overview of the nostrils

The nasal passage filters 95% of the particles with a diameter greater than 15 μm from the inspired air. The nose is extremely important in protecting the distal airways from the influence of gases, aerosols, and pathogens [20].

The anterior part of the nasal cavity (*vestibulum nasi*) is formed with stratified squamous epithelium, non-ciliated keratinized (60% of the strains of *S. aureus* originating from the nose are isolated in this part). It has also been shown that *S. aureus* can colonize and persist in ciliated nasal epithelial cells in the inner part of the nasal cavity (internal nostrils) with pseudostratified columnar ciliated epithelium [9, 14].

The epidermis and dermis are the two main layers that line the *vestibulum nasi*. The dermis is a connective tissue that contains both epidermal and lymphatic structures, and vascular ducts, nerves, nerve endings, collagen, and elastic fibers, as well as a wide variety of specialized immune cells [7].

The epidermis is made up of the basal, spiny, granular, lucid and corneal striatum [7]. These five main strata are characterized by cells in different stages of differentiation, during which the anterior nasal epithelial cells change their appearance to keratinized squamous anucleated cells called corneocytes, these cells form the stratum corneum (also called cornified layer) being the most external, they are also surrounded by a protein structure containing loricrin and involucrin (**Figure 2**) [7, 14]. The upper layers of the keratinized epithelium are constantly being replaced, which could contribute to the elimination of the attached bacteria, however, this does not happen [14].

2.1.1 Loricrin

Epithelial tissues are the main appendages that protect the internal organs of the body from environmental stress, chemical damage, and microbial infections. The stratified epithelia seen on the skin and oral mucosa are one of the most resistant and protective epithelia, as it resists severe physical and chemical forces and do so by producing a hardened structure: the cornified cell envelope (CE). Loricrin is an important component of keratins. These keratins are structural proteins and constitute approximately 85% of a fully differentiated keratinocyte (**Figure 3**) [21, 22].

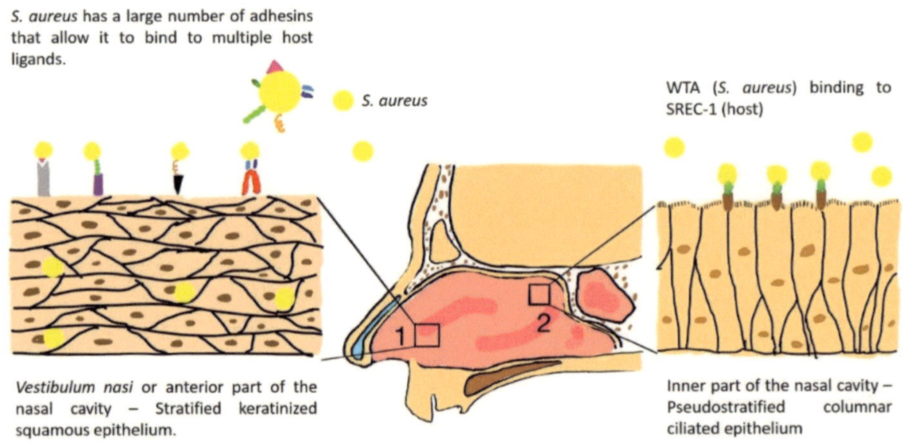

Figure 2.
Nasal colonization sites of S. aureus. *1.* Vestibulum nasi *or nasal cavity, is the ecological niche of* S. aureus *in humans.* S. aureus *Has a large amount of adhesins such as ClfB (light blue line), IcaA (strong blue line), Spa (orange line), SdrC (green dots), FnBPA (pink triangle), which can bind to various proteins of the nasal epithelial cells such as keratin and loricrin (red line), involucrin (purple line), unknown receptors (black triangle), fibronectin (gray rectangle). 2. The inner part of the nasal cavity can also be colonized by* S. aureus *and survive for a long time, at this site it binds by multiple load interactions by the teichoic acids of the bacterial wall (WTA) with the SREC-1 nasal cell receptor. (modified from Sakr et al. [16]).*

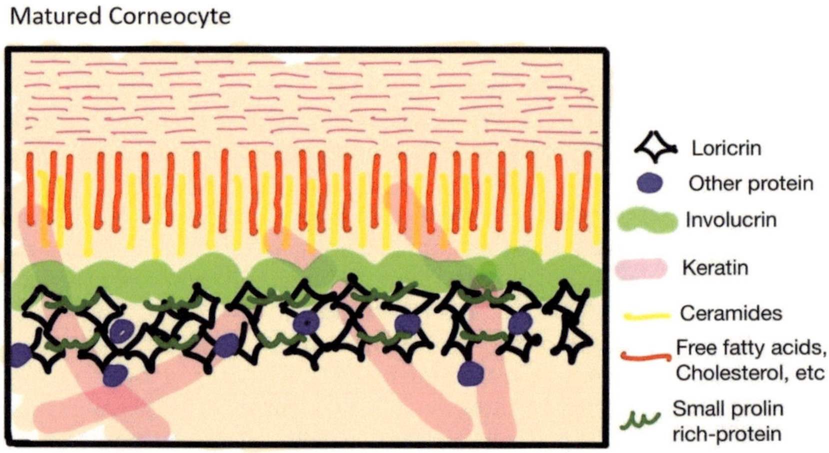

Figure 3.
Location of loricrin, involucrin, keratin and other macromolecules in mature corneocytes (modified from Ishitsuka and Roop. [21]).

Loricrin is an insoluble polypeptide with a molecular weight of 26 kDa. It has a conserved epitope and is a major cornified envelope protein seen in the cytoskeleton of the stratified parakeratinized epithelium. Being a late differentiating protein, it is introduced into the cornified envelope structure due to its cross-linking and binding property. It improves the function of the corneocyte protective barrier in differentiated keratinocytes [21].

Loricrin occupies an important part (70%) of the cornified epidermal envelope. Its concentration is reduced to approximately 30–50% in certain areas such as the palate and esophagus, while it is not expressed in many internal epithelia such as the oral mucosa. In *in vivo* studies in mammalian tissues, loricrin has a very high expression in all stratified epithelia, and is expressed even more in moist tissues of newborns such as the epidermis, foreskin, epidermal sweat ducts, in addition to the oral and anal mucosa and the esophagus [21, 22].

In vitro analysis and studies in animal models have revealed that the main colonization target ligand of *S. aureus* is loricrin, binding with clumpling factor B (ClfB) in squamous epithelial cells [23].

2.1.2 Involucrin

Involucrin is a soluble cytosolic protein that is the precursor of the cornified envelope, its main function is to donate a glutamyl or glutamine in the crosslinking reaction catalyzed by the enzyme transglutaminase and it disappears from the soluble phase after the activation of calcium-dependent transglutaminase. 20% of its structure is glutamate and 25% glutamine. An important biochemical characteristic of involucrin is that it contains a central domain composed of 39 tandem repeats of 10 amino acids each segment, this repetitive structure is conserved in the involucrins of all higher primates, only varying the number of repeats [24]. In the cornified structure, involucrin is adjacent to the cell membrane, when the cell membrane is replaced, involucrin is the main substrate to which lipids esterify, primarily ceramides, are covalently attached to form the outer surface of the cornified envelope (**Figure 3**) [25].

The iron-regulated surface determining protein (IsdA) promotes the adhesion of *S. aureus* to squamous cells that cooperate in binding to the cornified cell envelope with the host proteins loricrin, involucrin, and cytokeratin [26].

2.1.3 Cytokeratine 10 (K10)

In the epidermis, keratinocytes travel from the basal cell layer to the postmitotic spinous suprabasal cells, and during the process, there is a significant change in the expression of basal cell keratins (K5, K14, and K15) to suprabasal epidermal keratins first to type II K1 keratin and later to type I K10 keratin. The keratin filaments are structurally composed of the K1 / K10 pair and form dense bundles, characteristic of suprabasal epidermal keratinocytes, and this gives the cells and the entire epidermis mechanical integrity (**Figure 3**). However, there are more functionalities, as K10 has been shown to specifically inhibit the proliferation and progression of the keratinocyte cell cycle and the decrease in K10 leads to an increase in keratinocyte renewal [27, 28].

It has been shown that cytokeratin 10 is a receptor for ClfB of *S. aureus*, which facilitates the nasal colonization of this and other bacteria [29].

2.2 Interactions with the nasal cavity

Another ecological niche of *S. aureus* in addition to the *vestibulum nasi* is the internal part of the nasal cavity (**Figure 2**). The teichoic acids of the bacterial wall (WTA) are a principal factor for the colonization process. A study reported in an animal model that mutated strains deficient in the *tagO* and *tarK* genes that participate in WTA biosynthesis did not adhere to or colonize the nose cells of cotton rats compared to control bacteria [14].

Baur et al. [30] re-studied the adhesion to nasal cells of WTA and reported the expression of the SREC-1 receptor (from the family of Scavenger receptors type F) in the nose of cotton rats and in epithelial cell lines of the human internal nasal cavity. In addition, they found that SREC-1 interacts with WTA and verified it in cotton rats infected with a previous treatment with anti-SREC-1 antibodies, significantly decreasing colonization after 8 hours and 6 days after inoculation compared to the control group.

2.2.1 SREC-1 receptor

The key role that WTA plays in the early colonization stages of *S. aureus* has been demonstrated, however, until recently the ligand with which it binds to initiate adhesion and colonization with the host was found.

The Scavenger receptor superfamily can bind and endocyte many ligands, which causes the elimination of both exogenous and unnecessary endogenous molecules [31]. It is important to mention that the affinity for the ligands is shared by several Scavenger receptors, regardless of whether their classes (A-J) have little or no biochemical homology [31, 32].

The Scavenger 1 class F receptor (SREC-1, SCARF1 or SR-F1), is the most expressed by endothelial cells (of the Scavenger family). It is a type I transmembrane protein that weighs 86 kDa, contains some epidermal growth factors (EGF) with similarity to the extracellular region, a small transmembrane domain, and a long cytoplasmic tail rich in proline and serine [33].

The size of the cytoplasmic domains could have a role in intracellular signaling, however, this function has not been found. SREC-1 is an evolutionarily highly conserved receptor, particularly in the extracellular domain, and shows significant homology with the *Caenorhabditis elegans* Scavenger receptor CED-1, important in homeostasis and innate immunity of *C. elegans* [34].

SREC-1 was obtained from human umbilical vein endothelial cells (HUVEC), but its expression has been reported in multiple cells, including epithelial cells [30], sinusoidal endothelial cells [33, 35], dendritic cells, B-1 cells. [36] and macrophages [35, 36]. It is important to mention that almost all studies focused on the functionality of this receptor have used transfected cell lines, designed to express the receptor extracellularly in vitro, and some studies have used cells that naturally express the SREC-1 receptor in vivo [33]. Furthermore, the first reports of the expression of this receptor showed high transcriptional expression in multiple human tissues such as spleen, lung, heart, liver, and kidney and it has been corroborated in murine tissues [33, 36]. However, more studies are needed to investigate its expression and cellular distribution at the protein quantity in these tissues. So far, there is only one study that has fully characterized the cellular distribution and expression of the SREC-1 receptor in healthy and chronically ill human liver [35]; therefore, much remains to be studied to understand the activity of this receptor in human cells and tissues [33].

2.3 Individual host factors favoring nasal colonization of *S. aureus*

Some studies have found that *S. aureus* nasal carriers are more common in people infected with the Human Immunodeficiency Virus (HIV) [37] and obese patients [38], compared to healthy individuals. Nowak et al. [39] published the positive correlation between percentage of body mass and susceptibility to colonization by *S. aureus* in healthy male individuals. This high prevalence was also reported in diabetic dialyzed patients, compared with non-diabetic patients [16]. Other diseases such as granulomatosis with rheumatoid arthritis, skin and soft tissue infections [40], atopic dermatitis, and recurrent furunculosis have been associated with an increased carrier rate [16].

Contrary to what was reported by Nowak et al. [39], Liu et al. [41] found similar percentages of carriers in women and men, however, men had a higher density of bacteria. To date, it has not been confirmed that hospital workers are at increased risk of being nasal carriers of *S. aureus* compared to the rest of the population [42, 43]. The association between nasal carriers of *S. aureus* and smoking is controversial, Olsen et al. [44], reported that healthy active smokers are protected from becoming carriers of *S. aureus*, due to the possible antibacterial activity of tobacco. However, another experimental inoculation study showed that smokers are colonized more frequently than non-smokers and that quitting smoking improves clearance of *S. aureus* nasal [45]. Other host pathologies, such as hormonal contraception [46], have also been extensively studied, and the presence of hemoglobin in nasal secretions has been reported as an additional predisposing factor [16].

Regarding host genetics, no significant heritability data has been detected for nasal colonization of *S. aureus* in twins and family studies [47, 48]. However, some polymorphisms have been found in genes involved in inflammatory processes and have been associated with the carriage of *S. aureus* in the nose, for example, the phenotype of the histocompatibility antigen HLA-DR3 could be a predisposition [16].

The host cell presents modified carbohydrates and secretes surface proteins, such as blood group antigens, which are involved in bacterial adhesion and colonization. An investigation found that people with blood group O have a 6.5 times higher risk of being carriers of *S. aureus* in the pharynx, compared to people with blood group A [9].

2.4 Overview of the pharynx

The pharynx is a muscular chamber that serves the respiratory and digestive systems to receive air for the nasal cavity and food and water for the oral cavity [49]. The oropharynx consists of five layers: mucosa, submucosa, pharyngobasilar fascia, constrictor muscle, and oropharyngeal fascia [50]. The pharynx has stratified non-ciliated epithelium that secretes mucus with mucin. Specifically, the posterior wall of the oropharynx (and the soft palate) is lined by a nonkeratinized stratified squamous epithelium, supported by an underlying lamina propria and a muscular layer. In the palatal and lingual tonsil regions, there are nodules of lymphoid tissue located below the epithelium, each tonsil is in a fixed position, in other regions there are membrane-associated lymphoid tissue [MALT], found throughout the body. The structural support is mainly provided by reticular fibers composed of type III collagen. These fibers condense and combine with elastin fibers to form septa that dissect the tonsillar parenchyma [50]. *S. aureus* can bind to multiple ligands of the pharynx such as collagen, fibronectin, fibrinogen through adhesin proteins such as Cna, FnBa, FnBb, among others (**Figure 4**) [16].

The oropharynx links the mouth, nasopharynx, lower respiratory tract, and gastrointestinal tract and is always exposed to a large number of microorganisms, both exogenous and endogenous. The set of species to be studied is wide, since there are very diverse bacterial communities in both adults and the elderly. The pharynx is also a niche for pathogenic bacteria that can cause localized (pharyngitis) or disseminated disease (primarily lung disease or systemic if spread) [51].

2.4.1 Importance of the study of S. aureus *in the pharynx*

The pharynx has recently been identified as a potential colonization site for *S. aureus*, this colonization can occur in the presence or absence of nasal colonization [52]. Being a carrier of *S. aureus* in the pharynx has potentially important implications in decolonization strategies for populations at high risk of infection, it is unlikely that topical drugs aimed at eradicating nasal colonization affect transport in the throat, therefore which could be an important focus in future infections if *S. aureus* persists in the pharynx [53].

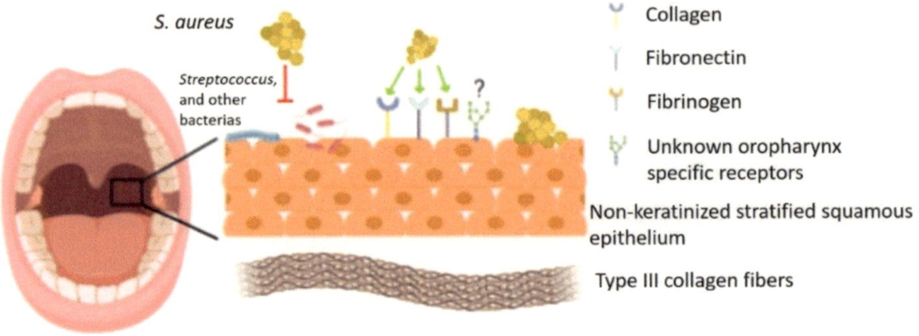

Figure 4.
Colonization of S. aureus *in the human pharynx.* S. aureus *Competes directly with bacteria that predominantly colonize the pharynx; it is known that bacteria such as* Streptococcus pneumoniae, Streptococcus mutans, Streptococcus mitis, *among others, inhibit the growth of* S. aureus. *Regarding the colonization mechanism, so far only the same ones as in the nose have been studied, for example, their binding to fibrinogen, fibronectin, collagen, among other proteins expressed in both anatomical sites, however, they have not been analyzed in depth its specific interactions with the pharynx.*

Most of the *S. aureus* detections, in particular MRSA, are only made from nasal swabs, since the pharyngeal swab is not considered a standard, Mertz et al. [54] mention that some drawbacks of pharyngeal exudate is causing discomfort to the patient and that it increases the cost to the health care system without significantly greater sensitivity. However, as mentioned above, pharyngeal colonization may be more common than nose colonization than has been published.

The rate of nasal carriers of MRSA in hospital patients has been found to be 5.9 to 15.6%, however, the rate of pharyngeal MRSA carriers is between 10 and 23.1%, which represents a greater number of carriers in the pharynx [55].

Cirkovic et al. [56] conducted a study of carriers and genetic diversity of MRSA in 195 hospitalized patients and 105 workers of a University Hospital in Serbia and reported a rate of 32.2% of exclusive MRSA carriers in the nose and another 32.2% of exclusive carriers of the pharynx, in addition of 35.5% of MRSA carriers in both sites, so the exclusion of pharyngeal exudates would result in a significant error in a substantial part of this work, since around a third are MRSA carriers exclusive to the pharynx [12, 13].

2.4.2 Interaction of S. aureus *with the microbiota*

Pathogenic bacteria can coexist with their host in two ways, as harmless microbiota microorganisms or as invading pathogens that enter healthy tissues after overcoming innate defense mechanisms or if the immune system is compromised [57]. Despite microbiology studies regarding infection mechanisms, ecological studies of pathogenic microorganisms present in the human microbiota are still lacking [58].

In vitro and in vivo studies that simulate colonization by *S. aureus*, as well as analysis of microbiomes and metagenomes reveal that the nose presents an intermediate level of bacterial diversity compared to the human oral cavity and intestine, but they present greater diversity than the vagina, which has less diversity. A percentage of the human population carries several bacterial species in the nose, such as *Finegoldia magna*, *Dolosigranulum pigrum* and *Salmonella* spp., are negatively correlated with colonization by *S. aureus* [41, 59]. It is not known how the nasal microbiota can prevent *S. aureus* colonization. Understanding this mechanism can help to understand why about 30% of the human population is persistently colonized by *S. aureus*, another 30% is highly resistant to nasal colonization by *S. aureus*, and the remainder are considered intermittent carriers [58].

DOI: http://dx.doi.org/10.5772/intechopen.95843

2.4.3 Nasal microbiota

The nasal cavity of humans harbors a diverse bacterial community that is in principle stable at the gender level [41, 59, 60], but may vary between individuals and with season [61] In the same way, other places in the human body that are exposed to the environment are the skin and the oropharynx [61–63]. The dynamics of the nasal microbiota have not yet been analyzed. The analysis of the nasal microbiota is performed by amplification and sequencing of the 16S rRNA gene, that in many cases it is not possible to distinguish between species, therefore should implement shotgun metagenome sequencing techniques [58].

Many species of nasal bacteria are anaerobic [64], indicating that part of the nasal epithelium is barely exposed to air in the nasal cavity. Many species cannot be cultivated in vitro, they require special growth conditions [58].

Bacteria in the nose belong mainly to three phyla (Actinobacteria, Firmicutes, and Proteobacteria) and 80% humans or more are colonized with *Corynebacterium* spp., *Propionibacterium* spp., and *Staphylococcus* spp. [62, 65, 66]. Other genera are found less frequently [41].

Based on the abundance of characteristic species in the human nose, seven types of community status (CST) have been defined. (CST), each of which represents a nasal bacterial community dominated by *S. aureus* (CST1), Enterobacteriaceae (*Escherichia* spp., *Proteus* spp., *Klebsiella* spp. and others; CST2), *S. epidermidis* (CST3), *Propionibacterium* spp. (CST4), *Corynebacterium* spp. (CST5), *Moraxella* spp. (CST6) or *Dolosigranulum* spp. (CST7) [41]. *S. aureus* was found in several CSTs, although much less frequently than in CST1 [58].

During the first years of life, the microbiota of the respiratory tract develops [67, 68]. The oral microbiota is similar to that of the skin, but is less similar to that of the oral cavity. So the nose could be an intermediate step between these two niches [62]. The microbiota of the sebaceous and moist areas of the skin is more similar to that of the nose than to the dry areas of the skin [61]. *Streptococcus spp.* is abundant in the oral cavity, but it is found in low numbers in the nose [69]. Species of Coagulase-negative *Staphylococcus* (SCN), such as *Staphylococcus capitis*, *Staphylococcus warneri*, *Staphylococcus hominis*, and *Staphylococcus lugdunensis*, are prevalent on the skin, but they are only found in the nasal cavity of some people, with the exception of *S. epidermidis*, which colonizes both the nose and the skin of most people [58].

2.4.3.1 Factors influencing composition of the nasal microbiota

Bacterial communities in the nose undergo seasonal variations, mainly during the change from winter to spring [70]. The environment plays an important role in the composition of the nasal microbiota as factors such as humidity, temperature, dust or pollen influence [41, 70]. Furthermore, smoking has been shown to prevent nasal colonization by *S. aureus* [44], although it is still under discussion [45]. Some studies have shown that the gender and genetic composition of the host have a moderate influence on the colonization of *S. aureus*, however the type of nasal microbiota seems to be an important factor for the colonization of this bacterium [41, 48]. Furthermore, nasal colonization by *S. aureus* hardly varies between humans of different ethnic and geographic origins [70]. The various regions of the nose, from the anterior vestibule to the sphenoethmoidal recess in the posterior nasal cavity, are lined with mucus, thus differing in the composition of the microbiota between individuals [60].

Metagenomic studies have shown the importance of the role of bacteriophages in the dynamics of the microbiota of the skin and intestine [71]. In the human nose the abundance and diversity of bacteriophages have not yet been analyzed, they can alter the nasal microbiota. Bacteriophages are one of the main mechanisms for horizontal transfer of virulence and antibiotic resistance genes between staphylococci and other bacteria, which can contribute to the appearance of new strains [72].

2.4.3.2 Competition for nutrients

Unlike the gastrointestinal microbiota, bacteria in the nasal cavity do not interact with food in the diet and can only acquire nutrients that are excreted by cells, so nasal secretions contain few nutrients [73] and are has hypothesized that bacteria in the nasal microbiota compete for scarce nutrients. Nasal secretions contain NaCl in physiological concentrations (~ 150 mM) and low levels of potassium, magnesium, and phosphate. Carbohydrates, amino acids, and other nutrients are found in nasal secretions in much lower amounts than those found in plasma [58]. There is a synthetic nasal medium (SNM), containing nutrients in the same amounts as in nasal fluid, allowing *S. aureus* to develop, but most SCNs cannot grow under these conditions or grow very slowly [73]. This would indicate that most of the SCNs present in the nose are only transitory and are not a permanent colonization site for these bacteria. Many of the genes involved in the nutrient absorption systems and anabolic metabolic pathways in *S. aureus* are highly expressed in NMS or in the nose [73]. *S. aureus* is successful when it competes with other nasal microorganisms as it depends on its ability to grow in low amounts of nutrients. Nasal bacteria do not always compete with other bacteria for nutrients, in certain cases they can also cooperate with others to obtain specific nutrients, such as *S. aureus* and *Corynebacterium accolens* that seem to have a mutualistic relationship [60].

The main carbohydrate in nasal fluids is glucose and it is found in low concentrations (between 35 μM and 1 mM, with an average value of ~370 μM) [73] which depends on the nutritional status of the person. The colonized by *S. aureus* is higher in diabetic people, perhaps due to high concentrations of nasal glucose. Sialic acids, which line the membrane of eukaryotic cells, can be an important source of energy for bacteria in the nasal cavity [58]. Many bacteria can metabolize sialic acids how *S. aureus* and some SCNs including *S. intermedius, S. lugdunensis*, and *S. saprophyticus*, but not *S. epidermidis*, can absorb and use sialic acid [74].

S. aureus is the only one of the staphylococci that can degrade the main phosphatidylcholine group that is released from eukaryotic cells, extracellular glycerophosphocholine (GroPC). *S. aureus* can grow with GroPC as the sole carbon source so it can survive in limited nutrient conditions [58].

Nasal fluids contain several of the 20 amino acids necessary for protein biosynthesis in concentrations between 10 μM and 250 μM; however, several such as methionine, tyrosine, aspartate, asparagine, glutamine, and isoleucine are found in very low concentrations [73] so they need to be synthesized by nasal bacteria. This was verified since a mutant of *S. aureus* that presents a deficiency in the synthesis of methionine was isolated and this affected its growth in the cotton rat nasal colonization model [14, 73]. In certain sites of the nose, the concentrations of amino acids and peptides may be higher, *S. aureus* and other nasal bacteria secrete proteases that can degrade host proteins, which are found in high concentrations in nasal fluids, such as albumin, lactoferrin, mucins, cytokeratin 10, and hemoglobin [75]. *S. aureus* produces approximately ten extracellular proteases, which makes it different from most other nasal bacteria that do not produce extracellular proteases or produce only a few [76].

Nasal discharge, in addition to being low in nutrients, is also poor in essential metal ions such as zinc, manganese, iron, and other host proteins such as calprotectin and lactoferrin, which sequester these ions from the nasal cavity to prevent bacterial growth [75]. Because of this, the microbiota needs specific mechanisms to compete with the host's defense, known as "nutritional immunity" [58].

When the growth of nasal bacteria slows due to a lack of nutrients, some bacteria produce antimicrobial substances to inhibit competing bacteria, these antimicrobial substances are normally ribosomally synthesized and post-translationally modified peptides (RiPP) or nonribosomal peptide-synthetase (NRPS) enzymes. Bacteria that produce these molecules are protected from specific immunity. Antimicrobial RiPPs (called bacteriocins) sometimes have a limited range of activity and are produced against specific groups of nasal bacteria. Most bacteriocins in nasal bacteria show changes such as thiazole heterocycles, lanthionine bridges (lantibiotics), and oxazole (microkines) or pyridine rings (thiopeptides) [77]. There are not many reports of bacteriocins in bacterial species isolated from the human nose [78].

Nasal strains of *Staphylococcus* spp. were studied for antimicrobial substances and found to be produced with a high frequency (86%) and a wide diversity of activities against groups of nasal bacteria. Due to this, bacteriocins can play a very important role in the formation of the nasal microbiota. Most members of Firmicutes and Proteobacteria are unaffected by the inhibitory activities of staphylococci, except *Dolosigranulum pigrum* and *Moraxella catarrhalis*. However, some bacteria of the phylum Actinobacteria, such as *Corynebacterium pseudodiphtheriticum* and *Micrococcus luteus*, were inhibited by staphylococcal bacteriocins [79]. These susceptible bacteria may be the main competitors of nasal staphylococci [58]. Most of the staphylococcal genes used in bacteriocin biosynthesis are found in mobile genetic elements forming part of plasmids or on the bacterial chromosome, which undergo extensive genetic rearrangements and horizontal gene transfer [79].

Bacteriocins have a wide variation in amino acid sequence, which can cause changes in the spectrum of activity [80, 81]. Due to this, the evolutionary process could have increased and changed the type of nasal bacteria, causing changes in the composition of the microbiota. This is the case with thousands of genes that produce secondary metabolites, many of which are potential antimicrobial substances. In investigations of the human metagenome of different surfaces of the human body, it was found that antimicrobial peptides can play an important role in the maintenance of the human microbiota [81]. In an investigation of nasal strains, *S. epidermidis* strains were found to be the main antimicrobial-producing bacteria, while *S. aureus* rarely produces these substances. The production of various antimicrobials is favored by stressful conditions during colonization, such as iron limitation or the presence of hydrogen peroxide (H_2O_2), indicating that many antimicrobials are tightly regulated [79].

Most staphylococcal bacteriocins are inactive for *S. aureus*. But, *S. lugdunensis* can synthesize an antimicrobial compound called lugdunin that inhibits and kills *S. aureus*. Lugdunin is encoded by the bacterial genome and is the first identified antimicrobial NRP produced by a human commensal bacterium, and represents a new class of cyclic peptide antibiotics containing thiazolidine. The lugdunin production operon is present in almost all nasal strains of *S. lugdunensis*, allowing this bacterium to compete with and kill *S. aureus*. People colonized by *S. lugdunensis* have a six times lower risk of being carriers of *S. aureus* than people who are not colonized [82]. Similarly, SCNs that produce certain bacteriocins can prevent *S. aureus* from colonizing the skin in patients with atopic dermatitis [83]. These results show the importance of the production of antimicrobial compounds by commensal bacteria that can prevent colonization by pathogenic bacteria such as *S. aureus* [58]. Another enzyme called lysostafin that is produced by *Staphylococcus simulans* could degrade the cell wall of multiple species of staphylococci, including *S. aureus*, by hydrolyzing the pentaglycine bonds that bind peptidoglycan [84].

Other bacteria in the nose use indirect methods to inhibit the growth of competing bacteria, such as *S. pneumoniae*, which is found mainly in the throat and rarely in the nose, but colonization by *S. pneumoniae* prevents colonization of the nose by *S. aureus* [58]. Possibly, this inhibition may be due to the release of hydrogen peroxide, a metabolite produced by *S. pneumoniae* that produces the generation of free radicals that damage DNA, and which also activates the prophages contained in the genome of *S. aureus* strains, which that causes the lysis of bacteria [85]. Also, *S. pneumoniae* can interfere with *S. aureus* in other ways, such as by inducing cross-reactive antibodies that prevent *S. aureus* colonization [86]. Viridans group streptococci (*S. mitis*, *S. sanguis*, *S. oralis*, *S. mutans*, and *S. sobrinus*) have also been found to prevent MRSA colonization of the pharynx in newborns, due to bacteriocin activity of peroxidase type [87].

2.5 Pharyngeal microbiota

In the nasal, oral and pharyngeal human cavities live hundreds of microbial species, including between 25 and 40 families archeas, bacteria, amoebae and fungi, as evidenced in a wide range of cultures. The number of newly discovered species has increased considerably due to the discovery of noncultivable species [88]. A data published in the Human Microbiome Project (HMP), 5 main bacterial phyla have been identified in the pharynx: Firmicutes, Proteobacteria, Bacteroidetes, Fusobacteria and Actinobacteria. Interestingly, the pharyngeal microbiome is distinguished from other parts of the body (intestines, skin and vagina) by having more Bacteroidetes. The proportion of bacterial phyla in the pharyngeal microbiome comprises 27% of Bacteroidetes and only 10% of Proteobacteria, compared to the salivary microbiome, whose proportion corresponds to 9% of Bacteroidetes and 51% of Proteobacteria. These two phyla are mentioned because they are the main pathogens in human infections, for example, periodontitis is caused by Bacteroidetes and the most common Gram-negative pathogens (*Acinetobacter*, *Moraxella*, *Pseudomonas*, *Haemophilus*, *Klebsiella*, and *Legionella* spp) [89]. However, the two genera that dominate the micro-ecosystem of the pharynx are *Streptococcus* and *Prevotella* [90].

2.5.1 The pharyngeal microecosystem

The most common bacterial genera in the human pharynx are *Prevotella*, *Capnocytophaga*, *Campylobacter*, *Veillonella*, *Streptococcus*, *Neisseria*, *Haemophilus*, which represent 9.72% to 1.26% of the bacteria in the normal microbiome, according to HMP data. [89, 90]. As there are few studies of the pharyngeal microbiome, many interactions between the components of the microecosystem are not clear, however, the interactions of microorganisms with factors of the local environment are characteristic of the microbiome. From the above, it can be assumed that the pharyngeal microbiome may share common characteristics of other human microbiomes [89].

2.5.2 Potential roles of the pharyngeal microbiome

Animals have developed strategies that allow them to evade the invasion of microbial pathogens and humans are no exception. Therefore, the one inhabited by commensal microorganisms that participate as defenders has a fundamental action to comply with these strategies. However, the role of the pharyngeal microbiome in respiratory tract infections (RTIs) is not fully understood, there is evidence to suggest a protective effect, like the gut microbiome [89].

The pharynx microbiome plays a crucial role in lining the mucosa of the respiratory tract by protecting against infections by airborne pathogens, in addition to the immune mechanisms of the host, particularly against emerging infectious agents [89, 91].

Homeostasis of the pharyngeal microbiome is necessary to prevent infections caused by native bacterial species, which allows the abundant development of each species. Many pathogenic species can adapt well to the pharyngeal ecosystem and become established in the resident microbiome, rendering the host asymptomatic (such as *S. aureus*, *H. influenza*, and *Mycoplasma pneumoniae*) [92]. In epidemiological studies it has been suggested that the proportion of resident pathogens varies seasonally, as does the incidence of RTIs attributed to them [93].

3. Conclusions

S. aureus is an important clinical pathogen for humans that has developed the ability to bind to various components of the extracellular matrix of a wide range of cells and has generated mechanisms that allow its survival and persistence in adverse conditions such as the formation of biofilms. and intracellular infection, which overwhelmingly evades the host's immune response in various human tissues.

On the other hand, it has also been possible to integrate with other important bacterial communities of the nose and skin to form part of the normal microbiome of these sites, but it can also survive in other tissues where it is not considered a normal microorganism, as is the case of the pharynx or intestines.

Although there are many studies of the colonization mechanisms and interactions of *S. aureus* in the nose, there is little information on the processes and interactions that it performs in the pharynx. Therefore, additional studies of the pharynx as a site of colonization of *S. aureus* are required.

Acknowledgements

This work was support by Special Research Support Program of UAM.

Conflict of interest

The authors declare no conflict of interest.

Author details

Samuel González-García[1], Aída Hamdan-Partida[2], Anaíd Bustos-Hamdan[3] and Jaime Bustos-Martínez[2]*

1 Doctorate in Biological and Health Sciences, Metropolitan Autonomous University, Mexico City, Mexico

2 Department of Health Care, Metropolitan Autonomous University-Xochimilco, Mexico City, Mexico

3 Children's Hospital of Mexico "Federico Gómez", Mexico City, Mexico

*Address all correspondence to: jbustos@correo.xoc.uam.mx

References

[1] Brown AF, Leech JM, Rogers TR, McLoughlin RM. Staphylococcus aureus colonization: modulation of host immune response and impact on human vaccine design. Front Immunol 2014;4:1-20. DOI: 10.3389/fimmu.2013.00507

[2] Mistretta N, Brossaud M, Telles F, Sanchez V, Talaga P, Rokbi B. Glycosylation of *Staphylococcus aureus* cell wall teichoic acid is influenced by environmental conditions. Sci Rep 2019;1:1-11. DOI: 10.1038/s41598-019-39929-1

[3] Kadariya J, Thapaliya D, Bhatta S, Mahatara RL, Bempah S, Dhakal N, et al. Multidrug-resistant *Staphylococcus aureus* Colonization in Healthy Adults Is more Common in Bhutanese Refugees in Nepal than Those Resettled in Ohio. Biomed Res Int 2019;2019:1-11. DOI: 10.1155/2019/5739247

[4] Tong SYC, Davis JS, Eichenberger E, Holland TL, Fowler VG. Staphylococcus aureus infections: epidemiology, pathophysiology, clinical manifestations, and management. Clin Microbiol Rev 2015;3:603-61. DOI: 10.1128/CMR.00134-14

[5] Khairalla AS, Wasfi R, Ashour HM. Carriage frequency, phenotypic, and genotypic characteristics of methicillin-resistant *Staphylococcus aureus* isolated from dental health-care personnel, patients, and environment. Sci Rep 2017;7:1-16. DOI: 10.1038/s41598-017-07713-8

[6] Rodríguez-Lázaro D, Oniciuc EA, García PG, Gallego D, Fernández-Natal I, Dominguez-Gil, et al. Detection and characterization of *Staphylococcus aureus* and methicillin-resistant *S. aureus* in foods confiscated in EU borders. Front Microbiol 2017;8:1-10. DOI: 10.3389/fmicb.2017.01344

[7] Hanssen AM, Kindlund B, Stenklev NC, Furberg AS, Fismen S, Olsen RS, et al. Localization of *Staphylococcus aureus* in tissue from the nasal vestibule in healthy carriers. BMC Microbiology 2017;17:1-11. DOI: 10.1186/s12866-017-0997-3

[8] van Belkum A, Verkaik NJ, De Vogel CP, Boelens HA, Verveer J, Nouwen JL, et al.. Reclassification of *Staphylococcus aureus* nasal carriage types. J Infect Dis 2009;199: 1820-6. DOI: 10.1086/599119

[9] Nurjadi D, Lependu J, Kremsner PG, Zanger P. Staphylococcus aureus throat carriage is associated with ABO−/secretor status. J Infect 2012;65:310-7. DOI: 10.1016/j.jinf.2012.05.011

[10] Sollid JUE, Furberg AS, Hanssen AM, Johannessen M. Staphylococcus aureus: determinants of human carriage. Infect Genet Evol 2014;21:531-41. DOI: 10.1016/j.meegid.2013.03.020

[11] Mertz D, Frei R, Jaussi B, Tietz A, Stebler C, Flückiger U, et al. Throat swabs are necessary to reliably detect carriers of *Staphylococcus aureus*. Clin Infect Dis 2007;45:475-7. DOI: 10.1086/520016

[12] Hamdan-Partida A, Sainz-Espuñes T, Bustos-Martínez J. Characterization and persistence of *Staphylococcus aureus* strains isolated from the anterior nares and throats of healthy carriers in a Mexican community. J Clin Microbiol 2010;48:1701-5. DOI: 10.1128/jcm.01929-09

[13] Hamdan-Partida A, González-García S, de la Rosa García, E, Bustos-Martínez J. Community-acquired methicillin-resistant *Staphylococcus aureus* can persist in the throat. Int J Med Microbiol 2018;308:469-75. DOI: 10.1016/j.ijmm.2018.04.002

[14] Weidenmaier C, Goerke C, Wolz C. Staphylococcus aureus determinants for nasal colonization. Trends Microbiol 2012;20:243-50. DOI: 10.1016/j.tim.2012.03.004

[15] Hanson BM, Kates AE, Mills E, Herwaldt LA, Torner JC, Dawson JD, et al.. The Oropharynx as a Distinct Colonization Site for *Staphylococcus aureus* in the Community. bioRxiv 2017;137901. DOI: 10.1101/137901

[16] Sakr A, Brégeon F, Mège JL, Rolain JM, Blin O. Staphylococcus aureus nasal colonization: an update on mechanisms, epidemiology, risk factors, and subsequent infections. Front Microbiol 2018;9:1-15. DOI: 10.3389/fmicb.2018.02419

[17] Maayan-Metzger A, Strauss T, Rubin C, Jaber H, Dulitzky M, Reiss-Mandel A, et al. Clinical evaluation of early acquisition of *Staphylococcus aureus* carriage by newborns. Int J Infect Dis 2017);64:9-14. DOI: 10.1016/j.ijid.2017.08.013

[18] Peacock SJ, Justice A, Griffiths D, De Silva GDI, Kantzanou MN, Crook, D, et al. Determinants of acquisition and carriage of *Staphylococcus aureus* in infancy. J Clin Microbiol 2003;41:5718-25. DOI: 10.1128/jcm.41.12.5718-5725.2003

[19] Reagan DR, Doebbeling BN, Pfaller MA, Sheetz CT, Houston AK, Hollis RJ, Wenzel R P. Elimination of coincident *Staphylococcus aureus* nasal and hand carriage with intranasal application of mupirocin calcium ointment. Ann Intern Med 1991;114:101-6. DOI: 10.7326/0003-4819-114-2-101

[20] Beule AG. Physiology and pathophysiology of respiratory mucosa of the nose and the paranasal sinuses. GMS Curr Top Otorhinolaryngol Head Neck Surg 2010;9:1-24. DOI: 10.3205/cto000071

[21] Ishitsuka Y, Roop DR. Loricrin: Past, Present, and Future. Int J Mol Sci 2020;21:1-28. DOI: 10.3390/ijms21072271

[22] Nithya S, Radhika T, Jeddy N. Loricrin–an overview. J Oral Maxillofac Pathol 2015;19:64-8. DOI: 10.4103/0973-029X.157204

[23] Mulcahy ME, Geoghegan JA, Monk IR, O'Keeffe KM, Walsh EJ, Foster TJ, et al. Nasal colonisation by *Staphylococcus aureus* depends upon clumping factor B binding to the squamous epithelial cell envelope protein loricrin. PLoS Pathog 2012;8:1-14. DOI: 10.1371/journal.ppat.1003092

[24] Yaffe MB, Beegen H, Eckert RL. Biophysical characterization of involucrin reveals a molecule ideally suited to function as an intermolecular cross-bridge of the keratinocyte cornified envelope. J Biol Chem 1992;267:12233-8. https://www.jbc.org/content/267/17/12233.long

[25] Candi E, Schmidt R, Melino G. The cornified envelope: a model of cell death in the skin. Nat Rev Mol Cell Biol 2005;6:328-40. DOI: 10.1038/nrm1619

[26] Foster TJ, Geoghegan JA, Ganesh VK, Höök M. Adhesion, invasion and evasion: the many functions of the surface proteins of *Staphylococcus aureus*. Nat Rev Microbiol 2014;12:49-62. DOI: 10.1038/nrmicro3161

[27] Moll R, Divo M, Langbein L. The human keratins: biology and pathology. Histochem Cell Biol 2008;129:705-33. DOI: 10.1007/s00418-008-0435-6

[28] Kumar A, Jagannathan N. Cytokeratin: A review on current concepts. Int J Orofac Biol 2018;2:6-11. DOI: 10.4103/ijofb.ijofb_3_18

[29] Trivedi S, Uhlemann AC, Herman-Bausier P, Sullivan SB, Sowash MG,

Flores EY, et al. The surface protein SdrF mediates *Staphylococcus epidermidis* adherence to keratin. J Infect Dis 2017;215:1846-54. DOI: 10.1093/infdis/jix213

[30] Baur S, Rautenberg M, Faulstich M, Grau T, Severin Y, Unger C, et al. A nasal epithelial receptor for *Staphylococcus aureus* WTA governs adhesion to epithelial cells and modulates nasal colonization. Plos Pathog 2014;10:1-13. DOI: 10.1371/journal.ppat.1004089

[31] Canton J, Neculai D, Grinstein S. Scavenger receptors in homeostasis and immunity. Nat Rev Immunol 2013;13:621-34. DOI: 10.1038/nri3515

[32] Zani IA, Stephen SL, Mughal NA, Russell D, Homer-Vanniasinkam S, Wheatcroft SB, et al. Scavenger receptor structure and function in health and disease. Cells 2015;4:178-201. DOI: 10.3390/cells4020178

[33] Patten DA. SCARF1: a multifaceted, yet largely understudied, scavenger receptor. Inflamm Res 2018;67:627-32. DOI: 10.1007/s00011-018-1154-7

[34] Means TK, Mylonakis E, Tampakakis E, Colvin RA, Seung E, Puckett L, et al. Evolutionarily conserved recognition and innate immunity to fungal pathogens by the scavenger receptors SCARF1 and CD36. J Exp Med 2009;206:637-53. DOI: 10.1084/jem.20082109

[35] Patten DA, Kamarajah SK, Rose JM, Tickle J, Shepherd EL, Adams DH, et al. SCARF-1 promotes adhesion of CD4+ T cells to human hepatic sinusoidal endothelium under conditions of shear stress. Sci Rep 2017;7:1-15. DOI: 10.1038/s41598-017-17928-4

[36] Ramirez-Ortiz ZG, Pendergraft III WF, Prasad A, Byrne MH, Iram T, Blanchette CJ, et al. The scavenger receptor SCARF1 mediates the clearance of apoptotic cells and prevents autoimmunity. Nat Immunol 2013;14:917-26. DOI: 10.1038/ni.2670

[37] Kotpal R, Bhalla P, Dewan R, Kaur R. Incidence and risk factors of nasal carriage of *Staphylococcus aureus* in HIV-infected individuals in comparison to HIV-uninfected individuals: a case–control study. J Int Assoc Provid AIDS Care 2016;15:141-7. DOI: 10.1177/2325957414554005

[38] Olsen K, Danielsen K, Wilsgaard T, Sangvik M, Sollid JU, Thune I, et al. Obesity and *Staphylococcus aureus* nasal colonization among women and men in a general population. PLoS One 2013;8:e63716. DOI: 10.1371/journal.pone.0063716.

[39] Nowak JE, Borkowska BA, Pawlowski BZ. Sex differences in the risk factors for *Staphylococcus aureus* throat carriage. Am J Infect Control 2017;45:29-33. DOI: 10.1016/j.ajic.2016.07.013

[40] Immergluck LC, Jain S, Ray SM, Mayberry R, Satola S, Parker TC, et al. Risk of skin and soft tissue infections among children found to be *Staphylococcus aureus* MRSA USA300 carriers. West J Emerg Med 2017;18:201-12. DOI: 10.5811/westjem.2016.10.30483

[41] Liu CM, Price LB, Hungate BA, Abraham AG, Larsen LA, Christensen K, et al. *Staphylococcus aureus* and the ecology of the nasal microbiome. Sci Adv 2015;1:e1400216. DOI: 10.1126/sciadv.1400216

[42] Elie-Turenne MC, Fernandes H, Mediavilla JR, Rosenthal M, Mathema B, Singh A, et al. Prevalence and characteristics of *Staphylococcus aureus* colonization among healthcare professionals in an urban teaching hospital. Infect Control Hosp Epidemiol 2010;31:574-80. DOI: 10.1086/652525

[43] Price JR, Cole K, Bexley A, Kostiou V, Eyre DW, Golubchik T, et al. Transmission of *Staphylococcus aureus* between health-care workers, the environment, and patients in an intensive care unit: a longitudinal cohort study based on whole-genome sequencing. Lancet Infect Dis 2017;17:207-14. DOI: 10.1016/S1473-3099(16)30413-3

[44] Olsen K, Falch BM, Danielsen K, Johannessen M, Sollid JE, Thune I, et al. *Staphylococcus aureus* nasal carriage is associated with serum 25-hydroxyvitamin D levels, gender and smoking status. The Tromsø Staph and Skin Study. Eur J Clin Microbiol Infect Dis 2012;31:465-73. DOI: 10.1007/s10096-011-1331-x

[45] Cole AL, Schmidt-Owens M, Beavis AC, Chong CF, Tarwater PM, Schaus J, et al. Cessation from smoking improves innate host defense and clearance of experimentally inoculated nasal *Staphylococcus aureus*. Infect Immun 2018;86:e00912-17. DOI: 10.1128/IAI.00912-17

[46] Zanger P, Nurjadi D, Schleucher R, Scherbaum H, Wolz C, Kremsner PG, et al. Import and Spread of Panton-Valentine Leukocidin–Positive *Staphylococcus aureus* Through Nasal Carriage and Skin Infections in Travelers Returning From the Tropics and Subtropics. Clin Infect Dis 2012;54:483-92. DOI: 10.1093/cid/cir822

[47] Roghmann MC, Johnson JK, Stine OC, Lydecker AD, Ryan KA, Mitchell BD, et al. Persistent *Staphylococcus aureus* colonization is not a strongly heritable trait in Amish families. PLoS One 2011;6: e17368. DOI: 10.1371/journal.pone.0017368

[48] Andersen PS, Pedersen JK, Fode P, Skov RL, Fowler Jr VG, Stegger M, et al. Influence of host genetics and environment on nasal carriage of *Staphylococcus aureus* in Danish middle-aged and elderly twins. J Infect Dis 2012;206:1178-84. DOI: 10.1093/infdis/jis491

[49] Sasegbon A, Hamdy S. The anatomy and physiology of normal and abnormal swallowing in oropharyngeal dysphagia. Neurogastroenterol Motil 2017;29:1-15 DOI: 10.1111/nmo.13100

[50] Fossum C, Beltran C, Ma DJ, Foote RL. Biological Model for Predicting Toxicity in Patients With Head and Neck Cancer Treated With Proton Beam Therapy. Int J Radiat Oncol Biol Phys 2016;96:E616-E617. https://www.redjournal.org/article/S0360-3016(16)32500-7/pdf

[51] de Steenhuijsen Piters WA, Sanders EA, Bogaert D. The role of the local microbial ecosystem in respiratory health and disease. Philos Trans R Soc Lond B Biol Sci 2015;370:20140294. DOI: 10.1098/rstb.2014.0294

[52] Bignardi GE, S Lowes. "MRSA screening: throat swabs are better than nose swabs." J Hosp Infect 2009;71:373-4. DOI: 10.1016/j.jhin.2009.01.003

[53] Lee CJ, Sankaran S, Mukherjee DV, Apa ZL, Hafer CA, Wright L, et al. *Staphylococcus aureus* oropharyngeal carriage in a prison population. Clin Infect Dis 2011;52:775-8. DOI: 10.1093/cid/cir026

[54] Mertz D, Frei R, Jaussi B, Tietz A, Stebler C, Flückiger U, et al. Throat swabs are necessary to reliably detect carriers of *Staphylococcus aureus*. Clin Infect Dis 2007;45:475-7. DOI: 10.1086/520016

[55] Nahimana I, Francioli P, Blanc DS. Evaluation of three chromogenic media (MRSA-ID, MRSA-Select and CHROMagar MRSA) and ORSAB for surveillance cultures of methicillin-resistant *Staphylococcus aureus*. Clin Microbiol Infect 2006;12:1168-74. DOI: 10.1111/j.1469-0691.2006.01534.x

[56] Cirkovic I, Stepanovic S, Skov R, Trajkovic J, Grgurevic A, Larsen AR. Carriage and genetic diversity of methicillin-resistant *Staphylococcus aureus* among patients and healthcare workers in a Serbian university hospital. PLoS One 2015;10:e0127347. DOI: 10.1371/journal.pone.0127347

[57] Tacconelli E, Foschi F. Does gender affect the outcome of community-acquired *Staphylococcus aureus* bacteraemia? Clin Microbiol Infect 2017;23:23-5. DOI: 10.1016/j.cmi.2016.09.011

[58] Krismer B, Weidenmaier C, Zipperer A, Peschel A. The commensal lifestyle of *Staphylococcus aureus* and its interactions with the nasal microbiota. Nat Rev Microbiol 2017;15:675-87. DOI: 10.1038/nrmicro.2017.104

[59] Wos-Oxley ML, Plumeier I, Von Eiff C, Taudien S, Platzer M, Vilchez-Vargas R, et al. A poke into the diversity and associations within human anterior nare microbial communities. ISME J 2010;4:839-51. DOI: 10.1038/ismej.2010.15

[60] Yan M, Pamp SJ, Fukuyama J, Hwang PH, Cho DY, Holmes S, et al. Nasal microenvironments and interspecific interactions influence nasal microbiota complexity and *S. aureus* carriage. Cell Host Microbe 2013;14:631-40. DOI: 10.1016/j.chom.2013.11.005

[61] Grice EA, Kong HH, Conlan S, Deming CB, Davis J, Young AC, et al. Topographical and temporal diversity of the human skin microbiome. Science 2009;324:1190-2. DOI: 10.1126/science.1171700

[62] Huttenhower C, Gevers D, Knight R, Abubucker S, Badger JH, Chinwalla AT, et al. Structure, function and diversity of the healthy human microbiome. Nature 2012;486:207-14. DOI: 10.1038/nature11234

[63] Segata N, Waldron L, Ballarini A, Narasimhan V, Jousson O, Huttenhower C. Metagenomic microbial community profiling using unique clade-specific marker genes. Nat Methods 2012;9:811-4. DOI: 10.1038/nmeth.2066

[64] Kaspar U, Kriegeskorte A, Schubert T, Peters G, Rudack C, Pieper DH, et al. The culturome of the human nose habitats reveals individual bacterial fingerprint patterns. Environ Microbiol 2016;18:2130-42. DOI: 10.1111/1462-2920.12891

[65] Mahdavinia M, Keshavarzian A, Tobin MC, Landay AL, Schleimer RP. A comprehensive review of the nasal microbiome in chronic rhinosinusitis (CRS). Clin Exp Allergy 2016;46: 21-41. DOI: 10.1111/cea.12666

[66] Kumpitsch C, Koskinen K, Schöpf V, Moissl-Eichinger C. The microbiome of the upper respiratory tract in health and disease. BMC Biol 2019;17:87. DOI: 10.1186/s12915-019-0703-z

[67] Biesbroek G, Tsivtsivadze E, Sanders EA, Montijn R, Veenhoven RH, Keijser BJ, et al. Early respiratory microbiota composition determines bacterial succession patterns and respiratory health in children. Am J Respir Crit Care Med 2014;190:1283-92. DOI: 10.1164/rccm.201407-1240OC

[68] Peterson SW, Knox NC, Golding GR, Tyler SD, Tyler AD, Mabon P, et al. A study of the infant nasal microbiome development over the first year of life and in relation to their primary adult caregivers using cpn60 universal target (UT) as a phylogenetic marker. PLoS One 2016;11:e0152493. DOI: 10.1371/journal.pone.0152493

[69] Lemon KP, Klepac-Ceraj V, Schiffer HK, Brodie EL, Lynch SV, Kolter, R. Comparative analyses of the bacterial microbiota of the

human nostril and oropharynx. mBio 2010;1:e00129-10. DOI: 10.1128/mBio.00129-10

[70] Camarinha-Silva A, Jáuregui R, Pieper DH, Wos-Oxley ML. The temporal dynamics of bacterial communities across human anterior nares. Environ Microbiol Rep 2012;4:126-32. DOI: 10.1111/j.1758-2229.2011.00313.x

[71] Mirzaei MK, Maurice CF. Ménage à trois in the human gut: interactions between host, bacteria and phages. Nat Rev Microbiol 2017;15:397-408. DOI: 10.1038/nrmicro.2017.30

[72] McCarthy AJ, Loeffler A, Witney AA, Gould KA, Lloyd DH, Lindsay JA. Extensive horizontal gene transfer during *Staphylococcus aureus* co-colonization in vivo. Genome Biol Evol 2014;6:2697-708. DOI: 10.1093/gbe/evu214

[73] Krismer B, Liebeke M, Janek D, Nega M, Rautenberg M, Hornig G, et al. Nutrient limitation governs *Staphylococcus aureus* metabolism and niche adaptation in the human nose. PLoS Pathog 2014;10:e1003862. DOI: 10.1371/journal.ppat.1003862

[74] Olson ME, Nygaard TK, Ackermann L, Watkins RL, Zurek OW, Pallister KB, et al. *Staphylococcus aureus* nuclease is an SaeRS-dependent virulence factor. Infect Immun 2013;81:1316-24. DOI: 10.1128/IAI.01242-12

[75] Tomazic PV, Birner-Gruenberger R, Leitner A, Obrist B, Spoerk S, Lang-Loidolt D. Nasal mucus proteomic changes reflect altered immune responses and epithelial permeability in patients with allergic rhinitis. J Allergy Clin Immunol 2014;133:741-50. DOI: 10.1016/j.jaci.2013.09.040

[76] Koziel J, Potempa J. Protease-armed bacteria in the skin. Cell Tissue Res 2013;351:325-37. DOI: 10.1007/s00441-012-1355-2

[77] Arnison PG, Bibb MJ, Bierbaum G, Bowers AA, Bugni TS, Bulaj G, et al. Ribosomally synthesized and post-translationally modified peptide natural products: overview and recommendations for a universal nomenclature. Nat Prod Rep 2013;30:108-60. DOI: 10.1039/c2np20085f

[78] Septimus EJ, Schweizer ML. Decolonization in prevention of health care-associated infections. Clin Microbiol Rev 2016; 29:201-22. DOI:10.1128/CMR.00049-15

[79] Janek D, Zipperer A, Kulik A, Krismer B, Peschel A. High frequency and diversity of antimicrobial activities produced by nasal Staphylococcus strains against bacterial competitors. PLoS Pathog 2016;12: e1005812. DOI:10.1371/journal.ppat.1005812

[80] Bierbaum G, Sahl HG. Lantibiotics: mode of action, biosynthesis and bioengineering. Curr Pharm Biotechnol 2009;10:2-18. DOI: 10.2174/138920109787048616

[81] Donia MS, Cimermancic P, Schulze CJ, Brown LCW, Martin J, Mitreva M, et al. A systematic analysis of biosynthetic gene clusters in the human microbiome reveals a common family of antibiotics. Cell 2014;158:1402-14. DOI: 10.1016/j.cell.2014.08.032

[82] Zipperer A, Konnerth MC, Laux C, Berscheid A, Janek D, Weidenmaier C, et al. Human commensals producing a novel antibiotic impair pathogen colonization. Nature 2016;535:511-6. DOI: 10.1038/nature18634

[83] Nakatsuji T, Chen TH, Narala S, Chun KA, Two AM, Yun T, et al. Antimicrobials from human skin commensal bacteria protect against

Staphylococcus aureus and are deficient in atopic dermatitis. Sci Transl Med 2017;9:eaah4680. DOI: 10.1126/scitranslmed.aah4680

[84] Mądry A, Jendroszek A, Dubin G, Wladyka B. Production of Lysostaphin by Nonproprietary Method Utilizing a Promoter from Toxin–Antitoxin System. Mol Biotechnol 2019;61:774-82. DOI: 10.1007/s12033-019-00203-4

[85] Selva L, Viana D, Regev-Yochay G, Trzcinski K, Corpa JM, Novick RP, et al. Killing niche competitors by remote-control bacteriophage induction. Proc Natl Acad Sci U S A 2009;106:1234-8. DOI: 10.1073/pnas.0809600106

[86] Lijek RS, Luque SL, Liu Q, Parker D, Bae T, Weiser JN. Protection from the acquisition of *Staphylococcus aureus* nasal carriage by cross-reactive antibody to a pneumococcal dehydrogenase. Proc Natl Acad Sci U S A 2012;109:13823-8. DOI: 10.1073/pnas.1208075109

[87] Uehara Y, Kikuchi K, Nakamura T, Nakama H, Agematsu K, Kawakami Y, et al. H2O2 produced by viridans group streptococci may contribute to inhibition of methicillin-resistant *Staphylococcus aureus* colonization of oral cavities in newborns. Clin Infect Dis 2001;32:1408-13. DOI: 10.1086/320179

[88] Ahn J, Chen CY, Hayes RB. Oral microbiome and oral and gastrointestinal cancer risk. Cancer Causes Control 2012;23:399-404. DOI: 10.1007/s10552-011-9892-7

[89] Gao Z, Kang Y, Yu J, Ren L. Human pharyngeal microbiome may play a protective role in respiratory tract infections. Genomics Proteomics Bioinformatics 2014;12:144-50. DOI: 10.1016/j.gpb.2014.06.001

[90] Jordán F, Lauria M, Scotti M, Nguyen TP, Praveen P, Morine M, et al. Diversity of key players in the microbial ecosystems of the human body. Sci Rep 2015;5:15920. DOI: 10.1038/srep15920

[91] Kim TH, Johnstone J, Loeb M. Vaccine herd effect. Scand J Infect Dis 2011;43:683-9. DOI: 10.3109/00365548.2011.582247

[92] Quintero B, Araque M, Van Der Gaast-de Jongh C, Escalona F, Correa M, Morillo-Puente S, et al. Epidemiology of *Streptococcus pneumoniae* and *Staphylococcus aureus* colonization in healthy Venezuelan children. Eur J Clin Microbiol Infect Dis 2011;30:7-19. DOI: 10.1007/s10096-010-1044-6

[93] Bogaert D, Keijser B, Huse S, Rossen J, Veenhoven R, Van Gils E, et al. Variability and diversity of nasopharyngeal microbiota in children: a metagenomic analysis. PloS One 2011;6:e17035. DOI: 10.1371/journal.pone.0017035

Chapter 12

The Evaluation and Treatment of Obstructive Sleep Apnea Syndrome

Abdullah Alhelali

Abstract

The pharynx is composed of complex soft structures such as muscles and lymphoid tissues. These soft tissues cause the pharynx to collapse during sleep, eventually causing narrowing and obstructive apneas. Recently, sleep obstructive apneas have received increasing attention because many serious consequences can occur. Systemic diseases such as hypertension, coronary artery diseases, and cognitive dysfunction can occur. Despite its low adherence rate, continuous positive airway pressure is considered the most recommended management strategy for adults. In children, adenotonsillectomy is the primary intervention. Many other surgical interventions have been utilized. This chapter will cover the most essential types of pharyngeal surgery used to manage obstructive sleep apnea syndrome.

Keywords: pharynx, sleep, obstructive, apnea, sleep surgery

1. Introduction

Obstructive sleep apnea syndrome (OSAS) is one of the common conditions encountered by otolaryngologists. During sleep, many episodic cessations or decreases in breathing (apnea or hypopnea) occur repeatedly in patients diagnosed with OSAS [1–4]. It affects all ages, with a higher incidence in adults [5]. The prevalence of sleep apnea ranges from 2% and 14% [6]. Many sequelae of this disease have been reported. Systemic diseases such as diabetes, hypertension, and heart diseases have been reported [7]. The treatment of OSAS has been associated with significant improvements in hypertension [8, 9], motor vehicle collisions [10], and many psychosocial functions [11]. Establishing the diagnosis of OSAS requires a combination of sleep studies (polysomnography PSG) and a record of daytime symptoms. An apnea-hypopnea index (AHI) equal to or greater than five events in one hour in adults [12] and equal to or more than one event per hour in children [13] is considered abnormal. During the day, individuals with OSAS may feel fatigued or unrested and may have vigilance and cognitive function impairments, as well as on-road and occupational accidents [14].

The pharyngeal airway plays the major role in airway narrowing during sleep. Many surgical and nonsurgical treatments have been proposed and used. Nonsurgical management includes behavioral changes, weight loss, the use of medications, continuous positive airway pressure (CPAP) and oral appliances. Surgical treatment includes tracheostomy, uvulopalatopharyngoplasty, mandibular advancement, and hypoglossal nerve stimulation [15].

In adults, CPAP is considered the first choice for management. It is useful in decreasing daytime sleepiness and improving quality of life measures [16]. CPAP works by splinting the airway, particularly the pharyngeal airway, during sleep. The main drawback of CPAP is poor adherence reported in the literature. Compliance was defined as a minimum of 4 hours of use per night. Nonadherence reports in the literature range from 46% to 83% [17].

2. Drug-induced sleep endoscopy, DISE

An endoscopic evaluation of the airway during sleep induced by anesthetic agents is a commonly used method to determine the area of obstruction. The ability to tailor the surgical intervention for each patient individually is paramount in determining the success rate. The main significant difference between awake and sleep endoscopic airway assessments is that the latter provides a thorough dynamic evaluation of airway and pharyngeal collapse in situations mimicking natural sleep. In one systematic review, over 50% of surgeries planned based on the awake examination were changed after DISE [18]. DISE is indicated before any sleep surgical intervention in adult patients with OSAS who is unable to tolerate CPAP [19], with socially impacting primary snoring [20], and in whom previous surgery was unsuccessful in curing OSAS [21]. The procedure can be performed safely in an office-based setting or operating room. The main requirements are a quiet and comfortable room with dim light simulating natural sleep. The procedure is performed by an endoscopist who inserts a thin flexible scope in the presence of an anesthetist with basic cardiac, oxygen saturation, and blood pressure monitoring [22]. The depth of sedation should mimic natural sleep. It can be assessed by observation and snoring. The bispectoral index, BIS, is currently a very commonly used tool to monitor the depth of sedation. The targeted depth of sleep is still a topic of debate. A range from 50 to 70 is recommended [20]. BIS monitoring and clinical observations must be combined to achieve the optimal depth of sedation. Many agents have been used for DISE. Midazolam, propofol, and dexmedetomidine are commonly used. Recent studies preferred dexmedetomidine in terms of safety and a lower induction of airway collapsibility during DISE [23–25]. The flexible endoscopic evaluation started from the nasal cavity, assessing the nasal airway, nasopharynx, velopharynx, lateral pharyngeal wall collapse, tonsils, tongue base, hypopharynx and larynx. A widely accepted classification to grade the obstruction is not available. Many classifications have been used [26, 27]. Most importantly, the chosen classification should document the level, degree, and configuration of the obstruction [20].

3. Pharyngeal surgeries for treating OSAS

3.1 Adenotonsillectomy

In children, hypertrophied adenoids and tonsils are the leading cause of OSAS [28]. Most children benefit from adenotonsillectomy. The cure rate (AHI < 1/hour) after adenotonsillectomy ranges from 25% to 71% [29–31]. Many factors affect the resolution of OSAS after adenotonsillectomy. Obesity, an older age, and severe preoperative AHI are among these factors [29, 31].

Adenotonsillectomy is one of the most widely performed surgeries. It is a safe, easy, and effective surgical intervention. Tonsillectomy is a very widespread procedure that is utilized to treat OSAS in adults alone or in combination with other surgical procedures. However, it is the first line of management in children with OSAS [29]. Despite a major improvement in OSAS in the majority of children who underwent tonsillectomy, some children might experience persistent OSAS. The incidence of persistent OSAS after adenotonsillectomy varies in the literature according to the definition of cure after adenotonsillectomy and the study population, ranging from 10 to 77% [32]. A clinician should consider persistent OSAS after tonsillectomy if symptoms of snoring, mouth breathing, restless sleep, enuresis, and daytime sleepiness do not improve. In patients with a suspicion of residual disease, PSG should be repeated [33, 34]. Other levels contributing to the obstruction should be re-evaluated. Regrowth of adenoids in children, the lingual tonsils, tongue base, soft palate and prolapsing epiglottis and supra-glottic structures are among the causes of unresolved OSAS after tonsillectomy. Awake endoscopy can help to re-evaluate the upper airway. Then, a dynamic assessment of the airway during sleep is recommended to tailor the surgical intervention accordingly. DISE and sleep cine-magnetic resonance imaging (MRI) are the most commonly used tools.

3.2 Lingual tonsillectomy

Large lingual tonsils can cause or contribute with other factors to cause OSAS. Lingual tonsillectomy can be performed as the primary surgery or for persistent OSAS after adenotonsillectomy in children. Different surgical techniques have been used, such as LASER, radiofrequency ablation, microdebrider, and suction electrocautery [35]. Many surgeons do not perform this procedure in combination with adenotonsillectomy because the desire to avoid creating a large, circular raw area that may subsequently cause oropharyngeal stenosis [36].

3.3 Uvulopalatoplasty, UPPP

Uvuloplatoplasty (UPPP), either with or without tonsillectomy, is one of the most frequently performed sleep surgeries. It was first described by Fujita et al. in 1979 [37–39]. The procedure is performed by cutting the edge of the soft palate and uvula with or without tonsillectomy [40, 41]. The main aim of this procedure is to decrease retropalatal obstruction and prevent pharyngeal collapse. The best candidate for this surgery is a patient with obstruction at the velum level. One meta-analysis from two randomized controlled trials (RCTs) found that UPPP was significantly more effective at reducing AHI than no treatment [39]. However, the results of long-term follow-up vary between studies [42–44]. The result tends to be better in a patient with a lower body mass index BMI [45–47]. A multiple staging system was established by Friedman et al. [48] based on the palate position, tonsil size and BMI, and the success rate in patients with Friedman stage 1 was 80.6%, but it decreased in patients with higher stages. In patients with stages 2, 3, and 4, the success rates were 37.9% and 8.1%, respectively [48]. One recent meta-analysis compared short-term to long-term outcomes and found that UPPP is an effective intervention, but the efficacy decreases over time [49].

3.4 Expansion pharyngoplasty

Lateral pharyngeal wall collapse is one of the most challenging issues for surgeons to address. In 2007, Pang and Woodson described expansion pharyngoplasty (EPP). The surgery starts with bilateral tonsillectomy, followed by antero-supero-lateral rotation of the superiorly based palatopharyngeus muscle to be attached to arching fibers of the soft palate [50]. Since then, many modifications have been proposed [51–53]. Many noncomparative studies reported its success in treating OSAS [54, 55]. One systematic review with a meta-analysis showed a significantly better EPP result than other traditional surgeries [56]. In 2009, Li et al. [57] described the relocation pharyngoplasty technique in 10 patients. This technique enables advancement of the soft palate and splinting of the lateral pharyngeal wall [57]. In 2012, Mantovani et al. [58] described the velo-uvulo-pharyngeal lift technique to lift, shorten, and advance the soft palate. The soft palate is lifted by threads anchored to fibro-osseous structure at the level of the posterior nasal spine and bilateral pterygoid hamuli [58].

4. Conclusions

Obstructive sleep apnea syndrome is a complex condition with many sequelae. Patient signs and symptoms must be combined with sleep studies to diagnose this condition. Nonsurgical treatments, such as weight reduction, oral application and CPAP, are the first treatments of choice in adults. Surgery such as adenotonsillectomy is the treatment of choice for clearly enlarged adenoids and tonsils in children. DISE is a very useful tool for directing surgical intervention to the most obstructed level. Many surgical interventions have been studied and used to address obstructions with good results.

Conflict of interest

The authors declare no conflict of interest.

Author details

Abdullah Alhelali
Otolaryngology Department, Aseer Central Hospital, Abha, Saudi Arabia

*Address all correspondence to: alhelaliii@hotmail.com

References

[1] Balk EM, Moorthy D, Obadan NO, Patel K, Ip S, Chung M, Bannuru RR, Kitsios GD, Sen S, Iovin RC, Gaylor JM, D'Ambrosio C, Lau J. Diagnosis and Treatment of Obstructive Sleep Apnea in Adults. Rockville (MD): Agency for Healthcare Research and Quality (US); 2011

[2] Greenstone M, Hack M. Obstructive sleep apnoea. BMJ. 2014;348:g3745. DOI: 10.1136/bmj.g3745

[3] Qaseem A, Dallas P, Owens DK, Starkey M, Holty JE, Shekelle P, Clinical Guidelines Committee of the American College of Physicians. Diagnosis of obstructive sleep apnea in adults: A clinical practice guideline from the American College of Physicians. Annals of Internal Medicine. 2014;161:210-220. DOI: 10.7326/M12-3187

[4] Bratton DJ, Stradling JR, Barbe F, Kohler M. Effect of CPAP on blood pressure in patients with minimally symptomatic obstructive sleep apnoea: A meta-analysis using individual patient data from four randomised controlled trials. Thorax. 2014;69:1128-1135. DOI: 10.1136/thoraxjnl-2013-204993

[5] Qaseem A, Holty JE, Owens DK, Dallas P, Starkey M, Shekelle P, Clinical Guidelines Committee of the American College of Physicians. Management of obstructive sleep apnea in adults: A clinical practice guideline from the American college of physicians. Annals of Internal Medicine. 2013;159:471-483. DOI: 10.7326/0003-4819-159-7-201310010-00704

[6] Myers KA, Mrkobrada M, Simel DL. Does this patient have obstructive sleep apnea? The Rational Clinical Examination systematic review. JAMA. 2013;310:731-741. DOI: 10.1001/jama.2013.276185

[7] Robichaud-Halle L, Beaudry M, Fortin M. Obstructive sleep apnea and multimorbidity. BMC Pulmonary Medicine. 2012;12:60. DOI: 10.1186/1471-2466-12-60

[8] Becker HF, Jerrentrup A, Ploch T, Grote L, Penzel T, Sullivan CE, Peter JH. Effect of nasal continuous positive airway pressure treatment on blood pressure in patients with obstructive sleep apnea. Circulation. 2003;107:68-73. DOI: 10.1161/01.cir.0000042706.47107.7a

[9] Martinez-Garcia MA, Gomez-Aldaravi R, Soler-Cataluna JJ, Martinez TG, Bernacer-Alpera B, Roman-Sanchez P. Positive effect of CPAP treatment on the control of difficult-to-treat hypertension. European Respiratory Journal. 2007;29:951-957. DOI: 10.1183/09031936.00048606

[10] George CF. Reduction in motor vehicle collisions following treatment of sleep apnoea with nasal CPAP. Thorax. 2001;56:508-512. DOI: 10.1136/thorax.56.7.508

[11] McFadyen TA, Espie CA, McArdle N, Douglas NJ, Engleman HM. Controlled, prospective trial of psychosocial function before and after continuous positive airway pressure therapy. European Respiratory Journal. 2001;18:996-1002. DOI: 10.1183/09031936.01.00209301

[12] Kapur VK, Auckley DH, Chowdhuri S, Kuhlmann DC, Mehra R, Ramar K, Harrod CG. Clinical practice guideline for diagnostic testing for adult obstructive sleep apnea: An American academy of sleep medicine clinical practice guideline. Journal of Clinical Sleep Medicine. 2017;13:479-504. DOI: 10.5664/jcsm.6506

[13] Sateia MJ. International classification of sleep disorders-third edition: Highlights and modifications.

Chest. 2014;146:1387-1394. DOI: 10.1378/chest.14-0970

[14] Jackson ML, Howard ME, Barnes M. Cognition and daytime functioning in sleep-related breathing disorders. Progress in Brain Research. 2011;190:53-68. DOI: 10.1016/B978-0-444-53817-8.00003-7

[15] Chang HP, Chen YF, Du JK. Obstructive sleep apnea treatment in adults. The Kaohsiung Journal of Medical Sciences. 2020;36:7-12. DOI: 10.1002/kjm2.12130

[16] Antic NA, Catcheside P, Buchan C, Hensley M, Naughton MT, Rowland S, Williamson B, Windler S, McEvoy RD. The effect of CPAP in normalizing daytime sleepiness, quality of life, and neurocognitive function in patients with moderate to severe OSA. Sleep. 2011;34:111-119. DOI: 10.1093/sleep/34.1.111

[17] Weaver TE, Grunstein RR. Adherence to continuous positive airway pressure therapy: The challenge to effective treatment. Proceedings of the American Thoracic Society. 2008;5:173-178. DOI: 10.1513/pats.200708-119MG

[18] Certal VF, Pratas R, Guimaraes L, Lugo R, Tsou Y, Camacho M, Capasso R. Awake examination versus DISE for surgical decision making in patients with OSA: A systematic review. Laryngoscope. 2016;126:768-774. DOI: 10.1002/lary.25722

[19] Vanderveken OM. Drug-induced sleep endoscopy (DISE) for non-CPAP treatment selection in patients with sleep-disordered breathing. Sleep and Breathing. 2013;17:13-14. DOI: 10.1007/s11325-012-0671-9

[20] De Vito A, Carrasco Llatas M, Vanni A, Bosi M, Braghiroli A, Campanini A, de Vries N, Hamans E, Hohenhorst W, Kotecha BT, Maurer J, Montevecchi F, Piccin O, Sorrenti G, Vanderveken OM, Vicini C. European position paper on drug-induced sedation endoscopy (DISE). Sleep and Breathing. 2014;18:453-465. DOI: 10.1007/s11325-014-0989-6

[21] Kezirian EJ. Nonresponders to pharyngeal surgery for obstructive sleep apnea: Insights from drug-induced sleep endoscopy. Laryngoscope. 2011;121:1320-1326. DOI: 10.1002/lary.21749

[22] Chong KB, De Vito A, Vicini C. Drug-induced sleep endoscopy in treatment options selection. Sleep Medicine Clinics. 2019;14:33-40. DOI: 10.1016/j.jsmc.2018.11.001

[23] Yoon BW, Hong JM, Hong SL, Koo SK, Roh HJ, Cho KS. A comparison of dexmedetomidine versus propofol during drug-induced sleep endoscopy in sleep apnea patients. Laryngoscope. 2016;126:763-767. DOI: 10.1002/lary.25801

[24] Chang ET, Certal V, Song SA, Zaghi S, Carrasco-Llatas M, Torre C, Capasso R, Camacho M. Dexmedetomidine versus propofol during drug-induced sleep endoscopy and sedation: A systematic review. Sleep and Breathing. 2017;21:727-735. DOI: 10.1007/s11325-017-1465-x

[25] Padiyara TV, Bansal S, Jain D, Arora S, Gandhi K. Dexmedetomidine versus propofol at different sedation depths during drug-induced sleep endoscopy: A randomized trial. Laryngoscope. 2020;130:257-262. DOI: 10.1002/lary.27903

[26] Kezirian EJ, Hohenhorst W, de Vries N. Drug-induced sleep endoscopy: The VOTE classification. European Archives of Oto-Rhino-Laryngology. 2011;268:1233-1236. DOI: 10.1007/s00405-011-1633-8

[27] Vicini C, De Vito A, Benazzo M, Frassineti S, Campanini A, Frasconi P,

Mira E. The nose oropharynx hypopharynx and larynx (NOHL) classification: A new system of diagnostic standardized examination for OSAHS patients. European Archives of Oto-Rhino-Laryngology. 2012;269:1297-1300. DOI: 10.1007/s00405-012-1965-z

[28] Marcus CL, Brooks LJ, Draper KA, Gozal D, Halbower AC, Jones J, Schechter MS, Ward SD, Sheldon SH, Shiffman RN, Lehmann C, Spruyt K, American Academy of Pediatrics. Diagnosis and management of childhood obstructive sleep apnea syndrome. Pediatrics. 2012;130:e714–e755. DOI: 10.1542/peds.2012-1672

[29] Bhattacharjee R, Kheirandish-Gozal L, Spruyt K, Mitchell RB, Promchiarak J, Simakajornboon N, Kaditis AG, Splaingard D, Splaingard M, Brooks LJ, Marcus CL, Sin S, Arens R, Verhulst SL, Gozal D. Adenotonsillectomy outcomes in treatment of obstructive sleep apnea in children: A multicenter retrospective studyQ. American Journal of Respiratory and Critical Care Medicine. 2010;182:676-683. DOI: 10.1164/rccm.200912-1930OC

[30] Tauman R, Gulliver TE, Krishna J, Montgomery-Downs HE, O'Brien LM, Ivanenko A, Gozal D. Persistence of obstructive sleep apnea syndrome in children after adenotonsillectomy. The Journal of Pediatrics. 2006;149:803-808. DOI: 10.1016/j.jpeds.2006.08.067

[31] Mitchell RB. Adenotonsillectomy for obstructive sleep apnea in children: Outcome evaluated by pre- and postoperative polysomnography. Laryngoscope. 2007;117:1844-1854. DOI: 10.1097/MLG.0b013e318123ee56

[32] Boudewyns A, Abel F, Alexopoulos E, Evangelisti M, Kaditis A, Miano S, Villa MP, Verhulst SL. Adenotonsillectomy to treat obstructive sleep apnea: Is it enough? Pediatric Pulmonology. 2017;52:699-709. DOI: 10.1002/ppul.23641

[33] Roland PS, Rosenfeld RM, Brooks LJ, Friedman NR, Jones J, Kim TW, Kuhar S, Mitchell RB, Seidman MD, Sheldon SH, Jones S, Robertson P, American Academy of Otolaryngology-Head Neck Surgery Foundation. Clinical practice guideline: Polysomnography for sleep-disordered breathing prior to tonsillectomy in children. Otolaryngology Head and Neck Surgery. 2011;145:S1-S15. DOI: 10.1177/0194599811409837

[34] Aurora RN, Zak RS, Karippot A, Lamm CI, Morgenthaler TI, Auerbach SH, Bista SR, Casey KR, Chowdhuri S, Kristo DA, Ramar K, American Academy of Sleep Medicine. Practice parameters for the respiratory indications for polysomnography in children. Sleep. 2011;34:379-388. DOI: 10.1093/sleep/34.3.379

[35] Cielo CM, Gungor A. Treatment options for pediatric obstructive sleep apnea. Current Problems in Pediatric and Adolescent Health Care. 2016;46:27-33. DOI: 10.1016/j.cppeds.2015.10.006

[36] Prager JD, Hopkins BS, Propst EJ, Shott SR, Cotton RT. Oropharyngeal stenosis: A complication of multilevel, single-stage upper airway surgery in children. Archives of Otolaryngology--Head & Neck Surgery. 2010;136:1111-1115. DOI: 10.1001/archoto.2010.197

[37] Kezirian EJ, Maselli J, Vittinghoff E, Goldberg AN, Auerbach AD. Obstructive sleep apnea surgery practice patterns in the United States: 2000 to 2006. Otolaryngology-Head and Neck Surgery. 2010;143:441-447. DOI: 10.1016/j.otohns.2010.05.009

[38] Kezirian EJ, Weaver EM, Yueh B, Deyo RA, Khuri SF, Daley J, Henderson W. Incidence of serious complications after

uvulopalatopharyngoplasty. Laryngoscope. 2004;114:450-453. DOI: 10.1097/00005537-200403000-00012

[39] Stuck BA, Ravesloot MJL, Eschenhagen T, de Vet HCW, Sommer JU. Uvulopalatopharyngoplasty with or without tonsillectomy in the treatment of adult obstructive sleep apnea - A systematic review. Sleep Medicine. 2018;50:152-165. DOI: 10.1016/j.sleep.2018.05.004

[40] Practice parameters for the treatment of obstructive sleep apnea in adults: The efficacy of surgical modifications of the upper airway. Report of the American sleep disorders association. Sleep. 1996;19:152-155. DOI: 10.1093/sleep/19.2.152

[41] Sundaram S, Bridgman SA, Lim J, Lasserson TJ. Surgery for obstructive sleep apnoea. Cochrane Database of Systematic Reviews. 2005:CD001004. DOI: 10.1002/14651858.CD001004.pub2

[42] Walker-Engstrom ML, Wilhelmsson B, Tegelberg A, Dimenas E, Ringqvist I. Quality of life assessment of treatment with dental appliance or UPPP in patients with mild to moderate obstructive sleep apnoea. A prospective randomized 1-year follow-up study. Journal of Sleep Research. 2000;9:303-308. DOI: 10.1046/j.1365-2869.2000.00210.x

[43] Browaldh N, Friberg D, Svanborg E, Nerfeldt P. 15-year efficacy of uvulopalatopharyngoplasty based on objective and subjective data. Acta Oto-Laryngologica. 2011;131:1303-1310. DOI: 10.3109/00016489.2011.616912

[44] Boot H, van Wegen R, Poublon RM, Bogaard JM, Schmitz PI, van der Meche FG. Long-term results of uvulopalatopharyngoplasty for obstructive sleep apnea syndrome. Laryngoscope. 2000;110:469-475. DOI: 10.1097/00005537-200003000-00027

[45] Dickson RI, Blokmanis A. Treatment of obstructive sleep apnea by uvulopalatopharyngoplasty. Laryngoscope. 1987;97:1054-1059. DOI: 10.1288/00005537-198709000-00011

[46] Laffont F, Lecendreux B, Minz M, Josse MO, Waisbord P, Fleury M, Chabolle F, Cathala HP. Efficacy of uvulopalatopharyngoplasty (UPPP) and modifications in sleep structure in the sleep apnea syndrome (SAS). Neurophysiologie Clinique = Clinical Neurophysiology. 1989;19:477-488. DOI: 10.1016/s0987-7053(89)80004-8

[47] Gislason T, Lindholm CE, Almqvist M, Birring E, Boman G, Eriksson G, Larsson SG, Lidell C, Svanholm H. Uvulopalatopharyngoplasty in the sleep apnea syndrome. Predictors of results. Archives of Otolaryngology–Head & Neck Surgery. 1988;114:45-51. DOI: 10.1001/archotol.1988.01860130049013

[48] Friedman M, Ibrahim H, Bass L. Clinical staging for sleep-disordered breathing. Otolaryngology—Head and Neck Surgery. 2002;127:13-21. DOI: 10.1067/mhn.2002.126477

[49] He M, Yin G, Zhan S, Xu J, Cao X, Li J, Ye J. Long-term Efficacy of Uvulopalatopharyngoplasty among adult patients with obstructive sleep apnea: A systematic review and meta-analysis. Otolaryngology—Head and Neck Surgery. 2019;161:401-411. DOI: 10.1177/0194599819840356

[50] Pang KP, Woodson BT. Expansion sphincter pharyngoplasty: A new technique for the treatment of obstructive sleep apnea. Otolaryngology—Head and Neck Surgery. 2007;137:110-114. DOI: 10.1016/j.otohns.2007.03.014

[51] Vicini C, Montevecchi F, Pang K, Bahgat A, Dallan I, Frassineti S, Campanini A. Combined transoral

robotic tongue base surgery and palate surgery in obstructive sleep apnea-hypopnea syndrome: Expansion sphincter pharyngoplasty versus uvulopalatopharyngoplasty. Head & Neck. 2014;36:77-83. DOI: 10.1002/hed.23271

[52] Sorrenti G, Piccin O. Functional expansion pharyngoplasty in the treatment of obstructive sleep apnea. Laryngoscope. 2013;123:2905-2908. DOI: 10.1002/lary.23911

[53] Ulualp SO. Modified expansion sphincter pharyngoplasty for treatment of children with obstructive sleep apnea. JAMA Otolaryngology–Head & Neck Surgery. 2014;140:817-822. DOI: 10.1001/jamaoto.2014.1329

[54] Plaza G, Baptista P, O'Connor-Reina C, Bosco G, Perez-Martin N, Pang KP. Prospective multi-center study on expansion sphincter pharyngoplasty. Acta Oto-Laryngologica. 2019;139:219-222. DOI: 10.1080/00016489.2018.1533992

[55] Pinto JA, Godoy LBM, Nunes H, Abdo KE, Jahic GS, Cavallini AF, Freitas GS, Ribeiro DK, Duarte C. Lateral-expansion pharyngoplasty: Combined technique for the treatment of obstructive sleep apnea syndrome. International Archives of Otorhinolaryngology. 2020;24:e107-e111. DOI: 10.1055/s-0039-1695026

[56] Pang KP, Pang EB, Win MT, Pang KA, Woodson BT. Expansion sphincter pharyngoplasty for the treatment of OSA: A systemic review and meta-analysis. European Archives of Oto-Rhino-Laryngology. 2016;273:2329-2333. DOI: 10.1007/s00405-015-3831-2

[57] Li HY, Lee LA. Relocation pharyngoplasty for obstructive sleep apnea. Laryngoscope. 2009;119:2472-2477. DOI: 10.1002/lary.20634

[58] Mantovani M, Minetti A, Torretta S, Pincherle A, Tassone G, Pignataro L. The velo-uvulo-pharyngeal lift or "roman blinds" technique for treatment of snoring: A preliminary report. Acta Otorhinolaryngologica Italica. 2012;32:48-53

Chapter 13

Assessment of Dysphagia as a Risk Factor of Chronic Cough

Barbara Jamróz, Magdalena Milewska, Joanna Chmielewska-Walczak, Magdalena Lachowska, Marta Dąbrowska-Bender, Magdalena Arcimowicz, Anna Staniszewska, Anna Brytek-Matera and Kazimierz Niemczyk

Abstract

Background: The aim of the study was to determine the prevalence of dysphagia in patients with chronic cough and its relationship with the long-term persistence of these symptoms. Methods: Thirty consecutive patients. All patients underwent physical examination, ENT assessment, videolaryngoscopy, functional phoniatric assessment at rest and speech, Water-Swallow Test, and Fiberoptic Endoscopic Evaluation of Swallowing disorders with Reflux Finding Score. Reflux Symptom Index questionnaire was performed. The study was approved by the local Ethics Committee Review Board (KB/39/A/2016). Results: The results of the RFS and the RSI questionnaire showed the risk of reflux in participating patients. The patients presented episodes of spillage, double swallows, penetration, aspiration and residue of food at the hypopharynx. The results of functional assessment correlated with the Water-Swallow Test. The correlation between Fiberoptic Endoscopic Evaluation of Swallowing disorders and Water-Swallow Test results was found for aspiration risk, spillage, and retention of saliva. Conclusion: The results of the study showed prevalence of dysphagia in most patients with chronic chough. It seems that phoniatric assessment in those cases should be expanded and the following tests should be performed: assessment of the laryngeal elevation, Water-Swallow Test, and Fiberoptic Endoscopic Evaluation of Swallowing disorders.

Keywords: dysphagia, chronic cough, phoniatric, water swallowing test, aspiration

1. Introduction

Chronic cough is commonly reported symptoms in clinical practice. However, there is no globally accepted definition. Chronic, disruptive, lasting more than eight weeks cough is a difficult diagnostic and therapeutic problem [1]. The other used in researches definition of chronic cough is a cough lasting ≥3 months [2] or "daily coughing for at least 3 months duration during preceding 2 years [3]. Recently, replacing term chronic term by cough hypersensitivity syndrome has been proposed to highlight different phenotypes of this condition [4]. We can distinguish also idiopathic chronic cough and refractory chronic cough [5].

In approximation, it can affect 10–40% of general population [1, 3, 6].

IntechOpen

The prevalence depend on sex, age and comorbidities. Recent observational study indicated that females, older adults, patients suffering from gastro-esophageal reflux disease, asthma, chronic obstructive pulmonary disease are at risk of chronic cough [3, 7]. Among additional risk factors are smoking [7] and drugs (e.g. angiotensin -converting enzyme inhibitors) [8].

People suffering from it require a multidisciplinary diagnostic panel like allergology tests, gastrological, pulmonary, otolaryngology and phoniatric counseling [1]. Despite enhanced diagnostics - the final diagnosis is difficult to be established, and the introduction of effective therapy sometimes impossible, which significantly reduces the quality of life in those patients [1, 9–11]. In practice, diagnosis of chronic cough raises difficulties cause cough can be symptom of disease from the one side, but from the other also consequence. Therefore carefully taken history provides information about potential causes. Clinical interview should aimed on exclusion malignancy, ongoing infection, body inhalation or using angiotensin converting enzyme inhibitors (ACE). Further question should focused on chronic pulmonary diseases, GERD, allergy [12]. The medical history should be deepen by different advanced methods like: chest CT or radiography, CT of sinusitis, spirometry, airway hypersensitivity test, allergic test, bronchoscopy, endoscopic examination of nose and paranasal sinuses, videolaryngostroboscopy, FEES, FVS, pH-metry, high resolution manometry, gastroscopy and functional assessment [5, 8]. Until recently, mainly pharmacological treatment was delivered. Results were promising although not free from side effects. The most often proposed pharmacological therapies include: proton pomp inhibitors and prokinetics agents, histamine H1 antagonists, inhaled corticosteroids and nasal steroids. In case of lack of therapeutic effect gabapentin, pregabalin are recommended. Other drugs like morphine, tramadol, codeine and dextromethorphan, amitriptyline are still controversial [12, 13]. Chronic cough treatment is still not well recognized, so the new pharmacological substance like Gefapixant are under investigation [14]. Recently physiotherapist and speech language therapist proposed several non-pharmacological treatment concentrated on breathing exercises and counseling. Following non-pharmacological components were indicated: education, psycho-educational counseling, vocal/laryngeal hygiene and hydration, cough control/suppression techniques [5].

Despite cough is a natural defense mechanism of the airway, a little is known about chronic cough long term implications. Our clinical experience shows that the from the one side increased neck muscle tension leads to lowering the elevation of the larynx and impedes swallowing thus favoring retention of food, and food penetration or aspiration into the respiratory tract. But from the other side, delay opening upper esophageal sphincter. This in turn may result in further worsening of the symptoms causing persistent cough. The association of GERD and swallowing problems implicate the risk of microaspiration into the lungs what can trigger persistent cough. The little is known about prevalence of microaspiration as a consequence of chronic reflux disease [8].

To our best knowledge, there are no published studies referring to dysphagia in patients with chronic cough. Clinical experience shows that the increased neck muscle tension leads to lowering the elevation of the larynx and impedes swallowing thus favoring retention of food, and food penetration or aspiration into the respiratory tract. This in turn may result in further worsening of the symptoms causing persistent cough.

2. Aim of study

The aim of the study was to determine the prevalence of dysphagia in patients with chronic cough and its relationship with the long-term persistence of these symptoms.

3. Materials and methods

3.1 Inclusion and exclusion criteria

Thirty consecutive patients were enrolled in this study. All of them underwent phoniatric counseling due to chronic cough. Inclusion criteria were as follow: cough lasting more than 8 weeks, the lack of response to standard antiallergic, antireflux and antiasthmatic therapy. The patients with previously diagnosed dysphagia, with stroke or trauma to the head and neck were excluded from the study. Medications that may cause dysphagia were also a part of the exclusion criteria.

3.2 Methods

All patients underwent physical examination, Ear, Nose and Throat (ENT) assessment with a detailed evaluation of the cranial nerves, in particular V, VII, IX, X, and XII cranial nerve, and Fiberoptic Endoscopic Evaluation of Swallowing disorders (FEES). Pulmonary counseling and allergy tests were also performed in each participating patient.

All patients completed a Reflux Symptom Index questionnaire (RSI). RSI consists of nine questions regarding extraesophageal symptoms of gastroesophageal reflux disease, assessed on a scale of 0–5. A score of over 13 points is interpreted as abnormal and indicates the need for further investigation e.g. gastroscopy, esophageal impedance test [15].

Phoniatric assessment included careful visual inspection of the oral cavity, pharynx and the larynx, videolaryngoscopic evaluation (VLS) and functional assessment of the larynx. The changes noticed in the larynx were assessed using the Reflux Finding Score (RFS) that rates objectively the laryngeal reflux changes. The scale ranges from 0 to 22 points where the result of 7 and more points indicates laryngopharyngeal reflux [16].

On physical examination, particular attention was drawn to: pharyngeal reflexes, strength, range and coordination of the oral cavity and pharyngeal muscles, and elevation of the larynx during swallows.

In the functional assessment the following was evaluated:

- posture - normal, increased or decreased lumbar and cervical lordosis
- breathing pattern - upper chest, chest-abdominal, and abdominal breathing
- tension of the sternocleidomastoid muscle (SCM), pharyngeal walls and submandibular area muscles - on a scale of 0-II$^{\circ}$ where 0° means normal tension, I$^{\circ}$ means medium increased, II$^{\circ}$ means significant tension
- thyrohyoid and the cricothyroid space - normal or reduced.

For the screening assessment of dysphagia the water-swallow test (WST) was used in following steps (liquid volume): 5, 10, 20, and 90 ml of non-carbonated water. After each step the presence of indirect signs of penetration/aspiration of the liquid into the larynx, i.e. coughing, change in voice quality, throat clearing, portioning or test termination [17].

Fiberoptic Endoscopic Examination of Swallowing (FEES) was used for a static and dynamic evaluation of the upper airways and upper digestive tract structures with the anatomy and physiology of the pharynx and larynx during swallows. FEES also gives opportunity to evaluate pharyngeal walls movements during phonation (squezee maneuver) and swallowing of different food consistency. Food consistency was gradually changed from liquid (non-carbonated water), puree (water thickened to the consistency of pudding), and solid food (rucks). In FEES the efficiency of swallowing and penetration/aspiration were assessed using Penetration-Aspiration Scale (PAS). According to Rosenbeck's criteria the scale ranges from 1 to 8, where 1 means no problem, 2–5 means different degree of penetration with or without cough, 6–8 means different degree of aspiration with or without the cough [18–21].

3.3 Ethical statements

The study was approved by the local Ethics Committee Review Board (KB/39/A/2016). All subjects gave their written informed consent to participation in the study.

3.4 Statistical analysis

Statistical analysis was performed using Statistica software (StatSoft, Inc., data analysis software system, version 10). The data were tested for normality, parametric and nonparametric criteria. To analyze the data, the Pearson test was used, and $p < .05$ was considered statistically significant.

4. Results

4.1 Patients characteristics

The study group included 25 women and 5 men, mean age 55.83 years (SD 15.17), reporting cough for the last 2 to 360 months (mean 48 months +/– 100.61) (**Table 1**).

The results of the RFS and the RSI questionnaire showed the risk of reflux in participating patients, RFS = 18.96 (SD 7.02) and RSI = 10.82 (SD 2.73) (**Table 1**). A statistically significant correlation was found between the age of patients and the result of RFS ($p = .03$).

4.2 Clinical assessment of dysphagia

The functional assessment at rest revealed increased submandibular and the pharyngeal walls tension in 19 patients, and SCM increased tension on the right

Analyzed parameter	Mean (+/– SD)
Females:Males	25:5
Age [years]	55,83 (+/– 15,17)
Body weight [kg]	73,86 (+/– 14,62)
Height [m]	164,50 (+/– 8,89)
Body mass index (BMI) [kg/m^2]	26,90 (+/– 5,05)
Duration of cough [months]	48,00 (+/– 100,61)
RSI [points]	18,96 (+/– 7,02)
RFS [pints]	10,82 (+/– 2,73)

RSI (Reflux Symptom Index); RFS (Reflux Finding Score).

Table 1.
Characteristics of the study group.

and left side in 23 and 24 patients, respectively. The reduced thyrohyoid and cricothyroid space was observed in 14 and 16 patients, respectively. The upper chest breathing pattern was observed in 19 subjects. In most of the patients, the increased cervical lordosis (22 patients) and decreased lumbar lordosis (23 patients) was observed. Disorders observed at speech were comparable or more intense to those found at rest (**Table 2**).

On physical examination the following was found: normal pharyngeal reflexes in 23 patients, normal soft palate activity during swallows in 29 patients, and impaired elevation of the larynx in 10 (**Figure 1**).

In case of water swallowing test (WST) results, the negative (no risk of aspiration) result was found in 28 patients (93.33%) for 5 ml amount of liquid, in 24 (80.00%) for 10 ml, in 21 (70.00%) for 20 ml, and in 15 (50.00%) for 90 ml (**Figure 2**). The remaining patients demonstrated positive WST result, which is associated with the risk of aspiration and requires verification by the objective diagnostic methods like FEES and/or videofluoroscopy [17].

Analyzed parameter		at rest number of patients (%)	at speech number of patients (%)
Submandibular tension	normal tension	10 (33.33%)	1 (3.33%)
	increased I^0	17 (56.67%)	12 (40.00%)
	increased II^0	2 (6.67%)	16 (53.33%)
Pharyngeal walls tension	normal tension	10 (33.33%)	5 (16.67%)
	increased I^0	17 (56.67%)	9 (30.00%)
	increased II^0	2 (6.67%)	15 (50.00%)
SCM tension right side	normal tension	6 (20.00%)	4 (13.33%)
	increased I^0	19 (63.33%)	9 (30.00%)
	increased II^0	4 (13.33%)	16 (53.33%)
SCM tension left side	normal tension	5 (6.67%)	2 (6.67%)
	increased I^0	13 (43.33%)	10 (33.33%)
	increased II^0	11 (36.67%)	17 (56.67%)
Thyrohyoid space	normal	15 (46.66%)	10 (33.33%)
	reduced	14 (46.67%)	19 (63.33%)
Cricothyroid distance	normal	13 (43.33%)	7 (23.33%)
	reduced	16 (53.33%)	22 (73.33%)
Breathing pattern	upper chest	10 (33.33%)	9 (30.00%)
	chest-abdominal	19 (63.33%)	20 (66.67%)
Cervical lordosis	decreased	3 (10.00%)	3 (10.00%)
	normal	4 (13.33%)	4 (13.33%)
	increased	22 (73.33%)	22 (73.33%)
Lumbar lordosis	decreased	23 (76.67%)	23 (76.67%)
	normal	4 (13.33%)	4 (13.33%)
	increased	2 (6.67%)	2 (6.67%)

SCM (Sternocleidomastoid muscle).

Table 2.
The results of functional examination.

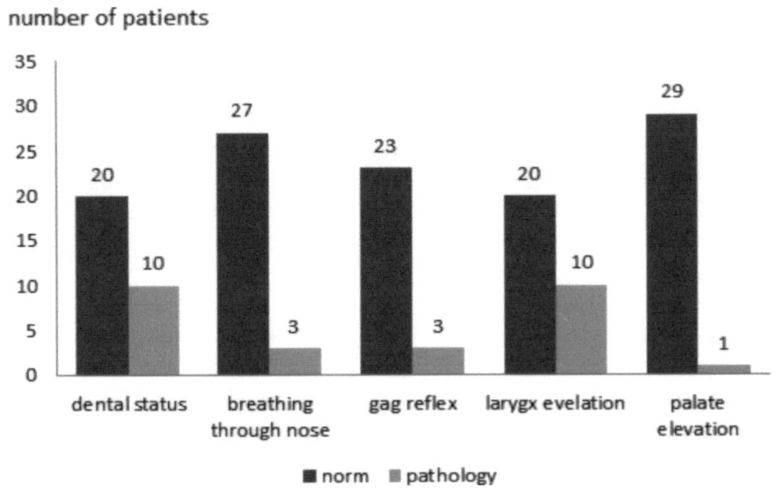

Figure 1.
Physical examination results.

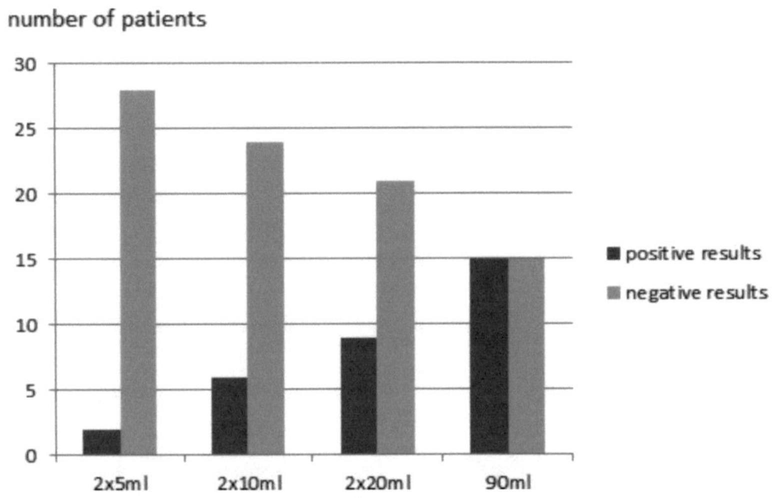

Figure 2.
Water-swallow test (WST) results. Positive result means risk of aspiration, negative result means no risk of aspiration.

4.3 Statistical correlations

Statistically significant correlation between some of the results of functional assessment at rest and speech and the WST results were found.

In case of the functional assessment at rest, a positive 5 ml WST result was found only in patients with increased submandibular and pharyngeal walls muscle tension (both $p = .03$), and for 10 ml WST in patients with increased SCM tension on the left side ($p = .03$) and for 10 and 20 ml WST in subjects with upper chest breathing pattern ($p = .04$ and $p = .01$, respectively).

In case of functional assessment at speech, the upper chest breathing pattern correlated with abnormal WST results. All patients with upper chest breathing pattern demonstrated positive WST result for 10 and 20 ml liquid test ($p = .06$ and $p = .01$, respectively).

On physical examination the following was found: normal pharyngeal reflexes in 23 patients, normal soft palate activity during swallows in 29 patients, and impaired elevation of the larynx in 10 (**Figure 1**). However, only the impaired elevation of the larynx was correlated with the abnormal 5 ml WST results ($p = .03$).

In case of WST results, the negative (no risk of aspiration) result was found in 28 patients (93.33%) for 5 ml amount of liquid, in 24 (80.00%) for 10 ml, in 21 (70.00%) for 20 ml, and in 15 (50.00%) for 90 ml (**Figure 2**). The remaining patients demonstrated positive WST result, which is associated with the risk of aspiration and requires verification by the objective diagnostic methods like FEES and/or videofluoroscopy

4.4 Other results

In FEES examination, in 5 patients (16.67%) small palato-pharyngeal insufficiency was found, and in almost all patients (29 subjects, 96.67%) enlarged lingual tonsil and laryngopharyngeal reflux symptoms. Laryngeal closure and squeeze maneuver (pharyngeal wall motions during phonation) were normal in most of the patients: vocal folds closure during cough (30 subjects, 100%), Valsalva maneuver (26 subjects, 86.67%), squeeze maneuver (28 subjects, 93.33%). Two patients (6,67%) did not show any of the spontaneous swallows. Retention of saliva at the level of the hypopharynx and larynx was found in 27 patients (90.00%).

The FEES evaluation of different food consistencies revealed (**Figures 3–6**):

- residue (bolus left in the pharynx after swallow) in 5 patients (16.67%) for liquid, 9 (30.00%) for puree, and in 7 (27.33%) for solid food

- spillage (bolus falls over the base of the tongue before the swallow begins) in 1 patient (3.33%) for liquid, and in 14 subjects (46.67%) for puree

- multiswallows in 7 patients (23.33%) for liquid, 2 (6.67%) for puree, and in 8 (26.67%) for solid food

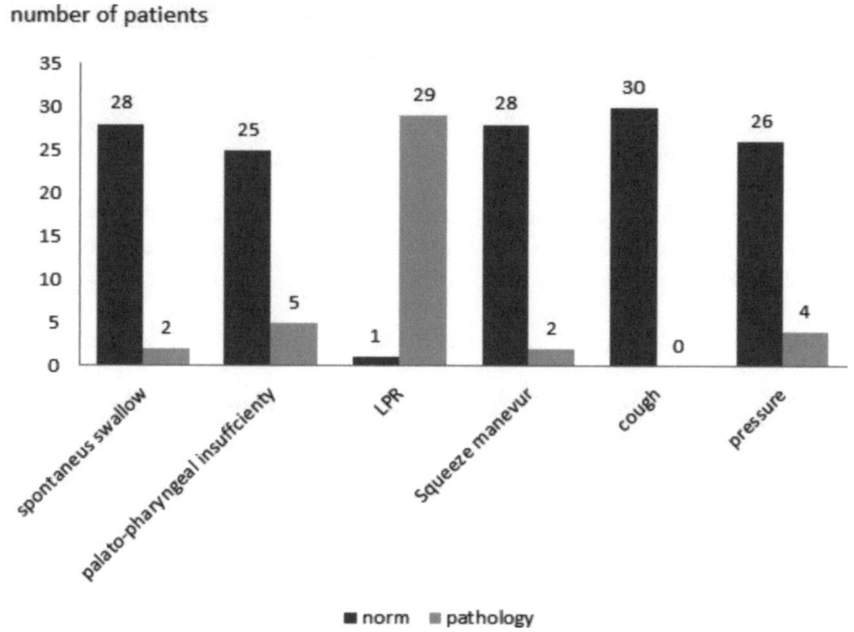

Figure 3.
Fiberoptic endoscopic examination of swallowing (FEES) - anatomy and physiology of the pharynx and larynx.

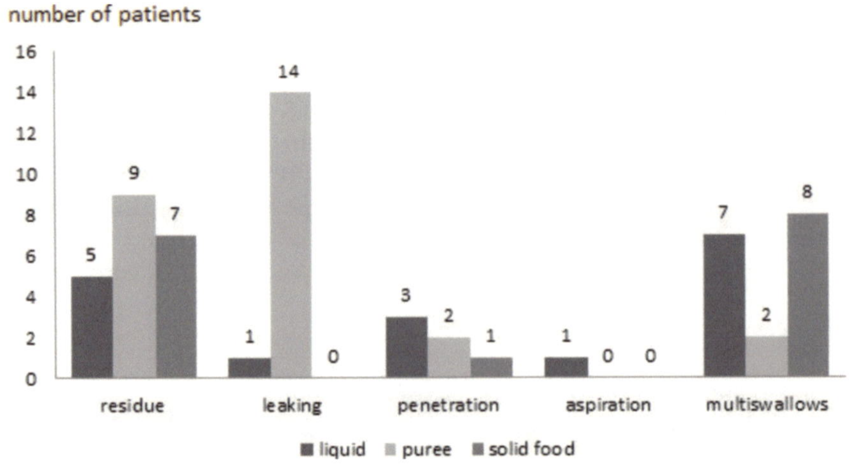

Figure 4.
Fiberoptic endoscopic examination of swallowing (FEES) - swallowing of different food consistency.

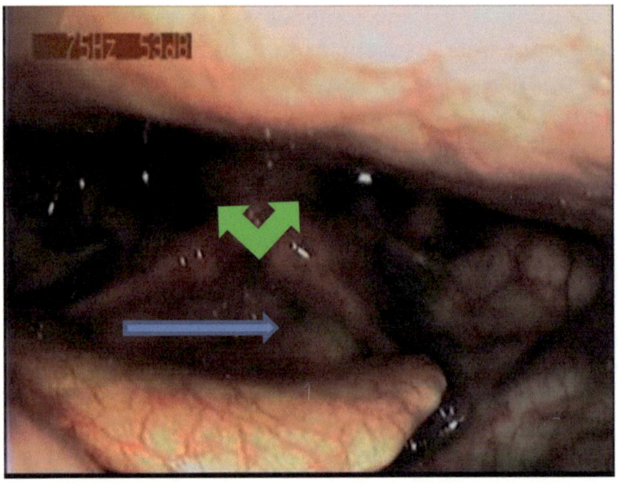

Figure 5.
Fiberoptic endoscopic examination of swallowing (FEES) - liquid penetration (blue arrow), residue in the piriform sinuses (green arrows).

- penetration (bolus enters the laryngeal vestibule, but does not cross the vocal folds) in 3 patients (10.00%) for liquid, 2 (6.67%) for puree, and in 1 (3.33%) for solid food

- aspiration (bolus passes below the vocal folds) of liquid in 1 patient (3,33%)

- in PAS scale, 5 patients (16.67%) reached second or third level, which means that bolus entered the laryngeal vestibule but remain above the vocal folds, with or without expectoration

- eight patients experienced episodes of upper esophageal sphincter opening

- in 13 subjects (20.00%) no swallowing disorders were found.

Also between the FEES and WST some associations were found. The 5 ml WST result was found to be positive only in patients with retention of thick mucus in

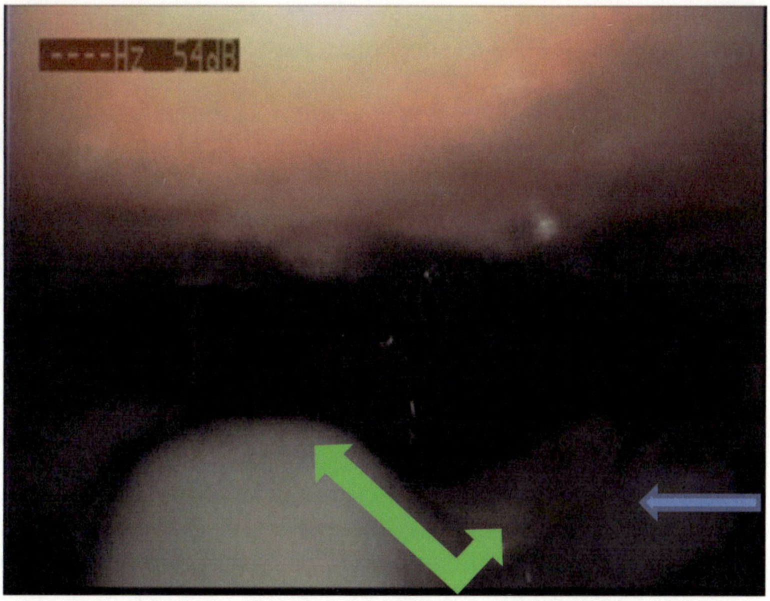

Figure 6.
Fiberoptic endoscopic examination of swallowing (FEES): Spillage (green arrows), residue in the piriform sinuses (blue arrow).

nasopharynx (p = .015). Half of the patients with 10 ml positive WST result presented risk of aspiration (p = .014), and only in 1 patient out of 18 with no FEES abnormal findings the 10 ml WST result was positive (p = .02). All patients with weakened squeeze maneuver presented positive 20 ml WST result (p = .025). For 90 ml WST no statistically significant results were found.

5. Discussion

According to various recommendations the diagnostic process of chronic cough usually begins with the exclusion of the pulmonary ailments (asthma, eosinophilic bronchitis, lung cancer, Chronic Obstructive Pulmonary Disease (COPD), inflammatory lung diseases, etc.), iatrogenic causes (drug-induced cough), and next gastrointestinal (gastroesophageal reflux), and laryngological or phoniatric problems [9–11, 22, 23]. There is also as a new disease called Chronic Cough Hypersensitivity Syndrome (CCHS), characterized by cough attacks lasting more than 8 weeks, aggravated upon exposure to specific factors i.e. cold fluids, poorly responsive to treatment, and with no links to the general health status of the patient [22]. In their study, Sandhu et al. [23] mentioned about the possible relation between chronic cough and dysphagia, in particular between presbyphagia and increased stiffness of the pharyngeal walls. Langmore et al. [18] described endoscopic examination of swallowing disorders in 1988, however, it was not until now routinely used to assess dysphagia as the cause of chronic cough.

The results of our study revealed dysphagia in little more than a half of the patients with chronic cough (56.67%). The patients presented episodes of spillage, double swallows, penetration, aspiration and residue of food at the hypopharynx, which are an indirect evidence of oral stage of swallowing disturbances, and direct evidence of pharyngeal phase of swallowing problems. The results of functional assessment correlated with the WST results, which seems logical – the external laryngeal muscles take part in the laryngeal elevation and their increased tension makes it difficult for the upper pharyngeal sphincter to open thus promoting retention (residue) at the level of the hypopharynx. Decrease in the elevation of the larynx was correlated with the 5 ml WST results.

The correlation between FEES and WST results was found for aspiration risk, spillage, and retention of saliva. It is known that pharyngeal retention of saliva is associated with impaired sensation in the critical region of the hypopharynx and larynx. The retention is slightly higher in patients with laryngopharyngeal reflux, which was found in all patients in the study group. It may be associated with an increased risk of serious swallowing disorders such as penetration or aspiration. In case of reduced sensation in the pharynx a chance of liquid or food penetration/aspiration to upper airways increases, especially when it resides in the hypopharynx and leads to multiswallows. However, more studies in larger group of patients should be conducted.

In their retrospective study, Drozd et al. [24] investigated the group of 15 patients with upper airways problems and found chronic cough in 40% of them. They used videofluoroscopy to assess dysphagia and showed correlation between degree of dysphagia and penetration, aspiration (the more severe dysphagia the higher score in PAS scale), and multiswallows. The authors believe that the dysphagia in this group of patients may be caused by incoordination between breathing and swallowing. In our study, the lower elevation of the larynx and increased muscle tension in the neck may confirm this hypothesis. Most authors involved in the problem of chronic chough highlights the difficulty not only with its diagnostics, but also with treatment [9, 11, 25–28]. There are a few reports in the literature about decrease of symptoms after speech therapy [4, 25]. It seems that the severity of dysphagia should be decreased after a treatment, which relaxes the external muscles of the larynx, however, it requires further study.

Taking into consideration that chronic cough can be harmful for larynx, the functions of the larynx will be more disturbed. The vocal folds oedema, hemorrhage, granuloma or other organic lesions can have an impact on vocal folds contraction (decreased defense reflex) [29]. Shorter maximal phonation time associated with dysphonia and chronic cough have an impact on swallowing and breathing function discoordination [30]. In that case non-pharmacological therapy can be applied, mainly forced/dry swallow, sipping water, chewing gum, sucking non-medical sweets, abdominal breathing pattern technique, cough control breathing technique exercise and physiotherapy which reduce upper body shoulder and neck tension, nasal breathing. Avoiding of irritants is also recommended. In case of risk of aspiration Mendelshon maneuver, suprahyoid muscle exercise (Shaker technique) [31] and lax vox technique is recommended [32].

The small group of patients and the lack of control group are the weak points of our study. However, to our best knowledge, this is the first study to assess the problem of dysphagia as a risk factor of chronic cough and we have been still working and collecting more data from patients and controls to analyze the results in much bigger group.

6. Conclusions

The results of the study showed prevalence of dysphagia in most patients with chronic cough. It seems that phoniatric assessment in those cases should be expanded and the following tests should be performed: assessment of the laryngeal elevation, WST, and FEES. It seems important to also investigate how rehabilitation techniques used by phoniatric specialists and speech therapists improve functional outcome and quality of life in patients with chronic cough.

Acknowledgements

Not applicable.

Funding sources

Funding information is not applicable. No funding was received.

Conflict of interest

The authors declare no conflict of interest.

Statement of ethics

The study was approved by the local Ethics Committee Review Board at the Medical University (no. KB/39/A/2016). All subjects gave their written informed consent to participation in the study.

Author details

Barbara Jamróz[1], Magdalena Milewska[2], Joanna Chmielewska-Walczak[1], Magdalena Lachowska[1], Marta Dąbrowska-Bender[2], Magdalena Arcimowicz[1], Anna Staniszewska[3*], Anna Brytek-Matera[4] and Kazimierz Niemczyk[1]

1 Department of Otolaryngology, Head and Neck Surgery, Medical University of Warsaw, Warsaw, Poland

2 Department of Clinical Dietetics, Medical University of Warsaw, Warsaw, Poland

3 Department of Experimental and Clinical Pharmacology, Medical University of Warsaw, Warsaw, Poland

4 Institute of Psychology, University of Wroclaw, Wroclaw, Poland

*Address all correspondence to: anna.staniszewska@wum.edu.pl

References

[1] Song WJ, Chang YS, Faruqi S, et al. Defining Chronic Couhg: A Systemic Review of the Epidemiological Literature. Allergy Asthma Immunol Res. 2016;8(2):146-155. DOI: 10.4168/aair.2016.8.2.146

[2] Tarlo SM, Altman KW, Oppenheimer J, et al. Occupational and environmental contributions to chronic cough in adults: chest expert panel report. Chest 2016; 150: 894-907.

[3] Arinze JT, de Roos EW, Karimi L, Verhamme KMC, Stricker BH, Brusselle GG. Prevalence and incidence of, and risk factors for chronic cough in the adult population: the Rotterdam Study. ERJ Open Res. 2020;6(2):00300-2019. Published 2020 Apr 19. doi:10.1183/23120541.00300-2019

[4] Morice AH, Millqvist E, Belvisi MG, Bieksiene K, Birring SS, Chung KF, Dal Negro RW, Dicpinigaitis P, Kantar A, McGarvey LP, Pacheco A, Sakalauskas R, Smith JA Expert opinion on the cough hypersensitivity syndrome in respiratory medicine.Eur Respir J. 2014 Nov; 44(5):1132-1148.

[5] Chamberlain Mitchell SAF, Ellis J, Ludlow S, Pandyan A, Birring SS. Non-pharmacological interventions for chronic cough: The past, present and future. Pulm Pharmacol Ther. 2019 Jun;56:29-38. doi: 10.1016/j.pupt.2019.02.006. Epub 2019 Feb 23. PMID: 30807836.

[6] Andersson C, Bonvini SJ, Horvath P, et al. Research highlights from the 2017 ERS International Congress: airway diseases in focus. ERJ Open Res. 2018;4(1):00163-02017. doi: 10.1183/23120541.00163-2017.

[7] Çolak Y, Nordestgaard BG, Laursen LC, Afzal S, Lange P, Dahl M. Risk Factors for Chronic Cough Among 14,669 Individuals From the General Population. Chest. 2017 Sep;152(3):563-573. doi: 10.1016/j.chest.2017.05.038. Epub 2017 Jun 15. PMID: 28625577.

[8] Ding H, Shi C, Xu X, Yu L. Drug-induced chronic cough and the possible mechanism of action. Ann Palliat Med. 2020 Sep;9(5):3562-3570. doi: 10.21037/apm-20-819. Epub 2020 Sep 2. PMID: 32921095

[9] Chung KF, Pavord ID. Prevalence, pathogenesis, and causes of chronic cough. Lancet. 2008;371(9621):1364-1374. DOI: 10.1016/S0140-6736(08)60595-4

[10] Aakash KP, Lee KK, Birring SS. Cough. Medicine. 2016;44(4):213-216. DOI: 10.1016/j.mpmed.2016.02.008

[11] Birring SS. New concepts in the management of chronic cough. Pulm Pharmacol Ther. 2011;24(3):334-338. DOI: 10.1016/j.pupt.2011.01.005

[12] Morice AH, Millqvist E, Bieksiene K, et al. ERS guidelines on the diagnosis and treatment of chronic cough in adults and children. Eur Respir J. 2020;55:1901136.

[13] Irwin RS, French CL, Chang AB, Altman KW. CHEST Expert Cough Panel. Classification of cough as a symptom in adults and management algorithms: CHEST guideline and expert panel report. Chest 2018;153:196-209.

[14] Smith JA, Kitt MM, Morice AH, Birring SS, McGarvey LP, Sher MR, Li YP, Wu WC, Xu ZJ, Muccino DR, Ford AP; Protocol 012 Investigators. Gefapixant, a P2X3 receptor antagonist, for the treatment of refractory or unexplained chronic cough: a randomised, double-blind, controlled, parallel-group, phase 2b trial. Lancet Respir Med. 2020 Aug;8(8):775-785. doi: 10.1016/S2213-2600(19)30471-0. Epub 2020 Feb 25. PMID: 32109425.

[15] Belafsky PC, Postma GN, Koufman JA. Validity and Reliability of the Reflux Symptom Index (RSI). J Voice. 2002;16(2):274-277. DOI: 10.1016 / s0892-1997 (02) 00097-8

[16] Belafsky PC, Postma GN, Koufman JA. The Validity and Reliability of the Reflux Finding Score (RFS). Laryngoscpoe. 2001;111(8):1313-1317. DOI: 10.1097 / 00005537-200108000-00001.

[17] Ickenstein W. Clinical Swallowing Examination (CSE). In: Ickenstein WG, Ambrosi D, Clave P, Dziewas R, Ekberg O, Ende F et al. editors. Dignosis and treatment of neurogenic oropharyngeal dysphagia. 2nd ed. Uni-MedVerlag AG, Bremen; 2014. p. 42-48.

[18] Langmore SE, Schatz K, Olsen N. Fiberoptic endoscopic examination of swallowing safety: a new procedure. Dysphagia. 1988;2(4):216-219. DOI: 10.1007 / BF02414429.

[19] Dziewas R. Swallowing endoscopy. In: Ickenstein WG, Ambrosi D, Clave P, Dziewas R, Ekberg O, Ende F et al. editors. Dignosis and treatment of neurogenic oropharyngeal dysphagia. 2nd ed. Uni-MedVerlag AG, Bremen; 2014. p. 48-52.

[20] Jamróz B, Sielska-Badurek E, Niemczyk K. Use of flexible endoscope for evaluation of swallowing. Pol Otorhinolaryngol Rev. 2015;4(2):1-5. DOI: 10.5604/20845308.1150791

[21] RosenbekJC, Robbins JA, Roecker EB et all. A penetration-aspiration scale. Dysphagia. 1996;11:93-98. DOI:10.1007/ BF00417897

[22] Chung KF. Chronic cough hypersensitivity syndrome: A more precise label for chronic cough. Pulm Pharmacol Ther. 2011;24(3):267-271. DOI: 10.1016/j.pupt.2011.01.012.

[23] Sandhu G, Kuchai R. The larynx in cough. Cough. 2013;9(1):16. DOI: 10.1186/1745-9974-9-16

[24] Drozdz DRC, Costa CC, de Oliveira Jesus PR et al.. Pharyngeal swallowing phase and chronic cough. Int Arch Otorhinolaryngol. 2012; 16(4):502-508. DOI: 10.7162/ S1809-97772012000400012

[25] Birring SS, Kavanagh J, Lai K, Chang AB. Adult and paediatric cough guidelines: ready for an overhaul? Pulm Pharmacol Ther. 2015;35:137-144. DOI: 10.1016/j.pupt.2015.01.007

[26] Chellini E, Lavorini F, Campi G, Mannini C, Fontana GA. Effect of an anti-reflux medical device in the control of deflation cough: A placebo-controlled comparative study with an antacid drug in chronic coughers. Pulm Pharmacol Ther. 2015;33:11-14. DOI: 10.1016/j. pupt.2015.05.002

[27] Patcharatrakul T, Gonlachanvit S. Gastroesophageal reflux symptoms in typical and atypical GERD: Roles of gastroesophageal acid refluxes and esophageal motility. J Gastroenterol Hepatol. 2014;29(2):284-290. DOI: 10.1111/jgh.12347

[28] Xu X, Yu L, Chen Q, Lv H, Qiu Z. Diagnosis and treatment of patients with nonacid gastroesophageal reflux-induced chronic cough. J Res Med Sci. 2015;20(9):885-892. DOI: 10.4103/1735-1995.170625

[29] Yeakel H, Balouch B, Vontela S, Alnouri G, Sataloff RT. The Relationship Between Chronic Cough and Laryngopharyngeal Reflux. J Voice. 2020 Nov 28:S0892-1997(20)30425-2. doi: 10.1016/j.jvoice.2020.11.011. Epub ahead of print. PMID: 33262000.

[30] Martinez-Paredes JF, Alfakir R, Thompson CC, Menton SM, Rutt A. Effect of Chronic Cough on Voice Measures in Patients With Dysphonia. J

Voice. 2021 Jan 8:S0892-1997(20)30484-7. doi: 10.1016/j.jvoice.2020.12.025. Epub ahead of print. PMID: 33431203.

[31] Speyer R, Baijens L, Heijnen M, Zwijnenberg I. Effects of therapy in oropharyngeal dysphagia by speech and language therapists: a systematic review. Dysphagia. 2010 Mar;25(1):40-65. doi: 10.1007/s00455-009-9239-7. Epub 2009 Sep 17. PMID: 19760458; PMCID: PMC2846331.

[32] Mendes ALF, Dornelas do Carmo R, Dias de Araújo AMG, Paranhos LR, da Mota CSO, Schneiberg S, Reis FP, Aragão JA. The Effects of Phonation Into Glass, Plastic, and LaxVox Tubes in Singers: A Systematic Review. J Voice. 2019 May;33(3):381.e1-381.e9. doi: 10.1016/j.jvoice.2017.12.005. Epub 2018 May 3. PMID: 29731378.

Chapter 14

Juvenile Nasopharyngeal Angiofibroma

Anukaran Mahajan and Karunesh Gupta

Abstract

Juvenile Nasopharyngeal Angiofibroma (JNA) remains one of the most enigmatic tumors encountered by laryngotologists-head neck surgeons. Its origin at a particular age in a particular sex has intrigued many. Histopathologically benign, JNAs are locally aggressive tumors with tendency to cause massive recurrent nasal bleeds. While surgery remains the gold standard treatment, a paradigm shift from open approaches to endoscopic approach is noted. Recent advances in genomic testing, radiodiagnosis and endoscopic nasal surgeries allow us to manage these tumors more efficiently. Introduction of intensity modulated radiotherapy (IMRT), stereotactic surgery, and interventional radiology (embolisation) has further helped in this cause. This chapter aims to give a brief overview of all these aspects related to JNA with the hope to initiate more ENT surgeons to contribute to further research on this benign but dangerous tumor.

Keywords: juvenile nasal angiofibroma, JNA, vascular tumor, epistaxis, pterygopalatine fossa, frog face deformity, pathways of spread of angiofibroma, staging of JNA, immunohistochemistry of JNA, open surgery for angiofibroma, endoscopic resection, treatment of angiofibroma, embolisation, CT angiography

1. Introduction

Juvenile nasopharyngeal angiofibroma (JNA) is a benign, non-encapsulated, highly vascular tumor, occurring almost exclusively in adolescent males. Although JNAs comprise of less than 0.05% of all head and neck tumors, their tendency to bleed torrentially makes them an interesting disease entity to study and treat [1].

Development of other medical fields has been instrumental in studying the origin, growth and other characteristics of this disease entity. Advancements in radiology, histopathology and endoscopic nasal surgeries have been particularly useful. We can now better diagnoses, stage and treat JNA than the previous decade.

2. History of juvenile nasopharyngeal angiofibroma

Earliest known documentation of juvenile nasopharyngeal angiofibroma is credited to Hippocrates in the 4th century BC [2]. The term "juvenile nasopharyngeal angiofibroma" was coined by Chaveau in 1906 and his works re-sparked the interest in JNA [3]. Shaheen et al. [4] reported the first female case of JNA (1930).

IntechOpen

Harma et al. in 1959 gave a detailed clinico-pathological insight into this tumor [5]. Works of Bensch, Ewing, Som, Neffson, Moore, Handousa, Denker etc. have been vital in understanding the natural history of disease and its surgical management [6–9].

3. Relevant anatomy

3.1 Nasopharynx

Nasopharynx is a near-cuboidal shaped space with an approximate volume of 30cm^3. It is located exactly below the middle cranial fossa.

Boundaries of Nasopharynx:

- **Anterior:** Choanae and posterior margin of nasal septum. Further anteriorly lie the right and left nasal cavities.

- **Posterior:** Fascia, prevertebral muscles, basiocciput and first two cervical vertebrae.

- **Superior:** Superior wall is continuous with the posterior wall. It is formed by basisphenoid and basiocciput.

- **Inferior:** Opens into oropharynx. When the soft palate is elevated, it makes contact with the Passavant's ridge (palatopharyngeus muscle fibers); and together these from the inferior boundary of nasopharynx.

- **Lateral:** Eustachian tube openings along with the torus tuboris is the prominent structure.

Posterior to the torus tuboris, lies a deep recess called **lateral pharyngeal recess** or **fossa of rosenmuller**. Foramen lacerum lies immediately superior to the fossa of rosenmuller. Foramen spinosum and ovale are present laterally. Petrous apex and carotid canal form its posterior relation (**Figure 1**).

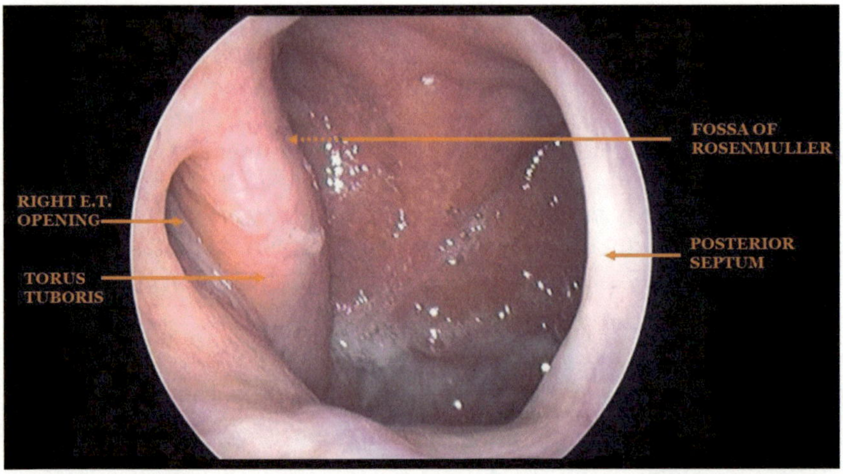

Figure 1.
Endoscopic anatomy of nasopharynx as seen through right nasal cavity (E.T.- Eustachian Tube).

3.2 Pterygopalatine fossa

Pterygopalatine fossa is a bilateral wedge-shaped space located below the orbital apex and behind the posterior wall of maxillary sinus. It communicates with other regions of skull through various canals and foramina.

Boundaries of Pterygopalatine Fossa:

- **Anterior:** Superomedial part of posterior wall of maxillary sinus.
- **Posterior:** Root of pterygoid process and anterior face of greater wing of sphenoid.
- **Medial**: Upper part of perpendicular plate of palatine bone with its sphenoidal and orbital process; sphenopalatine foramen leading to nasopharynx.
- **Lateral:** pterygomaxillary fissure leading to infratemporal fossa.
- **Superior:** Undersurface of body of sphenoid.
- **Inferior:** Pyramidal process of palatine bone with greater palatine canal.

Communications of Pterygopalatine Fossa:

- Via **sphenopalatine foramen** to nasopharynx
- Via **pterygomaxillary fissure** to infratemporal fossa
- Via **inferior orbital fissure** to orbit
- Via **greater palatine canal** to oral cavity
- Via **foramen rotundum** to middle cranial fossa
- Via **vidian (pterygoid) canal** to foramen lacerum to middle cranial fossa
- Via **palatovaginal canal** to pharynx

Contents of Pterygopalatine Fossa:

- Pterygopalatine ganglion with its branches
- Maxillary nerve (V2) and its branches
- Vidian Nerve (carrying secretomotor fibers of facial nerve from superior salivatory nucleus and sympathetic fibers from internal carotid artery via deep petrosal nerve)
- Third part of maxillary artery

4. Etiopathogenesis

Juvenile Nasopharyngeal Angiofibroma occurs almost exclusively in males and that too in adolescent period. Mean age of presentation is 14 years (range 7 years to

19 years) [10]. Isolated cases of JNAs in females or in younger/ older ages have been reported in literature [4, 11]. Exact etiology, although unknown, evidences point towards a hormonal influence on its occurrence and growth.

4.1 Theories of origin

1. **Ringertz Theory (1938):** JNA arises from the periosteum of the skull base [12].

2. **Som- Neffson Theory (1940):** If bones forming the skull base grow in a disproportionate manner, it results in the hypertrophy of underlying periosteum. Additional stimulation by hormones can result in formation of a tumor in nasopharynx [6].

3. **Bensch- Ewing Theory (1941):** Between the basi sphenoid and basi occiput, exists an embryonic fibrocartilage. This embryonic fibrocartilage proliferates to form a tumor [7].

4. **Brunner's Theory (1942):** JNA arises from conjoined buccopharyngeal and pharyngobasilar fascia [13].

5. **Martin's Theory (1948):** Imbalance between estrogens and androgens during adolescence causes JNA. Increased estrogen stimulation and/ or decreased androgen stimulation is suggested as the probable cause [14].

6. **Sternberg's Theory (1954):** JNAs are nothing but hemangiomas of nasal cavity and skull base [15].

7. **Handousa's Theory (1954):** JNA is a true neoplasm arising from periosteum of basi sphenoid [9].

8. **Osborn's Theory (1959):** Two theories were given by him. JNA is a fetal erectile tissue which proliferates under hormonal influence **(Pseudo-tumor theory)**. Or, JNA is a true hamartoma **(True tumor theory)** [16].

9. **Girgis- Fahmy's Theory (1973):** Histopathological resemblance between JNA and paragangliomas was noted by Girgis and Fahmy. The growing edge of JNA showed cell nests of undifferentiated epitheloid cells. They called this pattern "Zellballen" (German- ball of cells). JNAs belong to the same disease entity as paragangliomas [17].

10. **Hamartoma and Vascular Malformation Theory:** This is the most accepted theory at present. Although, the dilemma still exists between JNA being a hamartoma or a vascular malformation, influence of sex-hormones is an accepted notion. While some consider JNAs to be true neoplasms, other studies reveal these to be only vascular malformations [18–20].

11. **Branchial Arch Artery Theory (Bernhard Schick, 2004):** Incomplete regression of first branchial arch artery has been proposed. First branchial arch artery regresses near pterygoid base and sphenopalatine foramen, and is finally incorporated into sphenopalatine and maxillary artery. This explains

the anatomical location of the tumor at pterygoid base/ sphenopalatine foramen as well as its supply by maxillary artery. This also explains the need to drill pterygoid base to remove tumor remnants in this site of origin so as to avoid tumor recurrence. As first branchial arch artery is connected to C4-segment of internal carotid artery (ICA), its incomplete regression also explains how JNAs acquire blood supply from ICA despite no anatomical proximity [21].

4.2 Site of origin

Juvenile nasopharyngeal angiofibroma can arise from any one of the following sites:

1. *SPHENOPALATINE FORAMEN:* Upper margin of the sphenopalatine is considered as the most common site of origin of JNA. Sphenopalatine foramen is the point of trifurcation of 3 bones: palatine (perpendicular plate, orbital process and sphenoidal process), vomer (horizontal ala) and sphenoid (specifically root of pterygoid process).

2. *VIDIAN CANAL:* Vidian canal/ pterygoid canal arises from the anterior wall of foramen lacerum and opens into the posterior wall of pterygopalatine fossa. Literature states this as potential site of origin in cases with laterally extended JNAs having little/ no involvement of sphenopalatine foramen/ nasopharynx.

3. *PTERYGOID WEDGE:* Pterygoid wedge is found to be the most common site of recurrence [22]. Drilling of pterygoid wedge during primary surgery significantly reduces the risk of recurrence. First branchial arch artery theory for origin of JNA supports the same. Recent studies have been conclusively able to prove the same.

4.3 Factors for etiopathogenesis

Scientists are still looking out for exact etiological factors and how these affect the growth of the tumor. Following factors should be considered:

1. *Hormones:* Occurrence of tumor in males during adolescence phase strongly indicates hormonal influence on tumor growth initiation. An imbalance between testosterone, estrogen and progesterone has been theorized as an etiological factor. This allows the use of flutamide therapy as an adjuvant therapy for its treatment. Flutamide has been found to be effective in postpubertal patients as opposed to prepubertal patients [23].

2. *Genetic alterations:* gains and losses in the regions of 4q, 6q, 8q, 12, 17, 22q, X and Y –chromosomes are present in patients of juvenile nasopharyngeal angiofibroma [19, 24–26]. Over expression or under expression of p53 on chromosome 17 has been implicated in tumor cells [27–30]. Her-2/neu receptors (encoded by Her-2 gene on chromosome 17) have also a role in JNA [29].

3. *Molecular pathology:* Cytokines such as transforming growth factor beta-1 (TGFβ-1) and Insulin-like growth factor-2 (IGF2) are involved in the growth of this tumor. Vascular endothelial growth factor (VEGF) and platelet derived

growth factor (PDGF) have been implicated as most important factors for neoangiogenesis [28, 30]. AURKB, FGF18, and SUPT16H can act as potential molecular markers in JNA [31].

5. Pathology

MACROSCOPIC: On gross examination, the tumor appears as a polypoidal, non-encapsulated, red to gray colored mass with spongy appearance. Mean size is 4 cm.

MICROSCOPIC: The tumor has a fibrous stroma with abundant blood vessels. The blood vessels are of variable sizes without any organized layout. Elastin fibers in the blood vessels are typically absent while the muscle layer maybe absent, focal (pad-like) or circumferential. This accounts for profuse bleeding in these tumors as these blood vessels are unable to contract to achieve effective hemostasis.

The fibrous stroma has varying amounts of fine and coarse collagen fibers. Plump spindle, angular, or stellate-shaped cells are also seen. Rarely, mast cells may be present. The nuclei of stromal cells generally lack any characteristic features; although, multinucleated pleomorphic cells are not uncommon.

The vascular and fibrous elements vary in proportion within the same tumor and with the tumor age. While the fibrous component is more towards the centre of the tumor, peripheral areas have abundance of vascular elements. Also, newer lesions have predominantly vascular component while long standing tumors are enriched with fibrous tissue.

Embolised specimens show myxoid changes with areas of infarction. Embolic agent can be seen in the tumor vessels. Post flutamide therapy or radiotherapy specimens show a significant increase in fibrous component (**Figure 2**).

IMMUNOHISTOCHEMISTRY: Immunohistochemistry (IHC) tests act as ancillary tests for juvenile nasopharyngeal angiofibroma. Various IHC tests are described in the **Table 1**.

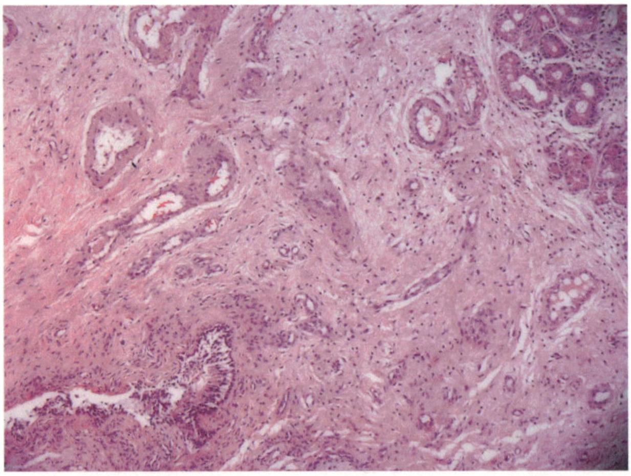

Figure 2.
Histopathological section of JNA as seen under a microscope. Multiple blood vessels of varying diameters are seen in a fibrous stroma.

IMMUNOHISTOCHEMISTRY			
TEST ANTIBODY	**TUMOR COMPONENT**	**TUMOR CELLS**	**STAINING PATTERN**
1. Vimentin	Vascular & Fibrous	All tumor cells	Cytoplasmic
2. Androgen receptor	Vascular & Fibrous	All stromal cells and endothelial cells	Nuclear
3. VEGF	Vascular & Fibrous	Stromal and vascular cells	Cytoplasmic
4. PDGF	Vascular & Fibrous	Stromal and vascular cells (+/−)	Cytoplasmic
5. IGF-2	Vascular & Fibrous	Stromal and vascular cells (+/−)	Cytoplasmic
6. TGF- β	Vascular & Fibrous	Stromal and vascular cells (+/−)	Cytoplasmic
7. SMA (Smooth Muscle Actin)	Vascular	Smooth muscle cells in blood vessels	Cytoplasmic
8. Desmin	Vascular	Cells in walls of larger blood vessels	Cytoplasmic
9. FVIIIRAg	Vascular	Endothelial cells	Cytoplasmic
10. CD31	Vascular	Endothelial cells	Cytoplasmic
11. CD34	Vascular	Endothelial cells	Cytoplasmic
12. ER	Vascular	Vascular cell nuclei (+/−)	Nuclear
13. PR	Vascular	Vascular cell nuclei (+/−)	Nuclear
14. CD117 (c-kit)	Fibrous	Stromal cells	Cytoplasmic
15. β Catenin	Fibrous	Stromal cells	Nuclear

Table 1.
Immunohistochemistry (IHC) tests for JNA.

6. Spread of JNA

JNA arises at the upper lip of sphenopalatine foramen. As it grows further, it spreads along the path of least resistance to involve many vital structures.

6.1 Medial extension

From sphenopalatine foramen, it extends into the nasopharynx and grows submucosally. It can occupy the entire nasopharynx to produce bilateral nasal obstruction and nasal intonation of voice (rhinolalia clausa). Recurrent epistaxis often starts at this stage only. The tumor mass may depress the soft palate or hang in the oropharynx. Blockage of eustachian tube(s) results in conductive hearing loss (otitis media with effusion).

6.2 Anterior extension

i. It enters the ipsilateral nasal cavity first to cause unilateral nasal obstruction and epistaxis. Here it may acquire secondary attachments.

ii. As the tumor grows further within the ipsilateral nasal cavity, it pushes the nasal septum towards the opposite side to produce contralateral nasal obstruction as well.

iii. Further tumor growth allows it to involve ethmoidal sinuses. This results in flattening of the nasal bridge and an increase in the intercanthal distance.

An associated proptosis gives a classical '**frog- face deformity**' to the patient.

iv. The tumor may encroach upon and erode anterior wall of sphenoid sinus. It may further invade the sphenoid sinus.

6.3 Lateral extension

Lateral growth of the tumor results in the involvement of pterygopalatine fossa. Pterygopalatine fossa is a small wedge-shaped cavity, which can be considered as a cross-section/ junction point of many important 'highways'.

i. As the mass lesion fills the pterygopalatine fossa, it causes anterior bowing of the posterior wall of maxillary sinus (**Antral Sign/ Holman- Miller Sign**).

ii. From pterygopalatine fossa, it can extend into the orbit via the inferior orbital fissure. This produces proptosis. Further involvement of orbital apex results in loss of vision. Involvement of extraocular muscles produces diplopia.

iii. From pterygopalatine fossa, tumor grows laterally to invade infratemporal fossa via the pterygomaxillary fissure. This causes facial swelling and fullness in the cheek region. Erosion of the anterior face of greater wing of sphenoid causes entry of tumor into the middle cranial fossa.

iv. From pterygopalatine fossa, it can grow along the vidian canal to reach foramen lacerum. Foramen lacerum opens in the middle cranial fossa, providing easy access to the tumor for intra cranial extension.

6.4 Posterior extension

i. The tumor can erode the pterygoid process posteriorly and spread downwards into the pterygoid fossa. It can reach as far as the parapharyngeal space.

ii. Tumor growth in the posterolateral part of nasopharynx can cause extension into the fossa of rosenmuller. Further posterolateral growth into the apex of this fossa results in intracranial extension by eroding the carotid canal and petrous apex.

6.5 Inraorbital extension

The tumor can involve the orbit through the following routes-

i. Sphenopalatine foramen ➔ pterygopalatine fossa ➔ via inferior orbital fissure ➔ enters orbit.

ii. Sphenopalatine foramen ➔ nasopharynx and nasal cavity ➔ erodes lamina papyracea ➔ enters orbit.

6.6 Intracranial extension

The tumor can have intracranial extension through the following routes:

i. Sphenopalatine foramen ➔ pterygopalatine fossa ➔ infratemporal fossa ➔ erosion of anterior face of greater wing of sphenoid AND/ OR through foramen ovale causing its widening ➔ middle cranial fossa. The tumor lies lateral to Internal Carotid Artery (ICA) and Cavernous Sinus (CS) in such cases.

ii. Sphenopalatine foramen ➔ pterygopalatine fossa ➔ via inferior orbital fissure ➔ orbit ➔ growth within orbit towards orbital apex and superior orbital fissure ➔ middle cranial fossa. The tumor lies anterolateral to ICA and lateral to CS.

iii. Sphenopalatine foramen ➔ nasopharynx and nasal cavity ➔ erosion of floor and anterior wall of sphenoid sinus to invade sphenoid sinus ➔ erosion of roof of sphenoid sinus ➔ intracranial spread. The tumor lies medial to ICA and lateral to pituitary gland.

iv. Sphenopalatine foramen ➔ pterygopalatine fossa ➔ pterygoid (vidian) canal ➔ foramen lacerum ➔ middle cranial fossa. Encasement of ICA is seen early.

v. Sphenopalatine foramen ➔ nasopharynx ➔ fossa of rosenmuller ➔ erodes carotid canal and petrous apex ➔ intracranial spread.

vi. Sphenopalatine foramen ➔ nasopharynx ➔ nasal cavity ➔ through cribriform plate ➔ anterior cranial fossa (rare route for intracranial extension).

7. Clinical features

7.1 Age/sex

The patient is almost invariably male in his second decade of life. Mean age of presentation is 14 years (reference).

7.2 Symptoms

The patient may have one or more of the following symptoms

i. *Nasal bleed:* any adolescent male presenting with recurrent nasal bleeds should always raise the suspicion of angiofibroma. Nasal bleeds are usually massive and often require an intervention to control them.

ii. *Nasal obstruction:* initially unilateral. Later, bilateral nasal obstruction develops owing to involvement of entire nasopharynx or pushing of nasal septum to the other side

iii. *Nasal discharge:* mucopurulent nasal discharge due to pent up secretions in the nasal cavity followed by secondary infection.

iv. *Hyposmia/ Anosmia*: mechanical obstruction due to tumor mass of olfactory area can cause decreased sense of smell.

v. *Weakness and irritability:* easy fatiguability and irritability due to frequent nasal bleeds causing chronic anemia.

vi. *Voice change:* Voice takes a nasal intonation owing to the tumor mass in the nasopharynx (rhinolalia clausa). Tumor mass depressing the soft palate causes 'plummy voice'.

vii. *Facial swelling:* ipsilateral cheek swelling results when JNA involves the infratemporal fossa.

viii. *Facial deformity:* flattening of dorsum of nose with increased intercanthal distance and proptosis results in 'frog face deformity'.

ix. *Headache:* headache may result from chronic rhinosinusitis, or chronic anemia, or intracranial extension of tumor.

x. *Otological/ Aural symptoms*: eustachian tube blockade in nasopharynx results in serous otitis media causing conductive hearing loss and heaviness in ears.

xi. *Ocular symptoms*: involvement of orbit causes proptosis, double vision, or even loss of vision.

xii. *Intracranial symptoms:* headache, seizures, loss of consciousness owing to intracranial spread of tumor.

7.3 Anterior rhinoscopy

Mucopurulent discharge in the involved side is seen. Tumor mass may also be visualized. Septum is often deviated towards contralateral side.

7.4 Posterior rhinoscopy

Mass lesion is visualized in the nasopharynx.

7.5 Diagnostic nasal endoscopy

Examination with a Hopkin's rigid rod lens 0° endoscope reveals a fleshy mass lesion. It is usually covered in mucopurulent secretions which require gentle suctioning. Probing is avoided as it can complicate into profuse nasal bleed.

8. Investigations

8.1 Biopsy

Though for any nasal mass, golden rule is that biopsy is preceded by radiological imaging to ascertain origin, extent, and nature of the disease; in vascular tumors such as JNAs, biopsy is contraindicated. Risk of bleeding during and/ or after the procedure outweighs any added advantage we may get out of preoperative biopsy.

8.2 X-ray PNS

Water's view (Occipitomental view)/ Peer's view (Occipitomental view with open mouth) shows haziness of the involved sinus. Lateral view shows anterior bowing of posterior wall of maxillary antrum (**Holman Miller sign**).

8.3 CT NOSE–PNS

Contrast enhanced computed tomographic imaging is the investigation of choice for JNA. Infact, the diagnosis of JNA is confirmed by presence of a mass in nasopharynx and pterygopalatine fossa that enhances after contrast administration on CECT. CECT is a non-invasive procedure that forms the basis for JNA diagnosis and staging.

Lloyd's criteria for diagnosis of JNA on CECT [32]:

i. mass lesion in the nasopharynx/ nasal cavity and pterygopalatine fossa

ii. erosion of posterior bony margin of sphenopalatine foramen with extension to the upper medial pterygoid plate.

Holman Miller sign/ Antral sign: anterior bowing of the posterior wall of maxillary antrum. This is due to the tumor mass completely filling the pterygopalatine fossa.

Hondousa Sign: widening of the gap between the maxillary body and ramus of mandible. This occurs when the tumor mass involves infratemporal fossa.

Ram Haran Sign: In JNA patients, coronal cuts of CT Nose- PNS show widening of the pterygoid wedge. It appears as a quadrilateral area rather than normal triangular area [33].

Chopstick Sign: CECT when used for post-operative surveillance to detect residual/ recurrent tumor, shows 'floating' medial and lateral pterygoid plates in cases where the root of pterygoid base is drilled. These pterygoid plates are visualized separately to give appearance of a pair of chopsticks.

8.4 MRI

Contrast enhanced MRI (CE-MRI) is the investigation of choice for advanced JNA tumors, particularly those with intracranial, intra-orbital, or parapharyngeal space involvement. It can accurately determine the extent of the tumor. 'Salt and pepper' appearance on contrast MRI is characteristic to any vascular tumor, resulting due to flow-void areas (T2WI and contrast enhanced T1WI) [22, 34].

Fat Suppression MRI: This has an immense potential in detecting bone invasion by tumor. In fat-suppression MRI sequence, a normal pterygoid wedge should be hypointense owing to fat-rich marrow. Any iso−/hyper-intensity in that area indicates invasion by the tumor, therefore, requiring bone drilling to avoid recurrence.

MRI is also the preferred modality for post-operative long-term surveillance because of its superior soft tissue differentiation quality without any radiation exposure.

8.5 CT-angiography

CT angiography is useful to identify the feeder vessel(s) to the tumor. Internal maxillary artery is the most common feeder vessel for JNA. JNA may additionally acquire blood supply from ascending pharyngeal artery, contralateral external carotid artery branches, ipsilateral or contralateral internal carotid artery and its branches (ophthalmic, meningohypophyseal, vidian artery).

Knowledge about the feeding vessel and its site of entry into the tumor is absolutely critical to decide the surgical approach for JNA excision. For example, where feeder vessels are located posterior to the main tumor mass without direct access, open approach is preferred to endoscopic approach.

8.6 Digital subtraction angiography (DSA)

DSA is used in preoperative phase to identify the feeder vessel and its preoperative embolization. Selective vessel angiography in DSA allows to determine the exact branch(es) supplying the tumor and its selective embolization. JNA shows a characteristic *'tumor blush'* in DSA of external carotid artery. This can also help in predicting the expected blood loss during tumor resection [35].

9. Staging of JNA

Various staging systems have been proposed over the years, each with its own merits and demerits.

9.1 Session's staging system, 1981

Table 2

SESSION'S STAGING SYSTEM	
STAGE	**TUMOR EXTENSION**
IA	Involvement of the nose or nasopharyngeal vault
IB	Extension into one or more sinuses
IIA	Minimal extension into the pterygopalatine fossa
IIB	Full occupation of the pterygopalatine fossa
IIC	Infratemporal extension (± involvement of the cheek)
III	Intracranial extension

Table 2.
JNA staging system by Sessions, 1981 [36].

9.2 Chandler's staging system, 1984

Table 3

CHANDLER'S STAGING SYSTEM	
STAGE	TUMOR EXTENSION
I	Involvement of the nasopharyngeal vault
II	Extension into nasal cavity or sphenoid sinus
III	Extension into maxillary sinus, ethmoid sinus, pterygopalatine fossa, infratemporal fossa, cheek, palate
IV	Intracranial extension

Table 3.
JNA staging system by Chandler, 1984 [37].

9.3 Andrews-Fisch's staging system, 1989

Table 4

ANDREWS-FISCH'S STAGING SYSTEM	
STAGE	**TUMOR EXTENSION**
I	Confined to nose or nasopharyngeal vault
II	Invasion of the pterygopalatine fossa or maxillary/ ethmoid/ sphenoid sinuses with bone destruction
IIIA	Extension into the infra- temporal fossa or orbit
IIIB	Intracranial but extradural extension (parasellar area)
IVA	Intracranial intradural extension **without** involving **c**avernous sinus/ **o**ptic chiasma/ **p**ituitary fossa (*mnemonic C-O-P)*
IVB	Intracranial intradural extension involving **c**avernous sinus/ **o**ptic chiasma/ **p**ituitary fossa

Table 4.
JNA staging system by Andrew- Fisch, 1989 [38].

9.4 Radkowski's staging system, 1996

Table 5

RADKOWSKI'S STAGING SYSTEM	
STAGE	**TUMOR EXTENSION**
IA	Involvement of the nose or nasopharyngeal vault
IB	Extension into one or more sinuses
IIA	Minimal extension into pterygopalatine fossa
IIB	Complete extension into pterygopalatine fossa
IIC	Extension into infratemporal fossa/ posterior to pterygoid plates
IIIA	Minimal skull base involvement (middle cranial fossa/ base of pterygoid plates)
IIIB	Extensive intracranial involvement $\pm$ involvement of cavernous sinus

Table 5.
JNA staging system by radkowski, 1996 [39].

9.5 Endoscopic system of staging

9.5.1 UPMC (University of Pittsburgh Medical Center)/ Snyderman, 2010

Only valid for tumors which are preoperatively embolised (**Table 6**).

UPMC/ SNYDERMAN'S STAGING SYSTEM	
STAGE	**TUMOR EXTENSION**
I	Nasal cavity, medial pterygopalatine fossa
II	Paranasal sinuses and lateral pterygopalatine fossa, no residual vascularity
III	Skull base erosion, orbit, infratemporal fossa, no residual vascularity

UPMC/ SNYDERMAN'S STAGING SYSTEM	
STAGE	**TUMOR EXTENSION**
IV	Skull base erosion, orbit, infratemporal fossa, with residual vascularity from ICA
V	Intracranial extension with residual vascularity from ICA
VM	Medial cavernous sinus
VL	Middle cranial fossa

Table 6.
JNA staging system by Snyderman/ UPMC, 2010 [40].

10. Treatment

Choice of treatment depends on the size and extent of the tumor. Treatment modalities include surgical excision (open v/s endoscopic approach) and non-surgical adjuvant therapy (embolization/hormonal/ radiotherapy) or their combination(s).

10.1 Surgical treatment of JNA

Complete excision of the entire tumor mass should be the aim of any surgical procedure and the approach selected accordingly. Though the advancements in endoscopic surgery have minimized the need for open approaches, the surgeon should be well versed with all the techniques.

10.1.1 Open surgical approach

In general, open approaches have the advantage of providing a wide exposure. But this comes at the cost of higher morbidity, increased hospital stay, and some degree of cosmetic deformity.

10.1.1.1 Transpalatal approach

This is the shortest and most direct approach for tumors limited to nasopharynx with/ without minimal extension into sphenoid sinus/ choana [41, 42].

A U-shaped incision (Wilson's incision) is made 2.5 cm anterior to the junction of hard and soft palate. Submucoperiosteal flap is elevated posteriorly till the soft palate to bare the underlying horizontal plate of palatine bone. Soft palate and hard palate are separated. Bone is removed from the posterior part of hard palate to visualize the entire nasopharynx along with the tumor.

This approach has the advantage of good post-operative healing with no visible scar.

10.1.1.2 Transnasal- maxillary approach

10.1.1.2.1 Lateral rhinotomy

Lateral rhinotomy was first described by Irwin Moore in 1917 [43].

The incision is started 5 mm anterior and superior to the medial canthus and continued inferiorly along the deepest portion of the nasomaxillary groove. At its inferior end, it is curved medially in the crease beneath the ala. Skin flaps are elevated over the maxilla and nasal bones. Medial wall of maxillary antrum is removed.

This provides adequate exposure for tumors extending into the nasal cavity and/ or sinuses with minimal extension into the pterygopalatine fossa.

Adequate healing allows for an inconspicuous scar mark, well hidden within the facial creases.

10.1.1.2.2 Extended lateral rhinotomy

The lateral rhinotomy incision is further extended inferiorly along the ipsilateral ridge of the philtrum and continued to split the upper lip in paramedian position. After dividing the upper lip, incision is continued laterally along the gingivobuccal sulcus upto the first molar. This approach is required in cases needing exposure beyond the infraorbital neurovascular bundle.

10.1.1.2.3 Extended subtoal maxillectomy

The main objective of this approach is to expose the maxillary antrum and remove its medial, anterior and posterolateral walls along with perpendicular plate of palatine bone. Orbital floor and alveolar arch are left intact. This converts the maxillary sinus, nasal cavity, nasopharynx, pterygopalatine fossa and infratemporal fossa into a single large accessible cavity.

This wide exposure is required for large tumors spilling in the infratemporal fossa. Lateral most aspect of these tumors is identified. Feeder vessel in the form of internal maxillary artery (most common feeder vessel) is identified as it enters the lateral aspect of the tumor in the infratemporal fossa and ligated before starting with the tumor dissection. Ascending pharyngeal artery maybe seen entering and supplying the tumor at its posterior aspect. It is also identified and ligated. This allows for minimal blood loss during the tumor dissection and delivery. Tumor delivery is done in-toto through transnasal/ transoral route or in a piecemeal fashion.

Two pathways for this approach have been described:

I. **Weber-Ferguson's Incision:** The incision starts just below the lateral canthus upto the medial canthus in the subciliary crease. It is continued inferiorly along the nasomaxillary groove and turned medially at alar crease. It is again curved inferiorly along the philtrum to split the upper lip. Gingivobuccal incision is extended laterally upto the first molar area. Ectropion, cheek anesthesia, and an unsightly scar are often encountered complications of this approach.

II. **Mid Facial Degloving:** A complete transfixation incision is placed in the anterior nasal septum followed by bilateral intercartilagenous incisions between upper and lower lateral cartilages. Incision over the pyriform aperture is made on both sides. A sublabial incision between the two upper second molars is made and dissection continued superiorly to join it with the nasal incisions. Entire skin and soft tissue flap is retracted superiorly to reveal the whole midface skeleton. Although more technologically challenging, this approach has the advantage of no visible scar. Cheek anesthesia is an almost inevitable complication. Nasal vestibular stenosis has also been reported with the use of this approach.

10.1.1.2.4 Le fort-I approach

An incision is made in the gingivobuccal sulcus between the two upper second molars. Periosteum is elevated to expose maxilla in its anterior and lateral aspect. Horizontal osteotomies from pyriform aperture to pterygomaxillary fissure and from pyriform aperture to palatine canals are made. Nasal septum is freed from anterior nasal spine and maxillary crest. Pterygoid dysjuctioning allows easy down fracturing of maxilla to achieve a wide exposure of the tumor extending into multiple paranasal sinuses, infratemporal fossa or intracranial space.
After tumor excision, fixation of mid facial skeleton is achieved using titanium plates. This approach provides the widest possible exposure without any external scar [44].

10.1.1.3 Transfacial approach

10.1.1.3.1 Maxillary swing

A Weber-Ferguson incision is combined with the splitting of the hard palate [45, 46]. Multiple osteotomies are done and maxilla is disarticulated. Overlying skin and muscles are NOT dissected. Rather they are raised as a single flap along with underlying maxillary and zygomatic bone (**cheek masseter maxillary flap**). After tumor excision, maxilla is repositioned and fixed with titanium plates followed by layered suturing of the skin incision.

This approach provides accessibility to nasopharynx, paranasal sinuses, infratemporal fossa, parapharyngeal space and intracranial space. Malocclusion of upper jaw and palatal fistula are some uncommon but difficult to manage complications associated with this procedure [47].

10.1.1.3.2 Maxillary removal and reinsertion (MRR)

MRR starts as a midfacial degloving approach through a sublabial incision [48]. Partial osteotomy at nasofrontal angle allows extended degloving of midface. Multiple osteotomies are made to resect and remove the maxillary bone. Tumor is resected. Maxilla is repositioned at its original anatomical position and secured with titanium plates/ absorbable plates.

Wide exposure for tumor resection from infratemporal fossa, parapharyngeal space, and middle and anterior cranial fossa is achieved. Such extensive resections can cause malocclusions, visual disturbances and disruption of growth centres in the maxillary bone, resulting in future cosmetic deformities.

10.1.1.4 Infratemporal fossa approach

Fisch Type C and **Fisch Type D** are the two most commonly used approaches for extensive JNAs. Infratemporal approaches are suitable for gaining excess to infratemporal fossa, middle cranial fossa and lateral cavernous sinus [49]. Good resection rates are achieved with low recurrence rates. Major complications of Fisch Type C approach are a permanent conductive hearing loss, cosmetic deformity and loss of facial sensation. Fisch Type D approach was later added with the advantage of avoiding a visible facial scar, hearing loss and ability to convert as Type C approach as and when required [50, 51]. However, these approaches fail to resect tumors extending medial to the abducent cranial nerve in the cavernous sinus [52].

10.1.1.5 Craniofacial resection

A combination of infratemporal fossa approach and transfacial approach is required in certain cases with advanced stage angiofibromas [52]. This approach allows access to the infratemporal fossa, middle and anterior cranial fossa, and entire cavernous sinus (both medial and lateral aspects). An added enhanced exposure to the nasopharynx, paranasal sinuses and pterygopalatine fossa facilitates complete tumor excision. Facial skeletal growth retardations and facial asymmetry is rare [53].

10.1.1.6 Combined open approach

Large primary tumors or recurrent tumors may necessitate the need for using more than one open approach in the same sitting. These combinations can be tailor –made depending on size of the tumor, involvement of vital structures, and surgeon's expertise in one or more approaches. Some commonly used combined approaches are-

i. **Transapalatal + Lateral Rhinotomy:** In large tumors, not amenable to single approach surgery, this was the most common approach used earlier.

ii. **Sardana's Approach:** Sublabial approach combined with a partial transpalatal approach (without removing bone from posterior part of hard palate) [54].

iii. **Midface Degloving + Transzygomatic Approach:** This achieves a wide exposure with radical tumor excision and good hemostasis [55].

iv. **Triple Approach of Hiranandani:** Combination of lateral rhinotomy with transpalatal approach with Caldwell-Luc's approach [56].

v. **Craniofacial Resections:** Infratemporal fossa approach combined with transfacial approach. Craniofacial resections can be included in this category as well [52].

10.1.2 Endoscopic approach

Last decade has seen a paradigm shift from open approach to transnasal endoscopic approach. In today's time, endoscopic surgery can be regarded as the most rapidly advancing surgical field. As the surgeon's familiarity with the endoscopes is increasing, hard to reach anatomical regions are also becoming more accessible, thereby, widening the horizon for this approach. Tumors, which were earlier labeled as operable via an open approach only, can now be easily and completely resected using endoscopic approach.

Endoscopic surgery has the advantage of better illumination and magnification, lower morbidity, and shorter duration of hospital stay which ultimately leads to cost saving. Advantage of no visible facial scar adds to the cosmetic viability of this approach.

10.1.2.1 Surgical considerations for endoscopic jna surgery

1. Tumor size and extent decides the exact endoscopic approach required. While smaller tumors are managed via an endonasal approach; medium to large sized tumors require an endoscopic Denker's / Sturman- Canfield or a more extensive transpterygoid approach [57, 58].

Extended anterior skull base approaches are recommended for intracranial lesions [59].

1. Exposure is the key to a successful surgery. Adequate exposure allows identification of tumor limits, delineation of feeder vessels, and assessment of tumor's relation with vital structures. Most of the surgical time is spent in achieving this exposure before starting off with the tumor resection.

2. It is always advisable to identify and ligate the feeding artery first (usually internal maxillary artery), before starting with tumor dissection.

3. Posterior septectomy, wherever required, is recommended. This greatly increases the access to the tumor.

4. Dissection is carried along the tumor pseudocapsule from lateral to medial direction. Any injury to tumor surface can provoke massive bleeding.

5. For larger tumors, a four-handed technique is recommended [22]. For large tumors with extensive lateral extension into infratemporal fossa/ parapharyngeal space, the four-port Bradoo's technique is a worthy option [60].

6. Drilling of pterygoid base at the end of the procedure should be a routine practice, so as to minimize the recurrence rates (**Figures 3–8**).

7. The operative room should have the availability of hemostatic materials like SURGICEL, FLOSEAL, TIS SEEL and a functioning bipolar cautery. Access to a blood bank is recommended.

8. Coblation is a plasma based device that can be used for surface coagulation of the tumor without causing any collateral thermal damage. This shrinks the tumor and also greatly reduces intra-op bleeding.

9. During preoperative planning stage, it is imperative to discuss with the patient, the possibility to convert an endoscopic approach into an open approach at any given time during the surgery.

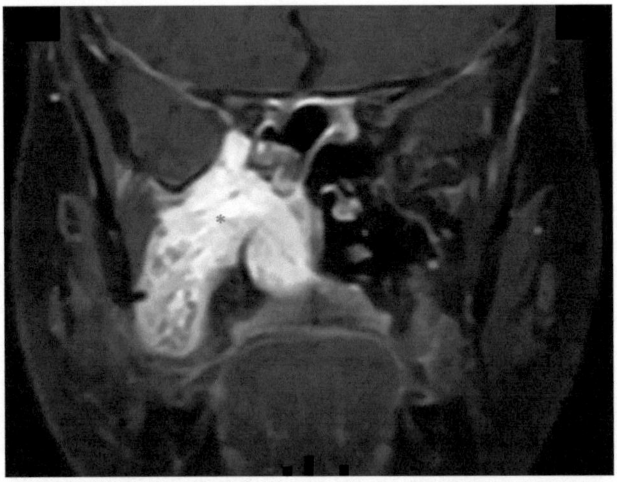

Figure 3.
CE-MRI showing hyperintense tumor (*) with massive lateral extension into infratemporal fossa.

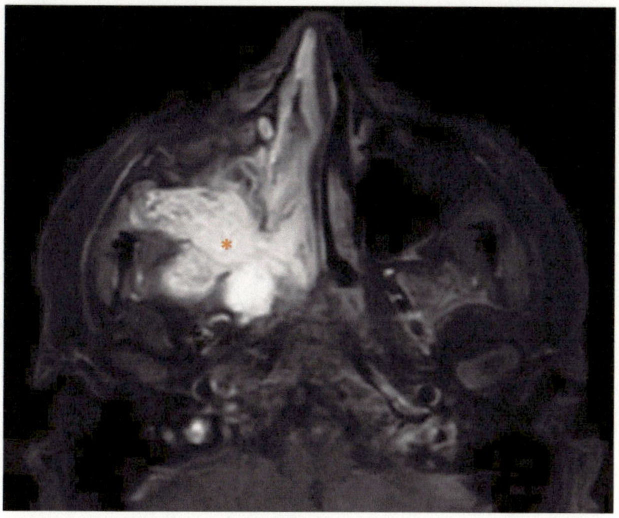

Figure 4.
CE-MRI showing hyperintense tumor (*) in the infratemporal fossa.

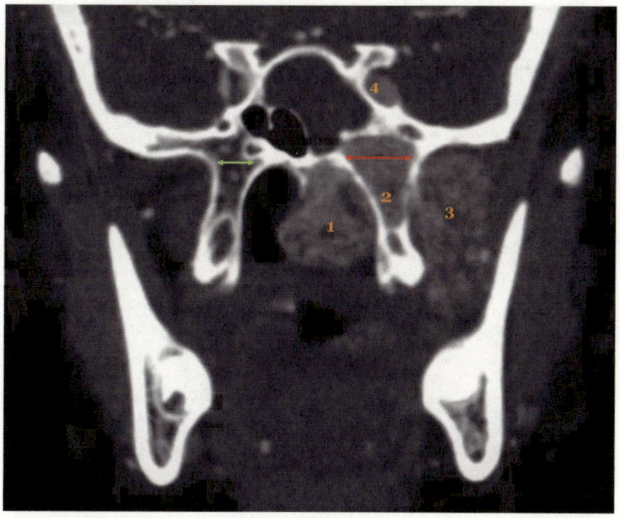

Figure 5.
CECT showing JNA occupying nasopharynx (1), pterygoid wedge (2), infratemporal fossa (3) and intracranial space (4). Notice the widening of left pterygoid wedge (red arrow) as compared to the right normal pterygoid wedge (green arrow)- Ram Haran Sign.

10.1.2.2 Contraindications to endoscopic approach

i. Broad skull base infiltration

ii. extensive blood supply from ICA

iii. encasement of ICA

iv. brain infiltration

Considering the pace of progress in endoscopic techniques, it would not be surprising if some more indications are added by the time this chapter reaches the readers.

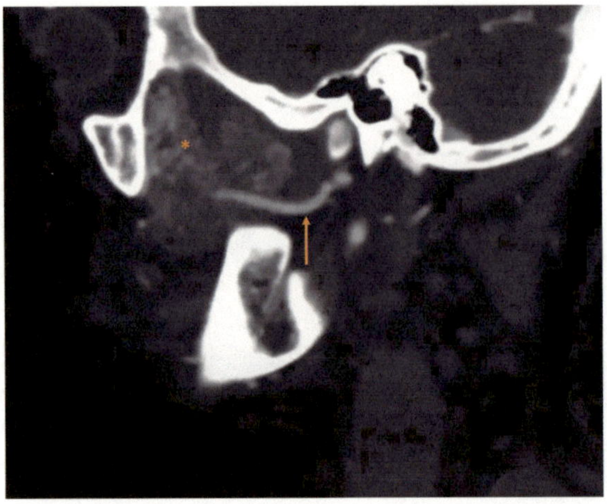

Figure 6.
CT angiography showing a vascular tumor (*). Notice the internal maxillary artery supplying this tumor (orange arrow).

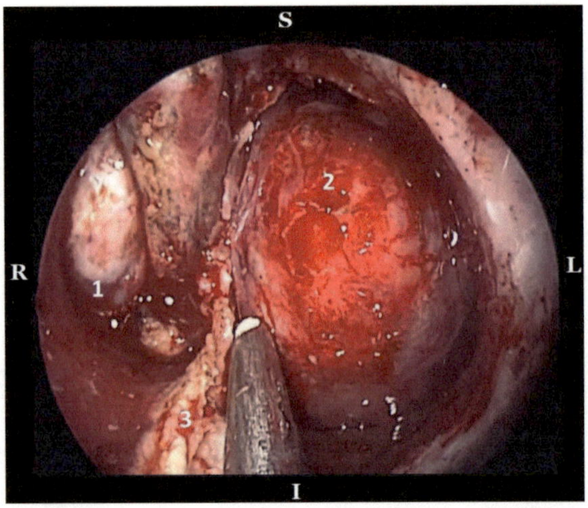

Figure 7.
Endoscopic view through left nasal cavity: Medial and posterior walls of left maxillary sinus and left inferior turbinate have been removed. 1-nasopharyngeal component of JNA; 2- pterygopalatine fossa + infratemporal fossa component of JNA; 3- remnants of left inferior turbinate; R- right, L- left, S- superior, I- inferior.

10.2 Non-surgical treatment of JNA: adjuvant treatment modalities

Though Juvenile angiofibroma is now an established surgical entity, there has been an era when medical management alone was the rule for extensive tumors especially those with intracranial extension. With paradigm shift towards more aggressive surgical procedures for all stages of the tumor, other treatment modalities are now valued as adjuvant therapy only.

10.2.1 Embolization

Transarterial embolization (TAE) is done preoperatively to decrease the blood flow to the tumor, thereby, reducing the intraoperative blood loss and need for blood transfusion. This is particularly useful for tumors with advanced stage.

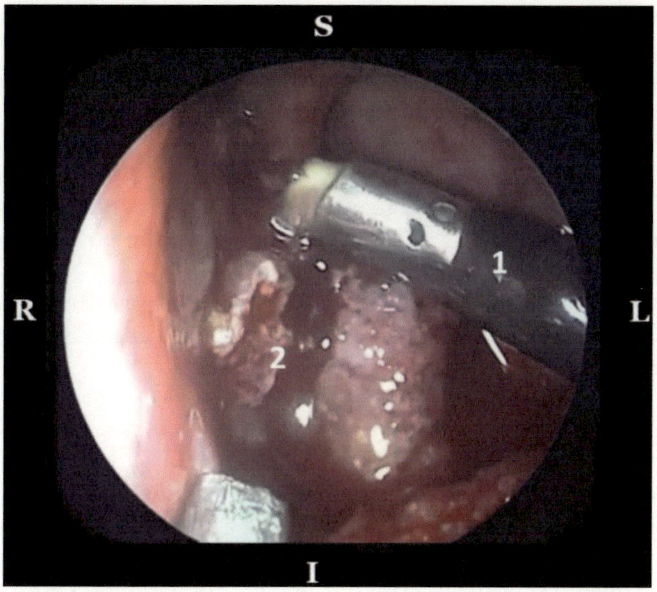

Figure 8.
Coblation wand being used in juvenile nasopharyngeal angiofibroma endoscopic surgery. 1- coblation wand, 2- tumor, R- right, L- left, S- superior, I- inferior.

Smaller tumors have less vascularity and can be resected easily even without preoperative embolization [61].

The procedure is usually done 24 to 48 hours before the scheduled surgery. Further surgical delay is not appreciated/recommended as tumor gains collateral blood supply through neoangiogenesis. A wide variety of materials are available as embolic agents: microspheres, gelatin sponge, Teflon particles, gel foam, poly-vinyl alcohol, polystyrene, silicone particles, silk, cyanoacrylate, sodium tetradacyl sulphate, autogenous clot, duramater, muscle fragments, etc. 300–500 micrometer spheres are preferred owing to greater blocking capacity of vascular lumen [62].

The procedure is not without complications. Cerebral ischemia and vision loss are known complications following embolic agent migrating to ICA system. Rare complications like cerebral edema, hemiplegia and aphasia have also been reported [63].

Direct Puncture Therapeutic Embolization (DPTE) is a new concept for tumor embolization. Embolizing agent is a mixture of n-butyl cyanoacrylate [NBCA], lipiodol, powdered tungsten with/without absolute ethanol. Under fluoroscopic visualization, embolizing agent is injected directly into the tumor through a percutaneous route or a transoral/ transnasal/transpalatal route [64].

This results in almost complete filling of tumor microvasculature with irreversible occlusion of embolized vessels. Tumor gains a dark color (due to tungsten powder with blue dye) which helps to better distinguish it from surrounding normal tissue. Direct cytotoxicity of absolute ethanol has shown good therapeutic effects.

DPTE alone or in combination with TAE has shown to have better devascularisation effects than TAE alone [65, 66].

10.2.2 Hormonal therapy

Hormonal influence on growth of JNA has been speculated since long. An interplay between estrogens and androgens has been associated with tumor proliferation and its spontaneous involution. Various hormonal therapies are recommended based on these concepts.

Estrogen therapy: exogenous estrogen has been tried traditionally with the aim of decreasing tumor size and vascularity. Lack of conclusive therapeutic advantage, feminizing side effects and propensity towards cardiovascular side effects have rendered its place to be of historical significance only.

Anti-androgen therapy: Flutamide is a non-steroidal androgen receptor blocker drug, primarily used in prostatic cancer. It binds with the androgen receptors, thereby blocking the action of testosterone. Recently, it has been proven that the response to flutamide therapy is much more pronounced in post-pubertal patients as compared to pre-pubertal patients [23].

Flutamide therapy is recommended as a six week preoperative adjuvant therapy for intracranial and intraorbital lesions, recurrent lesions and those with their blood supply primarily from ICA.

10.2.3 Radiotherapy

Low dose radiotherapy is used for angiofibromas extending intracranially, not amenable to primary surgery. Typically, total radiation dose of 3,500 cGy is given over 3 weeks. A successful response in terms of decreased tumor size and vascularity is seen over several months in 80% of the patients [67, 68]. Those showing no response/incomplete response by 2 years post radiotherapy are deemed as failures and taken up for salvage surgery.

There are numerous side effects to use of radiotherapy at a young age. Posterior capsular opacities, glaucoma, optic nerve atrophy, xerostomia, hypopituitarism, cerebral necrosis, osteoradionecrosis of mandible, skull base osteomyelitis, risk of developing new head–neck tumors later in life, potential malignant transformation of angiofibromas are few of the complications associated with the use of radiotherapy in head and neck region.

Intensity Modulated Radiotherapy (IMRT) allows higher doses to be given to the lesion without damaging adjoining normal tissues. Multiple beams from different directions converge onto the tumor shape so that the target area has the highest dose strength with relative sparing of surrounding vital structures.

Gamma Knife makes use of radiation beams from 201 sources, converging onto a single point. This causes retardation of further tumor growth. **Cyber Knife** is a type of stereotactic radiosurgery which uses a robotic arm to deliver radiations to a point source. These are being applied in association with other treatment modalities to achieve desired results in large angiofibromas [69, 70].

11. Conclusion

Juvenile nasopharyngeal angiofibroma, although an old disease entity, is still fascinating medical experts all over the world. Although still largely unknown, with advanced genetic and molecular studies, we have moved a step closer to find the origin and etiology of this disease. At present, surgery is the mainstay of treatment with endoscopic approach replacing the conventional open approach. Future considerations can be focused on therapeutic embolisation, stereotactic radiotherapy and targeted molecular therapy for a non-surgical cure.

Acknowledgements

I wish to express my sincere gratitude towards Dr. Anupama Mahajan, Dr. Stuti Mahajan and Dr. Anugeet Sethi for their constant moral support. I am fortunate to have worked with Dr. Rajesh Choudhary and Dr. Bikramjeet Singh on numerous juvenile nasopharyngeal angiofibroma cases. A special vote of thanks to Dr. Rohan Sardana and Dr. Karamjeet Singh Gill for providing valuable insight into the pathology of this disease. I shall always be indebted to ENT Department of my alma mater VMMC & Safdarjung Hospital, New Delhi.

Conflict of interest

The authors declare no conflict of interest.

Author details

Anukaran Mahajan* and Karunesh Gupta
Chikitsa ENT Hospital, Amritsar, India

*Address all correspondence to: anukaranmahajan@gmail.com

References

[1] Herman P, Lot G, Chapot R, Salvan D, Huy PT. Long-term follow-up of juvenile nasopharyngeal angiofibromas: analysis of re-currences. Laryngoscope 1999; 109:140–147

[2] Martin H, Ehrlich HE, Abels JC. Juvenile nasopharyngeal angiofibroma. Ann surg 1948; 127(3): 513–536

[3] Chaveau C. Histoire de maladies du pharynx. Vol 5. Paris, France: J.B. Bailliere et fils; 1906 (as in Janakiram, N., Wormald, P. and Sharma, S. Juvenile Nasopharyngeal Angiofibroma. Noida, India: Thieme; 2017:3)

[4] Shaheen HB. Nasopharyngeal fibroma. J Laryngol Otol 1930; 45: 259–264

[5] Harma RA. Nasopharyngeal angiofibroma; a clinical and histopathological study. Acta otolaryngol suppl 1959; 146: 1–74

[6] Som ML, Neffson AH. Fibromas of the nasopharynx: juvenile and cellular types. Ann Otol Rhinol Laryngol., 1940; 49: 211–218

[7] Bensch H, Ewing J. Neoplastic Disease. 4th edition, Saunders and Co., Philadelphia, 1941

[8] Moore I. Sarcoma of the right maxillary antrum; lateral rhinotomy performed (Moore's Operation). Proc R Soc Med 1917; 10: 29–31

[9] Handousa A, Farid H, Elwi AM. Nasopharyngeal fibroma; a clinico-pathological study of seventy cases. J Laryngol Otol 1954; 68(10): 647–666

[10] U. Srinivas Rao, CH. Venkata Subbaiah, K.S.R. Bargava. Juvenile nasopharyngeal angiofibroma in our experience. IAIM, 2017; 4(12): 107–112

[11] Delides A, Panayiotides JG, Kaberos A, Giotakis I. Nasopharyngeal angiofibroma in an adult with Proteus syndrome. First reported case. Hippokratia. 2017;21(3):147–149

[12] Ringertz N. Pathology of malignant tumors arising in nasal and paranasal cavities and maxilla. Acta Otolaryngol Suppl (Stockh) 1938; 27:158–161

[13] Brunner H. Nasopharyngeal fibroma. Ann Otol Rhinol Laryngol. 1942; 51: 29–65.

[14] Martin H, Ehrlich HE, Abels JC. Juvenile Nasopharyngeal Angiofibroma. Ann Surg. 1948;127(3):513–536. doi: 10.1097/00000658-194803000-00012

[15] Sternberg SS. Pathology of juvenile nasopharyngeal angiofibroma: a lesion of adolescent males. Cancer. 1954; 7: 15–28

[16] Osborn DA. The so-called juvenile angio-fibroma of the nasopharynx. J Laryngol Otol. 1959;73(5):295–316. doi: 10.1017/s0022215100055341

[17] Girgis IH, Fahmy SA. Nasopharyngeal fibroma: its histo-pathological nature. J Laryngol Otol. 1973;87(11):1107–1123. doi:10.1017/s002221510007804x

[18] Beham A, Beham-Schmid C, Regauer S, et al. "Nasopharyngeal angiofibroma: true neoplasm or vascular malformation?" Adv Anat Pathol 2000; 7: 36–46. 5.

[19] Schick B, Wemmert S, Willnecker V, et al. Genome-wide copy number profiling using a 100K SNP array reveals novel disease-related genes BORIS and TSHZ1 in juvenile angiofibroma. Int J Oncol 2011;39: 1143–51

[20] Zhang M, Sun X, Yu H, Hu L, Wang D. Biological distinctions between juvenile nasopharyngeal angiofibroma and vascular malformation: An immunohistochemical study. Acta Histochem 2011; 113:626–30

[21] Schick B. Juvenile nasopharyngeal angiofibroma. In: Watkinson JC, Clarke RW, 8. Scott-Brown's Otorhinolaryngology Head & Neck Surgery: Volume 1. Boca Raton, Florida: CRC Press; 2019:1265–68

[22] Janakiram, N., Wormald, P. and Sharma, S. Juvenile Nasopharyngeal Angiofibroma. Noida, India: Thieme; 2017:45, 54, 222

[23] Thakar A, Gupta G, Bhalla AS, et al. Adjuvant therapy with flutamide for presurgical volume reduction in juvenile nasopharyngeal angiofibroma. Head Neck. 2011;33(12):1747–1753. doi: 10.1002/hed.21667al

[24] Heinrich UR, Brieger J, Gosepath J, Wierzbicka M, Sokolov M, Roth Y, Szyfter W, Bittinger F, Mann WJ. Frequent chromosomal gains in recurrent juvenile nasopharyngeal angiofibroma. Cancer Genet Cytogenet 175(2):138–143, 2007

[25] Schick B, Brunner C, Praetorius M, Plinkert PK, Urbschat S. First evidence of genetic imbalances in angiofibromas. Laryngoscope 112(2):397–401, 2002

[26] Schick B, Wemmert S, Bechtel U, Nicolai P, Hofmann T, Golabek W, Urbschat S. Comprehensive genomic analysis identifies MDM2 and AURKA as novel amplified genes in juvenile angiofibromas. Head Neck 29(5):479–487, 2007

[27] Pandey P, Mishra A, Tripathi AM, Verma V, Trivedi R, Singh HP, Kumar S, Patel B, Singh V, Pandey S, Pandey A, Mishra SC. Current molecular profile of juvenile nasopharyngeal angiofibroma: First comprehensive study from India. Laryngoscope 127(3):E100-E106, 2017

[28] Nagai MA, Butugan O, Logullo A, Brentani MM. Expression of growth factors, proto-oncogenes, and p53 in nasopharyngeal angiofibromas. Laryngoscope 106(2 Pt 1):190–195, 1996.

[29] Schick B, Veldung B, Wemmert S, Jung V, Montenarh M, Meese E, Urbschat S. p53 and Her-2/neu in juvenile angiofibromas. Oncol Rep 13 (3):453–457, 2005.

[30] Mishra A, Pandey A, Mishra SC. Variable expression of molecular markers in juvenile nasopharyngeal angiofibroma. J Laryngol Otol 131(9): 752–759, 2017.

[31] Silveira SM, Custodio Domingues MA, Butugan O, Brentani MM, Rogatto SR. Tumor microenvironmental genomic alterations in juvenile nasopharyngeal angiofibroma. Head Neck 34(4):485–492, 2012

[32] Lloyd G, Howard D, Lund VJ, Savy L. Imaging for juvenile angiofibroma. J Laryngol Otol. 2000;114 (9):727–730. doi:10.1258/0022215001906642

[33] Janakiram TN, Sharma SB, Samavedam UC, Deshmukh O, Rajalingam B. Imaging in Juvenile Nasopharyngeal Angiofibroma: Clinical Significance of Ramharan and Chopstick Sign. Indian J Otolaryngol Head Neck Surg. 2017;69(1):81–87. doi:10.1007/s12070-016-1039-4

[34] Husrt RW, Rosenwasser RH. Interventional neuroradiology. Informa Healthcare; 2007

[35] Ballah D., Rabinowitz D., Vossough A., Rickert S., Dunham B., Kazahaya K. Preoperative angiography and external carotid artery embolization of juvenile nasopharyngeal angiofibromas in a tertiary referral paediatric centre. Clin Radiol. 2013;68 (November (11)):106–1097

[36] Sessions RB, Bryan RN, Naclerio RM, Alford BR. Radiographic

staging of juvenile angiofibroma. Head Neck Surg 1981;3(4):279–83.

[37] Chandler JR, Goulding R, Moskowitz L, Quencer RM. Nasopharyngeal angiofibromas: Staging and management. Ann Otol Rhinol Laryngol 1984;93(4 Pt 1):322–9

[38] Andrews JC, Fisch U, Valavanis A, et al. The surgical management of extensive nasopharyngeal angiofibromas with the infratemporal fossa approach. Laryngoscope 1989;99 (4):429–37

[39] Radkowski D, McGill T, Healy GB, et al. Angiofibroma. Changes in staging and treatment. Arch Otolaryngol Head Neck Surg 1996;122(2):122–9

[40] Snyderman CH, Pant H, Carrau RL, Gardner P. A new endoscopic staging system for angiofibromas. Arch Otolaryngol Head Neck Surg. 2010;136 (6):588–594. doi:10.1001/ archoto.2010.83

[41] Wilson~ Jol, 1951 c 65 : 738 Approach to Nasopharynx,

[42] Misra, R.N., Shardana, D.S. The transpalatal surgical approach for removal of nasopharyngeal fibromata. Indian J Otolaryngol 8, 1–15 (1956). doi: https://doi.org/10.1007/BF02996733

[43] Moore I. Carcinoma of the Right Maxillary Antrum; lateral Rhinotomy (Moure's Operation) performed. Proc R Soc Med. 1917;10(Laryngol Sect):60–63

[44] Girish Rao S, Sudhakara Reddy K, Sampath S. Le Fort I access for juvenile nasopharyngeal angiofibroma (JNA): a prospective series of 22 cases. J Craniomaxillofac Surg. 2012;40(2):e54-e58. doi:10.1016/j.jcms.2011.03.006

[45] Kalra GS, Midya M, Bedi M. Access to the skull base - Maxillary swing procedure - Long term analysis. Ann Maxillofac Surg [serial online] 2018 [cited 2020 Sep 11];8:86–90. doi: http://www.amsjournal.com/text.asp?2018/8/1/86/234302

[46] Amin AA. Maxillary swing approach for surgical resection of recurrent nasopharyngeal tumors. J Egypt Natl Canc Inst. 2007;19(3):219–223

[47] Roy Chowdhury S, Rajkumar K, Deshmukh T. Complications of Midface Swing for Management of Juvenile Nasopharyngeal Angiofibroma. J Maxillofac Oral Surg. 2017;16(1):96–100. doi:10.1007/s12663-016-0947-x

[48] Powell DM, Shah N, Carr A, et al. Maxillary Removal and Reinsertion in Pediatric Patients. Arch Otolaryngol Head Neck Surg. 2002;128(1):29–34. doi:10.1001/archotol.128.1.29

[49] Szymańska A, Szymański M, Czekajska-Chehab E, Szczerbo-Trojanowska M. Two types of lateral extension in juvenile nasopharyngeal angiofibroma: diagnostic and therapeutic management. Eur Arch Otorhinolaryngol. 2015;272(01):159–166. doi: 10.1007/s00405-014-2965-y

[50] Fisch, U . The infratemporal fossa approach for nasopharyngeal tumors. Laryngoscope. 1983;93(1):36–44

[51] Zhang, M, Garvis, W, Linder, T, Fisch, U. Update on the infratemporal fossa approaches to nasopharyngeal angiofibroma. Laryngoscope. 1998;108 (11 pt 1):1717–1723

[52] Bales C, Kotapka M, Loevner LA, et al. Craniofacial Resection of Advanced Juvenile Nasopharyngeal Angiofibroma. Arch Otolaryngol Head Neck Surg. 2002;128(9):1071–1078. doi: 10.1001/archotol.128.9.1071

[53] Lang DA, Neil-Dwyer G, Evans BT, Honeybul S. Craniofacial access in children. Acta Neurochir (Wien).1998; 140:33–40

[54] Sardana DS. Nasopharyngeal fibroma: extension into cheek. Arch Otolaryngol. 1965;81:584–588. doi: 10.1001/archotol.1965.0075005059901

[55] Antonelli AR, Cappiello J, Di Lorenzo D, Donajo CA, Nicolai P, Orlandini A. Diagnosis, staging, and treatment of juvenile nasopharyngeal angiofibroma (JNA). Laryngoscope. 1987;97(11):1319–1325. doi:10.1288/00005537-198711000-00014

[56] Hiranandani LH: Improved technique in operative removal of nasopharyngeal fibroma. J Laryngol Otol 82: 757, 1968

[57] Youssef Ahmed, Ricardo L. Carrau, Tantawy Ahmed, Aly Ibrahim Ahmed. Endoscopic approach to the infratemporal fossa. Alexandria Journal of Medicine, 50 (2) (2014), pp. 127–130, 10.1016/j.ajme.2013.12.001

[58] Hardillo JA, Vander Velden LA, Knegt PP. Denker operation is an effective surgical approach in managing juvenile nasopharyngeal angiofibroma. Ann Otol Rhinol Laryngol. 2004;113 (12):946–950. doi:10.1177/000348940411301202

[59] Snyderman CH, Gardner PA, Fernandez-Miranda JC, Wang EW. Extended anterior skull base approaches. In: Watkinson JC, Clarke RW, 8. Scott-Brown's Otorhinolaryngology Head & Neck Surgery: Volume 1. Boca Raton, Florida: CRC Press; 2019:1289–1303

[60] Bradoo R, Joshi A, Shah K, Patel T, Lohiya T. The Four-Port Bradoo Technique: An Alternative to the Modified Endoscopic Denker's Approach for Giant JNA. Indian J Otolaryngol Head Neck Surg. 2017;69 (3):277–281. doi:10.1007/s12070-017-1150-1

[61] Moulin G, Chagnaud C, Gras R, et al. Juvenile nasopharyngeal angiofibroma: comparison of blood loss during removal in embolized group versus nonembolized group. Cardiovasc Intervent Radiol. 1995;18(3):158–161. doi:10.1007/BF00204142

[62] Parikh V, Hennemeyer C. Microspheres embolization of juvenile nasopharyngeal angiofibroma in an adult. Int J Surg Case Rep. 2014;5(12): 1203–1206. doi:10.1016/j.ijscr.2014.10.019

[63] Janakiram N, Sharma SB, Panicker VB, Srinivas CV. A Drastic Aftermath of Embolisation in Juvenile Nasopharyngeal Angiofibroma. Indian J Otolaryngol Head Neck Surg. 2016;68 (4):540–543. doi:10.1007/s12070-016-1014-0

[64] Chaloupka JC, Mangla S, Huddle DC, et al. Evolving experience with direct puncture therapeutic embolization for adjunctive and palliative management of head and neck hypervascular neoplasms. Laryngoscope. 1999;109(11):1864–1872. doi:10.1097/00005537-199911000-00028

[65] Lv, M., Fan, X., Su, L. et al. Preoperative Direct Puncture Embolization of Advanced Juvenile Nasopharyngeal Angiofibroma in Combination with Transarterial Embolization: An Analysis of 22 Consecutive Patients. Cardiovasc Intervent Radiol 36, 111–117 (2013). https://doi.org/10.1007/s00270-012-0404-2

[66] Elhammady MS, Johnson JN, Peterson EC, Aziz-Sultan MA. Preoperative embolization of juvenile nasopharyngeal angiofibromas: transarterial versus direct tumoral puncture. World Neurosurg. 2011;76(3–4):328–265. doi: 10.1016/j.wneu.2010.11.011

[67] Cummings BJ, Blend R, Keane T, et al. Primary radiation therapy for

juvenile nasopharyngeal angiofibroma. Laryngoscope. 1984;94(12 Pt 1):1599–1605.

[68] Lee JT, Chen P, Safa A, Juillard G, Calcaterra TC. The role of radiation in the treatment of advanced juvenile angiofibroma. Laryngoscope. 2002;112 (7 Pt 1):1213–1220. doi:10.1097/00005537-200207000-00014

[69] Dare AO, Gibbons KJ, Proulx GM, Fenstermaker RA. Resection followed by radiosurgery for advanced juvenile nasopharyngeal angiofibroma: report of two cases. Neurosurgery. 2003;52(5): 1207–1211

[70] Parikh V, Hennemeyer C. Microspheres embolization of juvenile nasopharyngeal angiofibroma in an adult. Int J Surg Case Rep. 2014;5(12): 1203–1206. doi:10.1016/j.ijscr.2014.10.019